Phlebotomy
Essentials

Phlebotomy Essentials

SECOND EDITION

Ruth E. McCall, BS, MT(ASCP), CLS(NCA)
Director of Phlebotomy and Clinical Laboratory Assistant Programs
Instructor, MLT and Healthcare Technician Programs
Albuquerque Technical-Vocational Institute
Albuquerque, New Mexico

Cathee M. Tankersley, MT(ASCP), CLS(NCA)
Director of Phlebotomy and EKG Programs
Phoenix College
Phoenix, Arizona

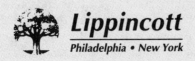

Lippincott
Philadelphia • New York

Acquisitions Editor: Lawrence McGrew
Assistant Editor: Holly Chapman
Project Editor: Gretchen Metzger
Production Manager: Helen Ewan
Production Coordinator: Sharon McCarthy
Design Coordinator: Nicholas Rook
Indexer: Ann Cassar
Compositor: Circle Graphics
Printer and Binder: R.R. Donnelley and Sons Company/Crawfordsville
Cover Printer: Lehigh Press

Edition 2

9 8 7 6 5 4 3 2

Library of Congress Cataloging in Publications Data

McCall, Ruth E.
    Phlebotomy essentials / Ruth E. McCall, Cathee M. Tankersley. —
2nd ed.
        p.   cm.
    Includes bibliographical references and index.
    ISBN 0-7817-9198-7 (alk. paper)
    1. Phlebotomy.   I. Tankersley, Cathee M.   II. Title.
    [DNLM: 1. Phlebotomy.   WB 381 M478p 1997]
    RB45.15.M33   1997
    616.07′561—dc21
    DNLM/DLC
    for Library of Congress   91-11637
                                                               CIP

Care has been taken to confirm the accuracy of the information presented and to describe generally accepted practices. However, the authors, editors, and publisher are not responsible for errors or omissions or for any consequences from application of the information in this book and make no warranty, express or implied, with respect to the contents of the publication.

The authors, editors, and publisher have exerted every effort to ensure that drug selection and dosage set forth in this text are in accordance with current recommendations and practice at the time of publication. However, in view of ongoing research, changes in government regulations, and the constant flow of information relating to drug therapy and drug reactions, the reader is urged to check the package insert for each drug for any change in indications and dosage and for added warnings and precautions. This is particularly important when the recommended agent is a new or infrequently employed drug.

Some drugs and medical devices presented in this publication have Food and Drug Administration (FDA) clearance for limited use in restricted research settings. It is the responsibility of the health care provider to ascertain the FDA status of each drug or device planned for use in their clinical practice.

To my husband John, my sons Chris and Scott, and my parents Charles and Marie Ruppert for their encouragement, patience, and support of this effort.

Ruth E. McCall

To my husband, Tank, who is always there with an encouraging word and two very special friends, Julie and Brigitte, for their continuous, unwavering support.

Cathee M. Tankersley

Preface

The goal of *Phlebotomy Essentials, 2nd edition* is to provide accurate, up-to-date, practical information and instruction in phlebotomy procedures and techniques, along with a comprehensive background in theory and principles. This book can be used as an instructional text in phlebotomy basics for students with no prior experience in the subject (including health care workers being cross-trained in phlebotomy), and as a current technique reference for practicing phlebotomists and other health care workers who wish to update their skills or pass a national phlebotomy certification exam.

The chapter format of the first edition has been maintained, including the list of key terms and objectives at the beginning of each chapter plus study questions and suggested laboratory activities at the end of each chapter. Color has been added to highlight these features and to enhance the art program for this new edition.

Outstanding features of the second edition include:

- An expanded chapter on phlebotomy equipment with lots of photos, including many examples of the latest safety devices
- A new section on pediatric venipuncture techniques
- The latest safety procedures, including the new Standard Precautions and Transmission-Based Precautions recommended jointly by the Hospital Infection Control Practices Advisory Committee (HICPAC) and Centers for Disease Control and Prevention (CDC)
- A section on point-of-care testing designed to address the expanding role of the phlebotomist, as well as meet the needs of the multiskilled health care worker

The content of the book is designed to fulfill competencies for phlebotomy training developed by the National Accrediting Agency for Clinical Laboratory Science (NAACLS). All procedures have been written to conform to Occupational Safety and Health Administration (OSHA) rules and regulations, and standards developed by the National Committee for Clinical Laboratory Standards (NCCLS) when applicable.

The authors wish to express their gratitude to Christopher and John McCall for their photography skills, and to all others who assisted and supported this effort.

Ruth E. McCall, BS, MT(ASCP), CLS(NCA)
Cathee M. Tankersley, MT(ASCP), CLS(NCA)

Contents

1 **Phlebotomy: Past and Present**   1
An Historical Perspective on Phlebotomy   2
Phlebotomy Today   4
The Role of the Phlebotomist in a Changing Health Care
   Environment   4

2 **The Health Care Setting**   19
Types of Health Care Facilities   20
Characteristics of Hospitals in the United States   21
Public Health Service   22
Financing Health Care   22
Departments Within the Health Care Facility or Hospital   27
Clinical Laboratory Personnel   41
Clinical Laboratory Improvement Act   43

3 **Medical Terminology**   45
Word Roots   45
Prefixes   46
Suffixes   47
Combining Vowels   48
Combining Forms   49
Plural Endings   49
Medical Terminology Reminders   49
Abbreviations and Symbols   50

4 **An Overview of the Anatomy and Physiology
of the Human Body**   57
Anatomic Position   58
Other Body Positions   58
Body Planes   58
Body Directional Terms   59
Body Cavities   60
Body Functions   61
Body Organization   61
Body Systems   62

5 **The Circulatory System**   87
The Heart   88
The Vascular System   92
The Blood   100
Hemostasis   107
The Lymphatic System   109

6 **Infection Control, Safety, and First Aid**   113
Infection Control   114
Safety   129
First Aid Procedures   145

7 **Blood Collection Equipment and Supplies**   151
General Blood Collection Equipment   151
Arterial Puncture Equipment   155
Skin Puncture Equipment   155
Venipuncture Equipment   155

8 **Factors to Consider Prior to Blood Collection**   175
Physiologic Factors   175
Test Status   178
Factors to Consider in Site Selection   180
Collection Devices   182
Complications Associated With Blood Collection   185

9 **Venipuncture Collection Procedures**   193
Initiation of the Test Request   194
Patient Contact   197
Patient Identification   199
Preparing the Patient for Testing   202
Routine Venipuncture Procedure   204
Failure to Obtain Blood   218
Procedure for Inability to Obtain a Specimen   220
Procedure for Using a Butterfly   221
Syringe Venipuncture Procedure   223
Pediatric Venipuncture   225

10 **Skin Puncture Equipment and Procedures**   233
Skin Puncture Equipment   234
Skin Puncture Principles   238
Skin Puncture Procedure   241
Special Skin Puncture Procedures   245

11 **Special Procedures and Point-of-Care Testing**   255
Special Procedures   256

Blood Bank Specimens   256
Point-of-Care Testing   273
Coagulation Monitoring   273
Arterial Blood Gas and Chemistry Panels   277
Skin Tests   285
Strep Testing   288
Urinalysis   289

12 **Arterial Blood Gases**   **293**
Personnel Who Perform Arterial Puncture   294
Site Selection   294
Equipment and Supplies   296
Preparation   298
Procedure for Radial ABGs   299
ABG Collection From Other Sites   303
Complications Associated With Arterial Puncture   303
Sampling Errors   303
Criteria for Specimen Rejection   304

13 **Nonblood Specimens and Tests**   **307**
Nonblood Specimen Labeling and Handling   308
Types of Nonblood Specimens   308

14 **Quality Assurance and Specimen Handling**   **319**
Quality Assurance in Health Care   320
Total Quality Management   321
Quality Assurance in Phlebotomy   322
Areas in Phlebotomy That Are Subject to Quality Control   325
Specimen Handling   329
Specimen Processing   333

15 **Communication and Computers**   **339**
Communication Defined   340
Communication in Health Care   344
Telephone Communication   346
Communication Through Computerization   346

16 **Laboratory Mathematics**   **359**
The Metric System   359
Military Time   362
Temperature Measurement   363
Roman Numerals   363
Percent   365
Dilutions   366
Blood Volume   366

Glossary   369

Appendix A   Answers to Study and Review Questions   A-1
Appendix B   Conversational Phrases in English and Spanish   A-3
Appendix C   A Patient's Bill of Rights   A-7
Appendix D   Listing of Departments and Tests   A-9
Appendix E   Conditions Requiring Work Restrictions for Health
                 Care Employees   A-19
Appendix F   Procedure Evaluation Checklists   A-21

Index   I-1

List of Color Plates Following Page 86

Color Plate 1   **Heart and great vessels**
Color Plate 2   **Common color-coded evacuated tube stoppers**
Color Plate 3   **Formed elements of the blood**

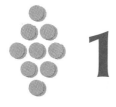

1

Phlebotomy: Past and Present

KEY TERMS

AAAHP	continuing education units	NCCLS
accreditation	(CEUs)	negligence
AMT	essentials	A Patient's Bill of Rights
approval	expressed consent	phlebotomy
ASCLS	fraud	professionalism
ASCP	implied consent	reciprocity
ASPT	informed consent	respondeat superior
assault	invasion of privacy	risk management
battery	licensure	standard of care
breach of confidentiality	malpractice	statute of limitations
certification	NAACLS	tort
civil law	NCA	vicarious liability

OBJECTIVES

Upon successful completion of this chapter, the reader would be able to:

1. Describe the evolution of phlebotomy to the present day.
2. List the duties of the phlebotomist.
3. Describe the traits that form the professional image.
4. Contrast certification, licensure, and accreditation.
5. Identify national organizations that support phlebotomy as a profession.
6. Describe the phlebotomist's role in public relations for the health care facility and list the important points in A Patient's Bill of Rights.
7. Define legal terminology associated with the health care setting, and describe how a phlebotomist can avoid litigation.

AN HISTORICAL PERSPECTIVE ON PHLEBOTOMY

Since very early times, man has been fascinated by blood and has believed in some connection between the blood racing through his veins and his well-being. From this belief, certain medical principles and procedures dealing with blood evolved, some surviving to the present day.

An early medical theory developed by Hippocrates (460–377 BC) stated that disease was the result of excess substance, such as blood, phlegm, black bile, and yellow bile, within the body. It was thought that removal of the excess would restore balance. The process of removal and extraction became the treatment and could be done either by expelling disease materials through the use of drugs or by direct removal during surgery. One important surgical technique was **phlebotomy**—the process of bloodletting. Bloodletting involved cutting into a vein with a sharp instrument and releasing blood in an effort to rid the body of evil spirits, cleanse the body of impurities, or, as in Hippocrates' time, bring the body into proper balance. Literal translation of the word phlebotomy comes from the Greek words *phlebos*, meaning veins, and *tome*, meaning incision.

Some authorities believe phlebotomy dates back to the last period of the Stone Age, when crude tools were used to puncture vessels to allow excess blood to drain out of the body. Bloodletting in Egypt around 1400 BC is evidenced by a painting in a tomb showing the application of a leech to a patient. Early in the Middle Ages, barber-surgeons flourished. By 1210, the Guild of Barber-Surgeons was formed and divided the surgeons into Surgeons of the Long Robe and Surgeons of the Short Robe. Soon the Short Robe surgeons were forbidden by law to do any surgery except bloodletting, wound surgery, cupping, leeching, shaving, extraction of teeth, and administering of enemas.

To distinguish his profession from that of the Long Robe surgeon, the barber-surgeon placed a striped pole from which a bleeding bowl (Fig. 1-1) was suspended outside his door. The pole represented the rod squeezed by the patient to promote bleeding and the white stripe on the pole corresponded to the bandages, which were also used as tourniquets. Soon, handsomely decorated ceramic bleeding bowls came into fashion and were passed down from one generation to the next. These bowls, which often doubled as shaving bowls, usually had a circular indention on one side to facilitate placing the bowl under the chin.

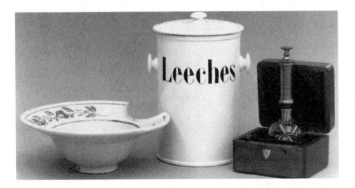

Figure 1-1 Early phlebotomy equipment (left to right): bleeding bowl, leech jar, and 19th century cupping glass and evacuating pump. (Courtesy Robert Kravetz, MD, FACP, FACG, Phoenix, AZ.)

During the 17th and early 18th centuries, phlebotomy was considered a major therapeutic (treatment) process and anyone willing to claim medical training could perform phlebotomy. In the late 18th and early 19th centuries, nonprofessional barbers and women were discouraged from bloodletting by well-known surgeons because of the dangers posed by the untutored. The lancet, a tool used for cutting the vein during a procedure called venesection, was perhaps the most prevalent medical instrument of the times. Antisepsis was unknown as lancets were often passed from patient to patient without cleansing. The usual amount of blood withdrawn was approximately 10 mL, but excessive phlebotomy was common. In fact, it was thought to have contributed to George Washington's death in 1799, when he was diagnosed with a throat infection and the physician bled him four times in 2 days. It was because of Washington's request to be allowed to die without further medical intervention that he was not completely exsanguinated.

During this same period, phlebotomy was also accomplished by cupping and leeching. The art of cupping required a great deal of practice to maintain the high degree of dexterity necessary so as not to appear clumsy and frighten the patient away. Cupping involved the application of a heated suction apparatus, called the "cup," to the skin to draw the blood to the surface before severing the capillaries in that area by making a series of parallel incisions with a lancet or fleam (Fig. 1-2). Around 1800, cups began to appear with brass syringes attached to remove air from the cup (see Fig. 1-1), eliminating the need to heat the cup in order to tumefy the area before cutting. This process was called dry cupping when performed prior to cutting the skin, and wet cupping if performed after cutting the skin.

Another procedure, called "leeching," involved enticing the *Hirudo medicinalis*, a European medicinal leech, to the spot needing bloodletting with a drop of milk or blood on the patient's skin. Once the leech was engorged with blood, which took about an hour, it was allowed to drop off by itself. Leechers, although not as high in status as professional cuppers, practiced in many large cities. In fact, in the early 1800s, leech farms were unable to meet the leech demand, making the little animals scarce and expensive.

With the popularity of bloodletting, improvement of the tools was inevitable. Two bloodletting instruments developed during this period were the schnepper and the

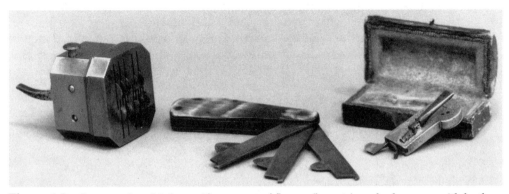

Figure 1-2   Octagonal multiple scarificator, set of fleams (lancets), and schnepper with leather-covered wooden case. (Courtesy Robert Kravetz, MD, FACP, FACG, Phoenix, AZ.)

scarificator (see Fig. 1-2). The crudely designed schnepper was an automatic or spring-action lancet which allowed the user to inject the blade into a vein without exerting manual pressure. This decorated or embossed tiny instrument was widely adopted for use on humans. The introduction of the scarificator in the 19th century represented a major change in the art of cupping. The scarificator had several crescent-shaped, spring-loaded blades concealed within a box-like case which, when activated, instantaneously created a series of parallel cuts. Like the spring lancet, the scarificator has its modern-day counterpart in the devices used for bleeding time tests.

PHLEBOTOMY TODAY

The practice of phlebotomy continues to this day; however, principles and methods have improved dramatically. Today, the main purpose of phlebotomy is to obtain blood for diagnostic testing. Phlebotomy procedures also are used to remove blood for transfusion purposes. Phlebotomy for therapeutic purposes is still practiced in certain instances, such as for a patient with polycythemia, a disease involving over-production of red blood cells, or hemochromatosis, a rare disease characterized by excess iron deposits throughout the body. The use of leeches has reemerged with a new pur-pose: that of reducing hemostatic swelling after microsurgery until reconnected tissue can grow new capillaries and veins to carry deoxygenated blood away, thus improving circulation in the replanted tissue.

Phlebotomy today is primarily accomplished by one of two procedures: (1) venipuncture, which involves collecting blood by penetrating a vein with a needle and syringe or other collection apparatus; and (2) skin puncture, which involves collecting blood after puncturing the skin with a lancet or similar skin puncture device.

THE ROLE OF THE PHLEBOTOMIST IN A CHANGING HEALTH CARE ENVIRONMENT

The term phlebotomist is applied to a person who has been trained to perform phlebotomy procedures. The primary responsibility of a phlebotomist is to collect blood for laboratory analysis, which is necessary for the diagnosis and care of a patient. Manual skills required are those necessary to obtain blood specimens by venipuncture and skin puncture techniques. Mental skills required are the ability to organize effi-ciently, perform under pressure, and follow written standardized procedures. Thorough knowledge of laboratory test requirements and departmental policies is also necessary.

THE TRADITIONAL DUTIES OF A PHLEBOTOMIST

1. Collect routine skin puncture and venous specimens for testing as required.
2. Prepare specimens for transport to ensure stability of sample.
3. Transport specimens to the laboratory.

THE TRADITIONAL DUTIES OF A PHLEBOTOMIST *(Continued)*

4. Comply with new and revised procedures instituted in the procedure manual.
5. Promote good public relations with patients and hospital personnel.
6. Assist in collecting and documenting monthly workload and recording data.
7. Maintain safe working conditions.
8. Perform laboratory computer operations.
9. Participate in continuing education programs.

Today, as the nation moves into managed care, the role of the phlebotomist is continually changing as roles and responsibilities for all health care providers undergo change. The development of teams and the sharing of tasks has become necessary as health care organizations attempt to find the balance between cost-effective treatment and quality care. As a result, the duties of health care workers are combined, for example, a respiratory therapist may collect the laboratory specimen or a phlebotomist may take care of the basic needs of a patient at the bedside. The job description for a phlebotomist can vary greatly from one facility to the next based on the needs of that particular organization. With the advent of point-of-care testing (POCT), centralized laboratory services are giving way to decentralized activities, forcing phlebotomists to become multiskilled or lose their jobs.

ADDITIONAL DUTIES OF THE MULTISKILLED PHLEBOTOMIST

1. Collect sample and perform point-of-care testing (POCT) eg, glucose monitoring.
2. Do quality control checks on POCT instruments.
3. Perform skin tests.
4. Do rapid strep and breath alcohol testing.
5. Perform electrocardiography.
6. Process specimens and perform basic laboratory tests.

During this time of transition, the profession of phlebotomy maintains a standardized educational curriculum with a recognized body of knowledge. Structured programs exist in hospitals, colleges, and vocational schools which incorporate classroom instruction and clinical practice to prepare the student for national certification. As the role of the phlebotomist expands, the knowledge base will also. It is expected that basic nursing skills, specimen processing, customer relations, and POCT instruction will become a part of the educational curriculum.

Professionalism

As part of a service-oriented industry, persons performing phlebotomy must practice professionalism. **Professionalism** is defined as the conduct and qualities that characterize a professional person.

The overall impression conveyed by a person creates an image. The professional image is the way in which an occupation or a member of that profession is perceived. This image is formed from several characteristics or traits. The first characteristic deals with the superficial aspects of a person, for example, the way a person dresses or his or her manner of speaking. In fact, general appearance and grooming reflect directly on whether the phlebotomist is perceived as a professional. Conservative clothing, proper personal hygiene, and physical well-being contribute to a professional appearance. Since protective clothing must be provided by the employer, the proper attire for the phlebotomist may be defined by institution guidelines, such as specified lab coats and shoes to conform with OSHA standards.

Professionalism also deals with personal behaviors or characteristics including integrity, compassion, motivation, dependability, and work ethic.

- A phlebotomist may function independently a large percentage of the time, and respecting the rules for collection is essential to the quality of the results. Professional standards of *integrity*, or honesty, require a person to do what is right regardless of the circumstances, especially when unsupervised.
- A phlebotomist may show *compassion* and still remain professional. Compassion simply means being sensitive to a patient's or customer's needs and being willing to offer reassurance in a caring and interested way.
- Phlebotomists with *motivation* find the workplace a challenge no matter what their tasks entail. Motivation is a direct reflection of a person's attitude about life. If phlebotomists have a positive attitude and a willingness to perform at their peak every day, the health care environment will consistently offer adventure and growth, especially during this exciting time of changing roles and responsibilities.
- *Dependability* and *work ethic* go hand-in-hand. An individual who is dependable and who takes personal responsibility for his or her actions is extremely refreshing in today's environment and is a very desirable candidate for job opportunities in the health care setting or anywhere.

Other factors that play a role in forming a professional image stem from public recognition of the education the individual has acquired and the assumption that this education constitutes a standardized curriculum and regulation of the profession. It is through national accrediting and certifying agencies that professions ensure adherence to expected standards. Because there are different philosophies concerning standards for phlebotomy curricula and certification, a number of agencies have evolved, offering the phlebotomist options for professional recognition.

CERTIFICATION

Recognition through **certification** is becoming more popular because of the need in today's climate for health care professionals to show evidence of proficiency in many different areas of practice. Certification is evidence that an individual has mastered fundamental competencies in a particular technical area. Not unlike licensure, certification is a process that indicates the completion of defined academic and training requirements and the attainment of a satisfactory score on an examination, usually from a national agency. This is verified by the awarding of a title, signified by initials which a phlebotomist is allowed to display after his or her name.

The purpose of certification is to protect the public through control of personnel working at a specified level of responsibility. Agencies that certify phlebotomists and the title each awards include the following:

- American Medical Technologists (AMT): Registered Phlebotomy Technician, RPT (AMT)
- American Society of Clinical Pathologists (ASCP): Phlebotomy Technician PBT(ASCP)
- American Society for Phlebotomy Technicians (ASPT): Certified Phlebotomy Technician, CPT(ASPT)
- American Association of Allied Health Professionals, Inc. (AAAHP): Certified Phlebotomy Technician, CPT(AAAHP)
- National Certification Agency for Medical Laboratory Personnel (NCA): Clinical Laboratory Phlebotomist, CLPlb(NCA)
- National Phlebotomy Association (NPA): Certified Phlebotomy Technician, CPT(NPA)

LICENSURE AND REGISTRATION

A license is a document or permit indicating that permission has been granted for a person to perform a certain service after he or she has met the education and experience requirements and successfully completed an examination. For example, barbers, beauticians, and nurses are licensed by the state in which they practice. A health professional who has successfully passed a national certification examination or a state licensure examination may be put on a list called a registry. This listing is maintained as long as the health professional pays the registration fee annually (*eg*, to the ASCP Board of Registry). Such registries may not reflect the level of the laboratory professional's knowledge since they may not require the registrant to maintain competency to be listed. If a nationally certified phlebotomist should wish to work in a state which has a **licensure** law, he or she could request that the state agency grant the license required in recognition of his or her certification. Such recognition is called **reciprocity**.

PROGRAM ACCREDITATION/APPROVAL

Accreditation, or **approval**, of an educational program for health professionals indicates the quality of the program. The accreditation process involves external peer review of the program, including an on-site survey to determine whether the program meets certain established educational standards referred to as **essentials.** Most medical technology, medical laboratory technician, and histology programs seek accreditation. For phlebotomy programs, approval, rather than accreditation, is offered. The approval process is similar to accreditation; however, programs must meet educational *standards* and *competencies* rather than essentials, and an on-site survey by the agency's approval team is not required. Examples of approval agencies for phlebotomy programs include the following:

- American Association of Allied Health Professionals, Inc. (AAAHP)
- American Medical Technologists (AMT)
- The American Society for Phlebotomy Technicians (ASPT)
- The National Accrediting Agency for Clinical Laboratory Sciences (NAACLS)
- The National Phlebotomy Association (NPA)

CONTINUING EDUCATION

To remain current in the increasingly complex field of laboratory medicine, it is important for a phlebotomist to participate in workshops and seminars to upgrade skills and knowledge on a continual basis. Some certification agencies require proof of such continuing education to renew certification. Employers may offer in-service education or funds to attend off-site programs. National organizations that offer the phlebotomist **continuing education units (CEUs)** are the following:

- American Association of Allied Health Professionals, Inc. (AAAHP)
- American Medical Technologists (AMT)
- The American Society for Clinical Laboratory Sciences (ASCLS)
- The American Society of Clinical Pathologists (ASCP)
- The American Society for Phlebotomy Technicians (ASPT)
- The National Phlebotomy Association (NPA)

NATIONAL STANDARDS

A national, nonprofit organization formed by representatives from the profession, industry, and government, called the National Committee for Clinical Laboratory Standards **(NCCLS)**, develops guidelines and sets standards for all areas of the laboratory. Phlebotomy program approval as well as certification examination questions are based on these important national standards.

Another agency that influences the standards of phlebotomy is the College of American Pathologists (CAP). This national organization is an outgrowth of the American Society of Clinical Pathologists (ASCP). The membership in this specialty organization is composed entirely of board-certified pathologist. CAP offers proficiency testing as well as a continuous form of laboratory inspection by a team made up of pathologists and laboratory managers. The CAP Inspection and Accreditation Program does not compete with the Joint Commission on Accreditation of Healthcare Organizations (JCAHO) accreditation for health care facilities because it is designed for pathology services only. A CAP-certified laboratory also meets Medicare/Medicaid standards because JCAHO grants reciprocity to CAP in the area of laboratory inspection.

Public Relations

As a member of the clinical laboratory team, the phlebotomist plays an important role in public relations for the laboratory. Positive public relations involves promoting good will and a harmonious relationship with staff, visitors, and especially patients. The phlebotomist is often the only real contact the patient has with the laboratory. A confident phlebotomist with a professional manner and a neat appearance helps to put the patient at ease and helps establish a positive relationship. In many cases, patients equate this encounter with the caliber of care they receive while in the hospital.

DIPLOMACY AND ETHICAL BEHAVIOR

A phlebotomist should demonstrate diplomacy and ethical behavior at all times. Diplomacy means the phlebotomist uses effective communication skills and tact while dealing with the patient, even in stressful situations. Ethical behavior entails conforming to a standard of right and wrong conduct to avoid harming the patient in any way. Based on a system of principles called ethics, the professional can identify conduct that is morally desirable. A code of ethics, while not enforceable by law, leads to uniformity and defined expectation by the members of that profession. Professional organizations, such as the American Society for Clinical Laboratory Scientists (ASCLS) and the National Phlebotomy Association (NPA), have developed codes of ethics for health care professionals.

Ethical decisions made every day in health care facilities inevitably focus on the most complex applications of modern medicine. As part of their mission statement, hospitals throughout the United States have established codes of ethics that deal specifically with a variety of management and patient concerns, including patient confidentiality, informed consent, treatment of the terminally ill, care for the poor, and allocation of funds for special procedures. The primary objective in any health care professional's code of ethics must always be the patient's welfare. As stated in the Hippocratic oath, "primum non nocere," or "first do not harm."

PATIENT RIGHTS

The phlebotomist, as any other member of the health care team, must recognize the rights and privileges a patient has while in a hospital or other health care facility. These rights have been clearly defined in a document originally published in 1975 by the American Hospital Association called **A Patient's Bill of Rights.** (See the complete Patient Bill of Rights in Appendix C.) This document, although not legally binding, is an accepted statement of principle that guides health care workers in their dealings with patients. It states that all health care professionals, including phlebotomists, have a primary responsibility for quality patient care, while at the same time maintaining the patient's personal rights and dignity. Some of the rights especially pertinent to the phlebotomist are as follows:

- The right of the patient to always be treated with respect
- The right to refuse to have blood drawn
- The right to have the results of laboratory work remain confidential
- The right to obtain from the physician the purpose of the testing and the results

Legal Considerations

Because of consumer awareness, lawsuits have increased in all areas of society. This is especially true in the health care industry, where physicians and providers were once considered above reproach. As health care providers go about their daily activities, there are many practices that, if performed without reasonable care and skill, could result in a lawsuit. It has been proven in past lawsuits that persons performing phlebotomy can and will be held legally accountable for their actions.

CRIMINAL VERSUS CIVIL LAW

In the United States, the legal system encompasses two areas of law: criminal and civil. Criminal law is concerned with acts committed in violation of laws established by state governmental agencies such as the legislature. Criminal laws are those rules that are designed to protect all members of society from injurious acts by others. Criminal cases are brought by the state (not an individual) against individuals. These crimes are either felonies or misdemeanors. The more serious crimes such as murder, assault, and rape are felonies. Misdemeanors, gross or small, are considered lesser offenses and usually carry a penalty of a fine or less than 1 year in jail.

Civil law is concerned with actions between two private parties, such as individuals, corporations, or organizations. They constitute the bulk of the legal actions dealt with in the medical office or health care facilities. An example of a civil case would be a patient who, while being assisted from a bed by a health care provider, slips and falls because of some liquid on the floor. The patient suffers a simple fracture of the lower arm from the fall. It is discovered that some water was spilled by another employee and not cleaned up. On the grounds that it is the health care facility's responsibility to provide a safe environment for those that enter, the patient takes action under civil law and sues for medical fees and loss of wages as a result of the injury.

TORT LAW

Civil law is based on tort. A **tort** is a civil wrong, other than breach of contract, committed against a person or property for which damages may be awarded in a court of law. It is an act that is committed without just cause. The act may be intentional (willful) or unintentional (accidental).

Examples of tort actions are as follows:

- **Assault** is defined as the act (threat) of intentionally causing another to be in apprehension (fear) of immediate harm to his or her person (battery). Battery does not necessarily have to follow an assault in order for the assault to be a tort. For it to be assault, the person that is committing the assault must have the ability to carry out the threat or the person being assaulted must believe the ability is there.
- **Battery** is the intentional harmful or offensive touching of another person without consent or legal justification. Legal justification would be, for example, when a mother gives permission to have her child examined or blood drawn from the child. Intentional harm may range from permanent disfigurement to merely removing a person's hat without permission or grabbing something out of another person's hand. A phlebotomist who attempts a procedure without the patient's consent is violating this right and can be charged with assault and battery.

- **Fraud** may be harm to a person, harm to property, or both. It is a type of deceitful practice or willful plan resorted to with the intent to deprive another person of his or her right or in some manner to cause that person injury. It is different than negligence in that it is always intentional.
- **Invasion of privacy** is the violation of one's right to be left alone and to live without being subject to unwarranted or undesired publicity. In the medical field, invasion of privacy by physical intrusion may be no more than walking through a closed door into a patient's room without asking the patient for permission. Invasion of privacy also involves the publishing or releasing of private information, even though true, which may be objectionable in nature. In the health care setting, this could be a breach of confidentiality of laboratory results causing great embarrassment for the patient or even greater consequences, such as loss of job.

NEGLIGENCE

In the majority of cases people do not deliberately try to inflict harm on another person. But if a person or business, such as a hospital, does unintentionally harm someone, that person has the right to sue under tort law for damages from improper treatment caused by **negligence**. Negligence can involve doing something carelessly or failing to do something that should have been done. There are various levels of negligence including slight (not much), ordinary (failing to act as a reasonable, careful person), or gross (reckless and willful). For negligence to be claimed the following must be present:

1. A legal duty or obligation owed by one person to another
2. A breaking or breach of duty
3. Harm done as a direct result of the action

Negligence is defined as the failure to exercise due care when there is a predictable risk of harm to another person. Due care is the duty that health care providers have to protect others from harm. It arises when a person can see that what he or she does may create an unreasonable risk of harm to others. For example, injuring a patient's arm or allowing the patient to get hurt if he or she should faint is not exercising due care as a phlebotomist. Due care also implies that the person performing the procedures possesses the qualifications and training to provide the necessary skilled care. This, in turn, requires that the physician or hospital provide competent personnel, thus making the physician or hospital ultimately liable under the law for the standard of care.

RESPONDEAT SUPERIOR

Respondeat superior is a Latin phrase that means "let the master respond." It is another way of saying that the employer must conform to a specific standard of care to protect patients and must answer for damages employees commit within the scope of employment, even though the employees may be at fault. This tort may be filed because of a neglectful act of an employee which results in physical harm or loss to someone else or because of an intentional act by the employee in connection with his or her employment that results in some type of physical injury to another person. The key points in the action of respondeat superior are that the employee is working within the scope of employment and that the employee has had the proper training to perform the required duties. If the employee is doing something that is outside of his or her scope of duties or training, the employee may be held solely responsible for that action because once a person reaches adulthood they are liable or legally responsible for their own acts.

In the past, the health care provider has not been a target for lawsuits because of the deep pocket theory (let the one with the most money pay) and the idea of respondeat superior (let the master respond). With managed care forcing the expansion of each individual's duties, workers are faced with more opportunities to practice beyond their scope of training. It has become more and more important for each individual to examine the possibility of a civil suit being brought against him or her. Consequently, the question arises: do health care workers other than physicians need financial protection in the form of insurance against lawsuits?

MALPRACTICE INSURANCE

One type of insurance that health care providers may wish to purchase is malpractice or liability insurance. The decision to purchase such an insurance should be based on financial considerations as well as legal ones. From the legal point of view, it may be desirable to be covered by a separate professional liability policy because the employer may give the insurer the right to recover damages from the employee if the employee is negligent. If the employee has his or her own policy, the insurer's primary duty is to the insured employee. Liability insurance can be found through professional organizations and is usually offered at a reasonable or reduced rate.

The most reasonable approach to lawsuits is to avoid them. A phlebotomist should consistently follow rules such as these:

1. Acquire informed consent before collection of specimens.
2. Strictly adhere to accepted procedures and practices.
3. Use proper safety containers and devices.
4. Listen and respond appropriately to the patient's requests.
5. Accurately and legibly record all information concerning patients.
6. Document incidents or occurrences.
7. Participate in continuing education to maintain proficiency.
8. Basically, perform at the prevailing standard of care.

STANDARD OF CARE

People working in the medical field are required to perform their duties in the same fashion that any other reasonable and prudent person with the same experience and training would. The performance of these duties is judged by a prevailing set of standards, called the **standard of care**. Standards of care are established by licensing and regulatory agencies, national standards, professional organizations, national publications, and state statutes.

MALPRACTICE

A patient who is injured because of the improper actions of a health care provider is entitled to compensation for the injury. Medical **malpractice**, a type of negligence, is a tort action brought against a health care provider by means of a civil lawsuit. To support the claim of malpractice it must be proven that actions by the health care provider were negligent or fell below the accepted standard of care, and were responsible for the plaintiff's injuries. An example would be injury to the cutaneous nerve caused by excessive probing during a venipuncture.

PATIENT CONSENT

Informed consent implies voluntary and competent permission for a medical procedure, test, or medication and requires that a patient be given adequate information regarding the method, risks, and consequences involved before consenting to it. An individual has a constitutional right to refuse medical treatment. A phlebotomist who attempts a procedure without the patient's consent is violating this right and can be charged with assault and battery. It is, therefore, mandatory for the health care provider to explain the procedure and obtain the patient's permission or consent before initiating any medical procedure. Information must be given to the patient in nontechnical terms and in his or her own language, if possible, meaning an interpreter may be necessary. Blood collection on minors requires consent of their parents or legal guardians.

HIV CONSENT

Legislation governing informed consent for HIV testing has been enacted in most states. The laws specify exactly what type of information must be given to inform the client properly. Generally speaking, the client must be advised on (1) the test and its purpose; (2) how the test might be used; and (3) the meaning of the test and its limitations.

EXPRESSED CONSENT

Expressed consent may be given verbally or in writing. Expressed consent is necessary for proposed treatment that involves surgery, experimental drugs, or high-risk procedures. Written consent gives the best possible protection for both the person providing the treatment and the one receiving the treatment. Written consent must be signed by the person providing the treatment and the patient and should be witnessed by a third party. If consent is given verbally, the provider giving the treatment should make an entry in the patient's chart covering what was discussed with the patient. The consent should cover what procedures are going to be performed and should not be in a general form that allows the physician carte blanche to do whatever he or she wants to do. If such a general consent goes to court, the court generally takes the word of the patient as to what he or she understood was to take place.

IMPLIED CONSENT

With **implied consent**, the patient need not make a verbal expression of consent. In the case of drawing blood from a patient, all that is needed is that the phlebotomist explain what he or she is going to do. If after the explanation is given, the patient holds out an arm, that alone is consent. Implied consent may be necessary in emergency procedures such as CPR to save a person's life. Health care providers need to recognize that laws for implied consent are enacted at the state level and may differ greatly from one state to another.

MEDICAL RECORDS

Without a medical record of some type, there would be no way of knowing the medical history of a patient. Patients cannot always recount what treatment they have received or when it was given. Often they do not know what types of medications they have been given over the years or what they are presently taking. For these reasons, it is a must that good medical records be kept on all patients. The law requires that medical records be kept on hospital patients but does not require physicians in their private practice to keep records on their patients, although most do.

The basic reasons for maintaining accurate, up-to-date medical records are as follows:

1. To provide an aid to practicing medicine. Through the use of a medical record, the physician can document treatment and give a written plan for continuation of the patient's care plan.
2. To provide an aid to communications between the physician and others involved with the patient's care. It can also serve as a communications tool between past, present, and future physicians that care for the patient.
3. To serve as a legal document that may be used in a court of law. It must be a factual, a legible, and an objective account of the patient, past and present.
4. To facilitate peer review and medical research, teaching, and statistics.
5. To serve as a very valuable tool for assisting the hospital in total quality management through utilization review, since the medical records include such information as a history of examinations, laboratory and other medical testing reports, prescriptions written, and supplies used.

Often the question comes up as to who owns the medical record. The record itself is the property of the physician or the hospital. This means that they have the right to restrict its removal. The information within the record is the patient's, and the patient has a right to that information if he or she should request it. All information in the medical record is confidential and must be protected even while in transit.

CONFIDENTIALITY

There must be a bond between the physician and his or her patients that allows the patients to speak freely about themselves, their mental health, and their medical condition overall. For this to happen, patients must know that what they say to their physician will not be made public. Physicians pledge when they take the Hippocratic oath that they will not disclose patient information. Today, all health care providers recognize and observe patient confidentiality.

Observance of the principle of confidentiality is seen by many as the ethical cornerstone of professional behavior in the health care field. It serves to protect both the patient and the practitioner. As a professional, the health care provider should recognize that all patient information is absolutely private and confidential. Confidentiality, or the right to privacy of information, whether patient or employee, must always be maintained, especially when dealing with sensitive areas such as drug screens or sexually transmitted disease.

Patient information, such as a patient's test results, treatment, or condition, is not to be discussed with a coworker on an elevator, in the lunchroom, or any place where the information might be overheard by friends or family of the patient. In addition, patient information should not be released to unauthorized persons or any person of celebrated status. Any questions relating to patient information, such as inquiries from a reporter in the case of a celebrity, should be referred to the proper person in administration. Unauthorized release of information concerning a patient can lead to a claim of **breach of confidentiality** or invasion of privacy, such as in the case of patient with HIV.

HIV Testing and Confidentiality

With a growing number of patients who are HIV positive now in our medical treatment facilities, an important concern is maintaining confidentiality. As long as privileged communications are maintained, this problem can be controlled. It is important to remember that none of the information concerning a patient can be given to a third party. Information should only be given out with the written consent of the patient or when a health care provider is legally obligated to release the information. Many court cases stem from breach of confidentiality and there are many more cases that are settled outside of court through arbitration.

STATUTE OF LIMITATIONS

Regardless of the type of tort, all civil suits, as well as criminal suits, have a limited amount of time after the alleged injury in which a person is permitted to file a lawsuit. The **statute of limitations** prescribes a time limit on how soon a plaintiff must file a lawsuit after an alleged injury has occurred. The question for all parties involved is when the clock starts. Some of the most common occurrences given for the beginning of a statutory period are as follows:

- On the day the alleged negligent act was committed
- When the injury resulting from the alleged negligence was actually discovered, or should have been discovered, by a reasonably alert patient
- The day the physician–patient relationship ended, or the day of the last medical treatment in a series

VICARIOUS LIABILITY

In today's health care facilities, consultants and independent contractors perform some of the services once considered the responsibilities of the employees of the particular facility. Should injury occur as a result of a negligent act committed by an independent contractor, the health care facility that hired the person is liable. This is called **vicarious liability** and is based on the fact that the contractor is acting on behalf of the facility by virtue of the facility's allowing the contractor to practice within the confines of the facility or under the auspices of that particular health care organization. The hospital, as the employer, would be deceiving the public if it were to escape liability for a patient's injury by simply subcontracting out various services to other persons and claiming it is not responsible because the party that caused the injury is not on its payroll.

RISK MANAGEMENT

Risk is defined as "the chance of loss or injury." Risks are inherent in the health care profession, and it is important for phlebotomists to know about these risks and how to minimize them. Careful planning, in the form of objectives, will reduce hazards and

LINCOLN   EMPLOYEE ACTION RECORD

_____   _____   _____
EMPLOYEE NAME   DEPARTMENT   DATE

THIS FORM IS USED TO DOCUMENT DISCUSSION CONCERNING A COMMENDATION OR ACTION TAKEN TO IMPROVE INAPPROPRIATE PERFORMANCE BY AN EMPLOYEE. THE INFORMATION CONTAINED ON THIS FORM WILL BE INCLUDED IN THE EMPLOYEE'S PERSONNEL FILE.

( ) COMMENDATION   ( ) CORRECTIVE ACTION   ( ) OTHER

I. DESCRIBE ISSUE OR INCIDENT (PROVIDE DATES AND DETAILS):
_____
_____
_____
_____

II. PROVIDE SPECIFIC INFORMATION DISCUSSED WITH THE EMPLOYEE REGARDING SECTION I.:
_____
_____
_____
_____

III. PROVIDE THE AGREED-UPON PLAN FOR TAKING CORRECTIVE ACTION, IF APPLICABLE (INCLUDE THE DATE FOR FOLLOW-UP AND NEXT ACTION TO BE TAKEN, IF NECESSARY):
_____
_____
_____
_____

IV. EMPLOYEE COMMENTS:
_____
_____
_____
_____

(ATTACH ADDITIONAL SHEETS IF NECESSARY)

_____   _____   _____   _____
DEPARTMENT MANAGER   DATE   EMPLOYEE (SIGNATURE DOES DATE
                                      NOT NECESSARILY
                                      INDICATE AGREEMENT.)

_____   _____
VICE PRESIDENT   DATE

WHITE COPY: HUMAN RESOURCES   YELLOW COPY: DIRECTOR   PINK COPY: EMPLOYEE

JCL: 04/91/N-115

Figure 1-3   Incident form. (Courtesy of John C. Lincoln Hospital, Phoenix, AZ.)

benefit the employee as well as the patient. Generic steps in **risk management** involve identification of the risk; treatment of the risk using policies and procedures already in place; education for employees and patients; and evaluation of what should be done in the future.

Reporting tools, such as incident or occurrence reports (Fig. 1-3), are a good way to identify situations that deviate from the normal so that proper investigation can be made. Risk is managed in two ways: controlling risk to avoid incidents and paying for occurrences after they have happened. As in any continuous quality improvement (CQI) program, the objective is to reduce unfavorable outcomes continuously. As new procedures are instituted to reduce risk, employees must be informed immediately and instructed on what to do. Throughout the operation of a risk management program, evaluation of occurrences, trends, and outcomes is essential so that appropriate changes can be made.

Study & Review Questions

1. Early equipment used for bloodletting includes all of the following *except* the
   - a. hemostat.
   - b. lancet.
   - c. schnepper.
   - d. scarificator.

2. A factor that contributes to the phlebotomist's professional image is
   - a. personal hygiene.
   - b. national certification.
   - c. a pleasant smile and a positive attitude.
   - d. all of the above.

3. The initials for the title granted after successful completion of the National Certification Agency phlebotomy examination are
   - a. CLPlb.
   - b. CLT.
   - c. CPT.
   - d. PBT.

4. The principles of right and wrong conduct as they apply to professional problems are called
   - a. certification.
   - b. ethics.
   - c. esteem.
   - d. tort.

5. Necessary elements of risk management are all of the following *except*
   - a. education.
   - b. evaluation.
   - c. identification.
   - d. obligation.

6. Which of the following is one of the expanded duties of a phlebotomist?
   - a. Collect routine capillary specimens
   - b. Promote good public relations with patients
   - c. Obtain blood pressures and temperatures of patients
   - d. Perform laboratory computer operations

7. Which of the following is a patient right?
   - a. To watch your test being performed in the laboratory
   - b. To read other patients' medical charts
   - c. To refuse treatment
   - d. To be disruptive to other patients

8. Informed consent means
   a. a phlebotomist tells the patient what is ordered and the implications of the test results.
   b. a patient agrees to a procedure after being told of the consequences associated with it.
   c. a patient has the right to look at all his or her medical records.
   d. a nurse has the right to perform a procedure on a patient even if the patient refuses.

Suggested Lab Activities

1. Write an article on phlebotomy history from a library resource.

2. Spend a day in a health care setting where phlebotomy is performed.

3. Review case studies involving patient's rights and discuss them in class.

BIBLIOGRAPHY AND SUGGESTED READINGS

Chamberlain, R. T. (1987). Professional negligence and the clinical laboratory. *Journal of Medical Technology*, May/June.

Cowdrey, M. D., & Drew, D. (1995). *Basic law for the allied health professions* (2nd ed.). Boston: Jones and Bartlett Publishers.

Davis, A., & Appel, T. (1979). *Bloodletting instruments in the National Museum of History and Technology*. Washington, DC: Smithsonian Institution Press.

Flight, M. (1993). *Law, liability, and ethics for medical office personnel* (2nd ed.). New York: Delmar Publishers.

Haller, J. (1973). The glass leech: Wet and dry cupping practices in the nineteenth century. *New York Journal of Medicine*, February 15.

Henry, J. B. (1996). *Clinical diagnosis and management by laboratory methods* (19th ed.). Philadelphia: W. B. Saunders.

Judson, K., & Blesie, S. (1996). *Law and ethics for health occupations*. New York: Glencoe/McGraw-Hill.

Lewis, M. A., & Tamparo, C. D. (1993). *Medical law, ethics, and bioethics in the medical office* (3rd ed.). Philadelphia: F. A. Davis.

Murdock, S., & Murdock, J. (1987). From leeches to luers: The history of phlebotomy. *Journal of Medical Technology*, September/October.

Oran, D. (1991). *Dictionary of law*. Los Angeles: West Publishing.

Reitzel, J. D., Lyden, D. P., Roberts, N. J., & Severance, G. B. (1990). *Contemporary business law: Principles and cases* (4th ed.). New York: McGraw-Hill.

Stanfield, P. S. (1990). *Introduction to the health professions*. Boston: Jones and Bartlett Publishers.

Wilbur, K. C. (1987). *Antique medical instruments*. West Chester, PA: Schiffer Publishing Ltd.

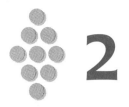

2

The Health Care Setting

KEY TERMS

accept assignment
capitation
CLIA '88
coinsurance
copayment
diagnostic-related groups
  (DRGs)
entitlement programs
gatekeeper

global capitation
health maintenance
  organizations (HMOs)
indemnity insurance
managed care
Medicaid
Medicare
outpatient/ambulatory
  care

preferred provider
  organization (PPO)
primary care
prospective payment
  system (PPS)
secondary care
service insurance
tertiary care
third-party payer

OBJECTIVES

Upon successful completion of this chapter, the reader should be able to:

1. List the types of health care offered in the United States and characteristics of health care facilities.

2. Contrast private health care with the public health service.

3. Compare types of third-party payers, coverage, and methods of payment to the patient, provider, and institutions.

4. Describe recent changes in the health care system and the driving forces behind them.

5. Describe traditional hospital organization and identify the health care providers in the acute care setting.

6. Contrast a typical hospital organizational chart with a non-traditional approach.

7. List the clinical analysis areas of the laboratory and the types of laboratory procedures performed in the different areas.

8. Describe the different levels of personnel found in the clinical laboratory.

9. Describe how the Clinical Laboratory Improvement Amendments of 1988 (CLIA '88) will affect laboratory medicine in the future.

Students in health care, as well as professionals, need to understand the organization of health care in the United States. Health providers, such as phlebotomists, benefit from this knowledge by recognizing different types of health care facilities, understanding how health care is financed, and recognizing the changing roles of personnel.

TYPES OF HEALTH CARE FACILITIES

Two general categories of facilities, inpatient and outpatient (or ambulatory) support all three levels (primary, secondary, and tertiary) of health care presently offered in the United States.

Outpatient or **ambulatory** is the principal source of health care services for most people. Ambulatory service is defined as "care for the walking patient" and ranges from simple and routine to complex and specialized. Examples of facilities offering **outpatient/ambulatory** care are doctor and dentist offices, surgical centers, health clinics, pharmacies, and hospitals. This type of service originates with the family physician, called the **primary care** physician, who offers the initial consult and related treatment. Other health care practitioners who may serve as primary caregivers are physician assistants (PAs) and nurse practitioners (NPs). Primary care assumes ongoing responsibility for maintaining patients' health and treating their disease states, which may involve referring patients for secondary (specialist) care. Today, there are physicians practicing ambulatory care as solo (single) practitioners or in group practice. Physicians in solo practice have referral arrangements and share on-call with other doctors. Group practice means the physicians share resources, such as facilities, staff, income, and expenses. In the United States, typical group practices are made up of 10 physicians or less.

Secondary care, defined as health care beyond primary, was essentially synonymous with inpatient care and services until recently. In today's health care environment, secondary and primary care are both being delivered in outpatient or ambulatory facilities where patients go home the same day. *Perhaps as many as 60% of all surgical services are performed on an ambulatory basis without overnight hospitalization* (Williams, 1995). Secondary care procedures, such as routine surgery, emergency treatments, and diagnostic or therapeutic radiology are available in freestanding ambulatory settings. Many hospitals, needing to provide comprehensive services for the purpose of contracting with insurers, now offer both inpatient and outpatient care. Over the past 20 years, hospitals have established fully staffed outpatient and urgent care facilities and clinics and formal ambulatory surgery centers.

Inpatient facilities, such as private and public hospitals, remain the key resource and center of the American health care system even as redesigning of health services forces hospitals to downsize. **Tertiary care** (highly complex services and therapy) is performed in inpatient facilities, such as acute care hospitals, and usually requires that patients stay overnight or longer. Acute care settings contain specialized instrumentation and technology to assist in unusual diagnosis and treatment. Other institutions that could provide tertiary care include nursing homes, intermediate and extended care facilities, and rehabilitation centers.

Hospitals can be classified based on one of three ways: length of stay, predominate type of service offered, and ownership or control. The categories of ownership and types of hospitals that fall under each classification are listed in Table 2-1.

Table 2-1
Classification of Health Care Institutions

Government, Federal [PUBLIC]	Government, Nonfederal
Air Force	State (mental institutions)
Army	County
Navy	City
Indian Health Services	
Veterans Administration	

Nongovernment, Not-for-Profit [PRIVATE]	Investor-Owned, For-Profit
Church operated	Individual
Community (university teaching hospitals)	Partnership
	Corporation

A private hospital is owned and operated by groups such as churches, businesses, or corporations. They can either operate as nonprofit or for-profit. The trend is toward large, for-profit corporations made up of a combination of smaller hospitals, such as Columbia Healthcare and Humana. Not-for-profit hospitals, such as university teaching hospitals and religious organizations, are typically community-based. These hospitals often make a profit, although it is not called "profit" because it is used for increasing services and further development of the facility. A public hospital is one that is financed and operated at the local, state, or federal level. Military, veterans, and Indian hospitals are federally owned and managed. State governments usually operate and financially support long-term hospitals, such as mental institutions.

CHARACTERISTICS OF HOSPITALS IN THE UNITED STATES

In the United States, there are roughly 6,000 acute care hospitals with approximately 1 million beds available. Most of the hospitals have under 200 beds; smaller hospitals only 50 or fewer beds. At present, the average hospital operates at only 66% occupancy, suggesting major changes will occur in the future due to looming cost constraints. The optimal size for a hospital is probably between 150 and 250 beds, and the ideal occupancy rate is most likely around 85% (Williams, 1995). The smaller the hospital, the less efficient, because of the necessity of maintaining the same range of basic services as a large hospital.

There are three sources of authority in the organization called a hospital: the board of directors, the hospital administration, and the medical staff. The board of directors is responsible for the overall operation of the hospital and delegates duties to the medical staff and the administrator or chief executive officer (CEO). It is the CEO that directs the overall management of the hospital and works in conjunction with the chief of staff or president of the medical staff to assure quality care. Occasionally, the hospital administration will have a vice president of medical affairs who is a physician–manager that handles medical issues originating from the physicians. The hospital board of directors delegates responsibilities to the medical staff; the medical staff invites community-based physicians to practice in their facility. In today's uncertain environment, many physicians have chosen to be employed by the hospital or contract with the hospital through physician organizations.

[handwritten margin: DHHS ↓ PHS local/state]

[handwritten: Top Public Health Official! Surgeon General]

PUBLIC HEALTH SERVICE

One of the principle units under the Department of Health and Human Services (DHHS) is the Public Health Service (PHS). PHS agencies at the local or state level offer defense against infectious diseases that might spread among the populace. They are constantly monitoring, screening, and educating the public (Table 2-2). Public health departments provide their services for little or no charge to the entire population of a region, with no distinction between rich or poor, simple or sophisticated, interested or disinterested. Public health facilities offer ambulatory care services through clinics, much like those in hospital outpatient areas, military bases, and Veterans Administration and Indian Health Service facilities. Because public health departments receive their financial support from federal grants and local or state governmental agencies, they reflect the economic and political moods of the country. The top public health official in the United States is the Surgeon General who can be influential in national policy making.

[handwritten margin: 1) offer defense against infectious diseases 2) constantly monitoring 3) screening 4) educating public 5) offer ambulatory care services through clinics]

As the country moves toward managed care, more integration between primary prevention and primary/ambulatory care is necessary. Since containment of health care costs is the driving force behind managed care, public health's programs may prove to be cost effective and contribute significantly to reductions in overall health care costs.

FINANCING HEALTH CARE

Health care is expensive and the cost continues to escalate. The consumer must make choices based on financial considerations as well as medical need and can no longer afford to be passive in the process. The health care professional, such as the phlebotomist, in addition to being a consumer, is also an employee of an institution that relies on third-party payers (health insurers) for a large portion of their income. Consequently, a health professional needs to understand the financing of health care.

[handwritten: Third Party Payers = health insurers / government program]

Table 2-2
Examples of Services Provided by Local Health Departments

Vital statistics collection
Health education
Cancer, hypertension, and diabetes screening
Public health nursing services
Tuberculosis screening
Immunization and vaccination
Operation of health centers
Venereal disease clinics

2 Primary Approaches! 1. Indemnity insurance = insurance co. Agrees to pay the health care provider A set Amt. of money (coinsurance = % of what pt pays)

2) Service Insurance = ins. co. Agrees to provide health care Services in place of money.

Third-Party Payers

Insurance is a way of pooling or distributing the risk (probability) of incurring a financial loss due to health problems and is made available through a third-party payer. A **third-party payer** can be an insurance company or government program that pays for health care services on behalf of a patient. Health insurance is a contract between the insurer and the patient which defines all aspects of the coverage. There are two primary approaches used by insurers to reimburse health care costs: **indemnity insurance** and **service insurance**. Indemnity reimbursement means the insurance company agrees to pay the health care provider a set amount of money. Under service insurance, the insurance company agrees to provide health care services in place of money to the patient. The obligation of patients to contribute toward their health care costs is called **coinsurance**. Coinsurance in an indemnity plan is a percentage of the bill anywhere from 10% to 20%. In HMOs, coinsurance is a fee (**copayment**) that is required at the time of service for an office visit and may be $5 to $10.

Methods of Payment

Third-party payers have greatly influenced the direction of medicine. In the past decade, major changes have come about in health care payments and third-party reimbursements.

PPS and DRGs. Due to the rapid rise in health care costs, the government put into place the **prospective payment system (PPS)**. The PPS, begun in 1983, attempted to limit and standardize the Medicare/Medicaid payments made to hospitals. This plan, originally designed by the American Hospital Association, reimburses hospitals a set amount for each patient procedure using established disease categories called **diagnostic-related groups (DRGs)**. When a patient is admitted to a hospital, he or she must be assigned a DRG from a list of approximately 500 DRGs. This DRG then defines the amount of reimbursement the facility will receive for that particular admission. This means the third-party payer (Medicare), rather than paying on the basis of services actually used by the patient, reviews the patient's diagnosis and gives the provider a predetermined amount based on that diagnosis. Additional costs must be covered by the patient or supplemental insurance or absorbed by the health care facility.

Accepting assignment. Private insurers have followed this example and now have fixed amounts they are willing to reimburse for given services. A provider who is willing to take the amount offered as payment in full is said to **accept assignment.** Providers who will not accept assignment reserve the right to bill the patient for the difference in what the provider's fee is and what the insurer pays. This is termed an out-of-pocket expense for the patient.

Reimbursing the Providers

Providers, such as physicians, are paid in several different ways, including fee-for-service, capitation, and salary. Each has its own set of incentives. The most traditional approach to reimbursement is that of **fee-for-service**, which is very clear-cut. Providers are paid a single fee for each office visit, procedure, or set of procedures. The amount of payment is based on the established or customary fee in the community and, consequently, does not support the managed care philosophy of cost containment and efficiency.

Capitation is another method of reimbursement in which the provider is paid an established fee for each patient in a panel (group of assigned patients). Under capitation (payment per head), the provider's fee is not tied to the number of services delivered, but to the number of patients in the panel. Therefore, the provider's reimbursement remains the same regardless of the amount of time and supplies required by a patient. This type of reimbursement discourages excessive use of the facilities and services and supports the philosophy of managed care. **Global capitation** refers to a payment system (one fee/head/month) offered to the provider for all the services provided to all the patients who are admitted to a facility.

The third type is **salaried reimbursement**. This type is used by government facilities and some managed care organizations. The provider or physician is paid a fixed salary which is not dependent on the number of patients, quantity of services delivered, or number of procedures performed. This type of reimbursement may foster inadequate effort on the part of the provider and should be monitored and evaluated.

Reimbursing the Institutions

The history of institutional reimbursement is tied to **entitlement** programs such as Medicare and public welfare in the form of Medicaid. These government social programs have not historically paid in ways that promoted efficiency. Prior to 1983, hospitals were paid retrospectively and reimbursed for all services performed on Medicare and Medicaid patients. Other insurers paid hospitals in the form of fee-for-service and allowed uncontrolled utilization of procedures and services.

Medicare, first enacted in 1965, is a federally funded entitlement program for providing health care to people over the age of 65, regardless of their financial status, and the disabled. It is called an entitlement program because it is a right earned by individuals through employment. This means the employee, employer, or both consistently contributed a portion of earnings to a government fund to take care of future unforeseen costs. Medicare is financed through Social Security payroll deductions and copayments. Benefits provided through Medicare are divided into two categories: Part A, called hospital services, and Part B, called supplementary medical insurance (SMI). Virtually all of the aged population of the United States is included in Part A.

Medicaid is a federal and state program that provides medical assistance for the indigent. It has no entitlement features; recipients must prove their eligibility. The funds used for reimbursement purposes come from federal grants and are administered by the state. Medicaid payments are closely associated to the economic status of the beneficiary. Benefits cover inpatient care, outpatient and diagnostic services, skilled nursing facilities, and home health and physician services. Medicare and Medicaid provide more than half the funding for health care for the older population. Since these programs are administered by individual states, they vary from one state to another. Arizona is the only state that has devised its own system outside of Medicaid, called **Arizona Health Care Cost Containment System (AHCCCS)**. It differs in that the providers (private physician groups) must bid annually for contracts to serve this population and patients are able to choose their health care provider through annual open enrollment. All other states use their governmental facilities and physicians; consequently, the consumer has no options.

The Changing Health Care System

Health care systems are currently undergoing major revisions. The driving force behind these changes is the government's move from retrospective payments (payments made to the health provider after care is completed) to the PPS and the use of DRGs. With the implementation of the PPS, the length of patient stay is decreasing and there are fewer admissions, causing an obvious reduction in income for hospitals. Other payers, using managed care plans, continually negotiate discounts on the amount they will reimburse the hospitals, forcing the hospitals to cut costs and downsize operations.

HMOs.   Group practices that are reimbursed on a prepaid, negotiated, and discounted basis of admission are an increasingly popular alternative design in health care plans. These practices are called **health maintenance organizations (HMOs)**. Members usually pay a flat amount for all defined services, regardless of usage. Basic elements of HMOs include a legal responsibility for financing and arranging to deliver a defined, complete package of health care services to members of the HMO. HMOs compete for members, therefore they have incentives to provide efficient and economical services. If expenditures exceed revenues, the HMO may incur a loss, which is often shared with its participating doctors and hospitals.

HMOs have been on the health care scene for some time, recently moving to center stage. Large numbers of employees and their dependents are drawn to HMO company benefits options with no deductibles. HMOs are capable of commanding sizable discounts on hospital beds and service. Besides their emphasis on preventive care, HMOs control member hospital usage by encouraging outpatient surgery for certain procedures, screening proposed hospital admission, closely monitoring length of stay, and providing alternative care at home or in skilled nursing facilities (nursing homes). Some very large HMOs, such as Kaiser-Permanente, even operate their own hospitals.

PPOs.   Another form of alternative delivery system, a **preferred provider organization (PPO)**, is an independent group of physicians or hospitals that offers its services to employers at discounted rates in exchange for a steady supply of patients. PPOs differ from HMOs in that they do not offer the employer their services for an annual capitation fee. Instead, PPOs tend to be more like a traditional insurance plan. The member is frequently offered a financial incentive for using the preferred providers, that is, his or her out-of-pocket expense will be greater if he or she chooses a provider who is not participating in the PPO.

Managed Care

Prepaid health care plans, such as HMOs and PPOs, are the precursor to today's **managed care** system. The idea of managed care evolved because the act of prepayment basically changed the relationships between the consumer and the provider. Now, the financial risk lies with the provider and not the insurer. This change in the fundamental principle of reimbursement has resulted not only in a reworking of financial incentives, but a restructuring of the whole system. Since managed care centers on the association of provider, payer, and consumer, several concepts have been developed to control this relationship, including gatekeepers and network services systems.

Primary care gatekeepers.   One of the most important concepts in managed care is that of the primary care physician filling the role of **gatekeeper**. This person's responsibilities as the patient's advocate are to advise and coordinate the patient's health care needs. Responsibilities of the gatekeeper also include providing early detection and treatment for disease, which should reduce the total cost of care.

Provider networks.   Managed care organizations contract with local providers to establish a complete network of services. Providers are reimbursed based on the number of enrollees served (capitation)—not on the number of services delivered. In fact, each service is an expense charged against revenue already collected that was based on a fixed prepayment amount per patient. The goal of the organization is to reduce the total cost of care while maintaining patient satisfaction.

Medical specialties.   In managed care, the primary physician is most often a family practitioner, a pediatrician, or an internist, but managed care will not do away with the medical specialist. The gatekeeper must refer to the appropriate specialist as needed. Some of the many health care areas in which a doctor of medicine (MD) or doctor of osteopathy (DO) can specialize are listed in Table 2-3.

Other Doctors.   There are other health care practitioners and specialists who do not hold the degrees of MD or DO, but are called "doctor." Some of these are listed in Table 2-4.

DEPARTMENTS WITHIN THE HEALTH CARE FACILITY OR HOSPITAL

Hospitals are often large organizations whose internal structure is complex. Traditionally, the delivery system in hospitals is arranged by departments or medical specialties. People who do similar tasks are grouped into departments, the goal being to perform each task as efficiently and accurately as possible. This style of management segregates the departments and their processes (Fig. 2-1). Consequently, it is difficult to look at the final result—patient outcome and satisfaction.

With the advent of managed care, the number of personnel in health care facilities has been reduced while the number of services remains the same. This downsizing has resulted in the formation of teams of cross-trained personnel and the consolidation of services. Such reengineering, as it is called, is designed to make the health care delivery system more process oriented by combining related groups of tasks into a system that is customer focused. This management of process is reflected in the new hospital organization, which blends former distinct departments into service or process areas (Fig. 2-2). The intent is to create a "gentle hand off" for patients between service areas, instead of the abrupt "toss and catch" approach that can occur in traditional settings with distinct and separate departments. Although the lines between former departments are becoming blurred, the following basic service areas still exist.

Patient Care Services
- Nursing: One of the major services in the hospital involves direct patient care. This includes careful observation to assess condition, and administering of medications

Table 2-3
Medical Specialties

Anesthesiology	Administers anesthetic agent, usually by injection or inhalation for partial or complete loss of sensation.
Cardiovascular diseases	A subspecialty of internal medicine dealing with diseases of the heart and blood vessels and cardiovascular surgery.
Dermatology	Treats diseases and injuries of the skin; more recently, concerned with skin cancer prevention.
Endocrinology	Diagnoses and treats disorders of the endocrine glands, such as sterility, diabetes, and thyroid problems.
Gastroenterology	Treatment of digestive tract diseases, a subspecialty of internal medicine.
Hematology	Treats disorders of the blood and blood-forming organs.
Internal medicine	Performs many of the same things as the general practitioner, with the exception of surgery and obstetrics.
Neonatology	Specializes in the study, care, and treatment of the newborn infant up to 6 weeks of age.
Nephrology	Treats diseases related to structure and function of the kidney.
Neurology	Concerned with disorders of the brain, spinal cord, and nerves.
Obstetrics and Gynecology	Deals with the reproductive tract disorders of women, prenatal care, childbirth, gynecologic surgery, and menopausal disorders.
Ophthalmology	Treats eye diseases; performs eye examinations and surgery.
Otolaryngology	Division of medical science that includes otology, rhinology, and laryngology.
Orthopedics	Deals with disorders of the musculoskeletal system.
Pediatrics	Diagnoses and treats diseases of children from birth to adolescence; does wellness checks and gives vaccinations.
Pulmonology	Concerned with the function of the lungs and respiratory system.
Rheumatology	Concerned with rheumatic diseases (acute and chronic conditions characterized by inflammation and joint disease).
Urology	Treats urinary tract disease and male reproductive organ disorders.

Table 2-4
Non-MD, Non-DO Doctors

Podiatrist (DPM, Doctor of Podiatric Medicine)	Specialist in care of feet, including radiograph, surgery, various therapies, and medication
Chiropractor (DC, Doctor of Chiropractics)	Treats with manipulation only (chiro = hand)
Naturopath (DN, Doctor of Naturopathy)	Treats with natural forces or substances, such as vitamins, diets, light, heat, air, and water
Psychologist (PhD, Doctor of Philosophy)	Group and individual counseling and testing; treats emotional disorders but cannot prescribe medication

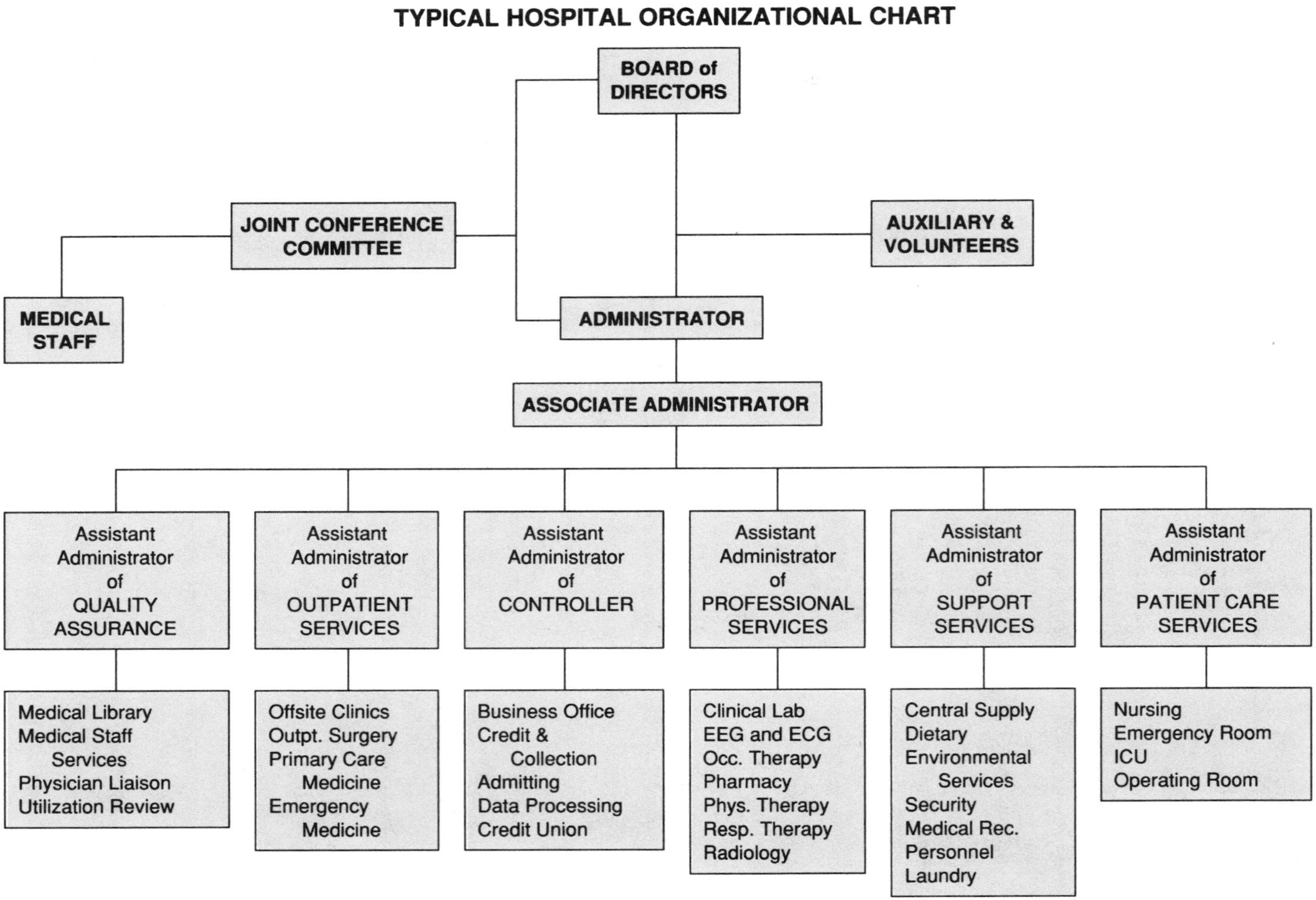

TYPICAL HOSPITAL ORGANIZATIONAL CHART

Figure 2-1   Typical hospital organizational flow chart.

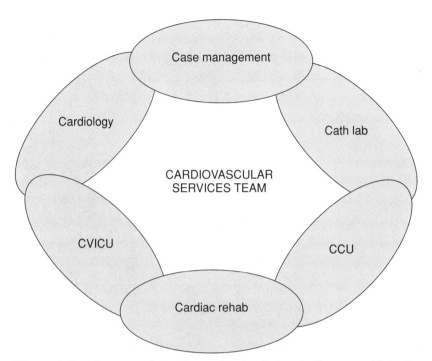

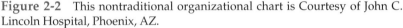

Figure 2-2 This nontraditional organizational chart is Courtesy of John C. Lincoln Hospital, Phoenix, AZ.

and treatments as prescribed by the physician. Types of nurses found in a hospital setting include:

- CNA: Certified nursing assistant
- LPN: Licensed practical nurse
- ADN: Associate degree nurse
- RN: Registered nurse
- BSN: Bachelor of science nurse
- NP: Nurse practitioner
- CNS: Clinical nurse specialist
- CRNA: Certified registered nurse anesthetist

    A newly emerging category of personnel in the nursing service area is the patient care technician (PCT) or patient care assistant (PCA), usually a CNA who has been trained to do phlebotomy and electrocardiograms (ECGs).
- Emergency Room (ER)/Emergency Department (ED): The department that is designed to handle medical emergencies that call for immediate assessment and management of injured or acutely ill patients, staffed by specialists such as emergency medical technicians (EMTs) and MDs who specialize in emergency medicine.
- Intensive Care Unit: An area of the hospital designed for increased bedside care due to the fragile condition of the patient. Intensive care units (ICUs) are found in many

areas of the hospital and are named for the patient care they provide (*eg*, trauma ICU, pediatric ICU, medical ICU).

- Surgery: An area concerned with operative procedures to correct deformities and defects, repair injuries, and cure certain diseases. All work is performed by a medical practitioner who specializes in surgery.

Support Services

- Central Supply: This unit prepares and dispenses all the necessary supplies required for patient care, including surgical packs for the operating room, intravenous pumps, bandages, syringes, and other inventory controlled by computer for close accounting.
- Dietary: Selects foods and supervises food services so as to coordinate diet with medical treatment.
- Environmental Services: Includes housekeeping and grounds keepers whose services maintain a clean and attractive facility.
- Health Information Technology: Maintains accurate and orderly records for inpatient medical history, tests results and reports, and treatment plans and notes from doctors and nurses to be used for insurance claims, legal actions, and utilization reviews.

Professional Services

- Cardiodiagnostics (EKG or ECG): Performs electrocardiograms (an actual record of the electrical currents that are detectable from the heart), Holter monitoring, and stress testing for diagnosis and monitoring therapy in cardiovascular patients (Fig. 2-3).
- Clinical Laboratory: Performs laboratory testing on blood and other body fluids to detect and diagnose disease, monitor treatments, and, more recently, assess health. Highly automated, the laboratory performs complicated testing. There are several specialized areas of the laboratory called departments (see Departments in the Clinical Laboratory).
- Electroneurodiagnostic Technology (ENT or EEG): Performs electroencephalograms (tracings that measure electrical activity from the brain). Uses techniques,

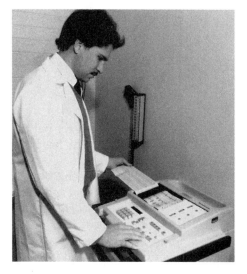

Figure 2-3 ECG technician reviews a patient tracing.

such as ambulatory EEG monitoring, evoked potential, polysomnography (sleep studies), and brain wave mapping to diagnose and monitor neurophysiologic disorders (Fig. 2-4).

- Occupational Therapy (OT): Uses techniques designed to develop or assist patients who are mentally, physically, or emotionally disabled to maintain daily living skills.
- Pharmacy: Prepares and dispenses drugs ordered by physicians; advises the medical staff on selection and harmful side effects of drugs, therapeutic drug monitoring, and drug use evaluation.
- Physical Therapy (PT): Diagnoses impairment to determine the extent of the disability and provides therapy to restore mobility through individually designed treatment plans.
- Respiratory Therapy (RT): Diagnoses, treats, and manages patient's lung deficiencies, *eg*, analyzes arterial blood gases (ABGs), tests capacity of the lungs, and administers oxygen therapy.
- Medical Imaging: Diagnoses medical conditions by taking x-ray films of all parts of the body. Uses latest procedures including powerful forms of imaging that do not involve radiation hazards, such as ultrasound machines, magnetic resonance (MR) scanners, and positron emission tomography (PET) scanners.
- Radiation Therapy: Treats disease, particularly cancer, by administering prescribed doses of ionizing radiation to specific parts of the body.

Departments in the Clinical Laboratory

There are two major divisions in the clinical laboratory: clinical analysis, and anatomical and surgical pathology. The clinical analysis area is divided into subunits called specimen processing, hematology, chemistry, microbiology, blood bank or immunohematology, immunology/serology, and education. In the larger facilities, specimens of blood and body fluids are analyzed using automation and advanced technology. Anatomic and surgical pathology procedures include performance of autopsies, tissue analysis, cytologic examination, surgical biopsy, and frozen sections.

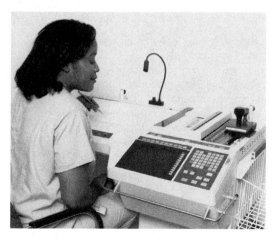

Figure 2-4   Technologist monitors an EEG.

CLINICAL ANALYSIS AREAS

Hematology.   The hematology department performs laboratory analysis to identify diseases associated with blood and the blood-forming tissues. Hematology tests aid the physician in diagnosing infections, leukemia, polycythemia, anemia, and other blood dyscrasias (abnormalities). The most commonly ordered hematology test is the complete blood count (CBC), which requires a whole blood sample collected in ethylene-diaminetetraacetate (EDTA), found in a lavender top tube. The CBC is routinely performed using automated instruments, such as the Coulter counter, that electronically count the cells and calculate results (Fig. 2-5). A complete blood count is actually a multi-part assay that is reported on a form called a hemogram (Tables 2-5 and 2-6).

Table 2-5
Hemogram for CBC Assay

Test	*Clinical Significance*
Complete Blood Count (CBC)	
Hematocrit (Hct)	Values correspond to the red cell count and hemoglobin level; when decreased, indicate anemic conditions.
Hemoglobin (Hgb)	Decreased values indicate anemic conditions; values normally differ with age, sex, altitude, and hydration.
Red blood cell (RBC) count	Measure of erythropoietic activity; decrease in numbers related to anemic condition.
White blood cell (WBC) count	Abnormal leukocyte response indicative of various conditions, such as infections and malignancies; when accompanied by WBC, differential test becomes more specific.
Platelet count	Decreased number indicative of hemorrhagic diseases; values may be used to monitor chemotherapy or radiation treatments.
Differential white count (Diff)	Changes in appearance or number of specific cell type signifies specific disease conditions; values also used to monitor chemotherapy or radiation treatments.
Indices	Changes in RBC size, weight, and Hgb content indicate certain types of anemias.
Mean corpuscular hemoglobin (MCH)	Decreased hemoglobin content indicative of iron deficiency anemia; increased hemoglobin content found in macrocytic anemia.
Mean corpuscular volume (MCV)	Decreased MCV associated with thalassemia and iron deficiency anemia; increased MCV due to folic acid or vitamin B_{12} deficiency and chronic emphysema.
Mean corpuscular hemoglobin concentration (MCHC)	Below-normal range means red cells are deficient in hemoglobin as in thalassemia, overhydration, or iron deficiency anemia; above-normal range will be seen in severe burns, prolonged dehydration, and hereditary spherocytosis.

Table 2-6
Other Common Hematology Tests

Body fluids	Cell type and number significant in diagnosing condition; Hct on fluid indirectly measures fluid volume.
Bone marrow	Provides diagnostic information about blood cell production.
Eosinophil count	Increased numbers in direct count indicate parasitic infections and allergies.
Erythrocyte sedimentation rate (ESR)	Increased rate at which RBCs settle out is indicative of inflammatory conditions or necrosis of tissue.
Lupus erythematosus (LE prep)	Presence of typical LE cells is diagnostic of SLE.
Osmotic fragility	Increased red cell fragility is indicative of hemolytic and autoimmune anemias; decreased fragility is indicative of sickle cell and thalassemia.
Reticulocyte count (retic count)	Increased number of retics in circulating blood attest to bone marrow hyperactivity.
Sickle cell	Sickling of red cells indicates presence of abnormal hemoglobin variant, Hgb S.

Coagulation.   This department is often housed in the hematology area. Coagulation deals with the study of defects in the blood clotting mechanism and the monitoring of medication given to people as "blood thinners" or anticoagulant therapy. (An anticoagulant is a chemical that prevents the blood from clotting.) The two most common coagulation tests are the prothrombin time (PT), used to monitor warfarin, and the activated partial thromboplastin time (APTT or PTT), for evaluating heparin therapy

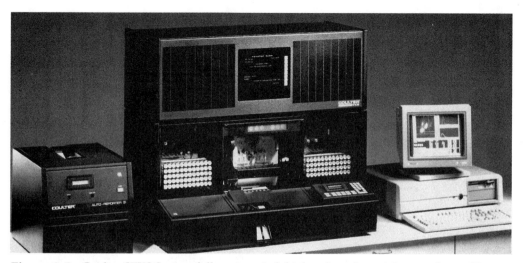

Figure 2-5   Coulter STKS System fully automated, high-volume hematology analyzer. (Courtesy Coulter Electronics, Inc., Hialeah, FL.)

(Table 2-7). The type of specimen on which the test is performed is plasma from a light blue tube containing whole blood with the anticoagulant sodium citrate added.

Chemistry.   The chemistry department analyzes the majority of laboratory tests. The computerized instruments found in this area are capable of performing panels (multiple tests) from one sample or discrete (individualized) tests. Examples of panels frequently ordered to evaluate a single organ or specific body system are given in Table 2-8.

The type of specimen primarily used for testing is serum collected in serum separator tubes, but other types of specimens are also used and can be collected in gray, green, blue, or lavender tubes. Some tests may require urine or other body fluids. Subsections of clinical chemistry are **special chemistry**, where tests such as lipoprotein and hemoglobin electrophoresis are performed, and **immunoassay**, which utilizes the techniques of radioimmunoassay (RIA) and enzyme immunoassay (EIA). RIA uses radioactively labeled antibodies or antigens, whereas EIA uses enzymes in color reactions to test for hormones, hepatitis, and drugs. Chemistry tests impact on other areas of the laboratory analysis and are commonly involved in confirming diagnoses as well as assessing health. Examples of tests normally performed in the automated clinical laboratory section are provided in Table 2-9.

Serology or immunology.   Serology literally means the study of serum. Serology tests deal with the body's response to the presence of bacterial, viral, fungal, or parasitic diseases that stimulate antigen–antibody reactions and can easily be demonstrated in the laboratory (Table 2-10). Autoimmune reactions, in which autoantibodies produced by B lymphocytes attack normal cells, are becoming more prevalent and are frequently analyzed in this area. Testing is done by EIA, agglutination, complement fixation, or precipitation to determine the antibody or antigen present and to assess the concentration or titer. Serological testing is performed on blood collected in a plain red tube. Collection

Table 2-7
Common Coagulation Tests

Test	Clinical Significance
Activated partial thromboplastin time (APTT)	Prolonged times may indicate stage one defects; values reflect adequacy of heparin therapy.
Bleeding time (BT)	Increased BT indicates hemorrhagic disorders associated with decreased platelet activity and lack of elasticity of capillary walls.
Fibrin degradation products (FDP)	High levels result in FDP fragments that interfere with platelet function and clotting.
Fibrinogen	Fibrinogen deficiency suggests hemorrhagic disorders and is used most frequently in obstetrics.
Prothrombin time (PT)	Prolonged times may indicate stage two and three defects; values used to monitor warfarin therapy.
Thrombin time (TT)	Prolonged clotting indicates deficiency of fibrinogen; values correlate with heparin therapy.

Table 2-8
Common Chemistry Test Panel Groupings

Panel Grouping	Battery of Selected Diagnostic Tests
Cardiovascular system	AST, CK, CK-MB, LD, HBDH, cholesterol, triglycerides, potassium, sodium, digoxin, PT, APPT, CT, ESR, WBC, blood gases
Hematologic system	CBC, RBC indices, platelet, reticulocyte, Hgb electrophoresis, sickle cell screen, BT, iron, folic acid, bilirubin, ESR, osmotic fragility, immunoglobin assay
Pulmonary system	ABGs, AFB on sputum, C&S on sputum, pleural fluid exam, theophylline
Musculoskeletal system	Adolase, ALP, CK, AST, calcium, RF, EST, CPR, synovial fluid

Table 2-9
Common Chemistry Tests

Test	Associated Body System	Examples of Clinical Significance
Acid phosphatase	Prostate	Elevated values may signify prostatic carcinoma.
Alanine aminotransferase (ALT)	Liver	Marked elevations point to liver disease; used for monitoring liver treatment.
Alpha-fetoprotein	Liver	Increased values in hepatic carcinoma; elevation of AFP in prenatal screening indicates neural tube disorder.
Aldolase	Muscle	Elevated level of this enzyme due to muscle disease.
Alkaline phosphatase (ALP)	Liver or bone	Elevated ALP levels due to biliary obstruction and bone disease.
Ammonia	Liver	Increased blood levels indicate cirrhosis and hepatitis.
Amylase	Pancreas & liver	Increased levels of this enzyme diagnostic of acute pancreatitis; decreased values associated with liver disease, cholecystitis, and advanced cystic fibrosis.
Aspartate aminotransferase (AST)	Liver or heart	Increase in enzyme indicative of liver dysfunction; significant increase following myocardial infarction.
Bilirubin	Liver	Increased levels in the bloodstream point to red cell destruction and liver dysfunction.
Blood urea nitrogen (BUN)	Kidney	Elevated values due to impaired renal function from toxins, inflammation, or obstruction.

(continued)

Table 2-9 (Continued)

Test	Associated Body System	Examples of Clinical Significance
Calcium	Bone	Increased levels associated with diseases of the bone; used in monitoring effects of renal failure.
Cholesterol	Heart	Indicative of high risk for cardiovascular disease.
Cortisol	Adrenals	Elevated levels signify adrenal hyperfunction (Cushing's syndrome); decreased levels indicate adrenal hypofunction (Addison's disease).
Creatine kinase (CK)	Heart or muscle	Elevated values point to muscle damage, *ie*, myocardial infarction, muscular dystrophy, or strenuous exercise.
Creatinine	Kidney	Increased levels indicate renal impairment; decreased levels associated with muscular dystrophy.
Digoxin	Heart	Drug values monitored so as to avoid toxic levels.
Electrolytes (sodium, potassium, chloride)	Kidney, adrenals, heart	Sodium values increased in disorders of the kidney and adrenals; decreased values of potassium seen in irregular heart beat; chloride values are increased in kidney and adrenal disorders and decreased in diarrhea.
Glucose	Pancreas	Elevated levels signify diabetic problems; decreased values support liver disease and malnutrition.
Iron	Circulatory system	Decreased levels indicate iron deficiency and malabsorption; increased levels significant in hemolytic disorders.
Lactic acid dehydrogenase (LD)	Heart, lungs, liver	Elevated levels confirm acute myocardial infarction; chronic lung, kidney, and liver dysfunction.
Lipase	Pancreas	Increased levels in acute pancreatitis, pancreatic carcinoma, and obstruction.
Lithium	CNS	Drug values monitored so as to avoid toxic levels and renal damage.
Magnesium	Kidney	Decreased levels point to chronic alcoholism and cirrhosis; increased levels occur in renal failure.
Total protein	Liver or kidney	Low levels point to liver and kidney disorders; elevated levels may occur with multiple myeloma and dehydration.

(continued)

Table 2-9 (Continued)

Test	Associated Body System	Examples of Clinical Significance
Triglycerides	Heart	Increased values indicate lipid metabolism disorders and serve as an index for evaluating atherosclerosis possibilities.
Uric acid	Kidney	Elevated values found in renal disorders and gout.
Vitamin B_{12} & folate	Liver	Decreased levels indicate anemias and disease of the small intestine.

tubes containing serum separator gel cannot be used because the gel interferes with the reaction between the antibody and antigen.

Urinalysis (UA). This department may be housed in the hematology or chemistry area or may be a completely separate section. Urine may be analyzed on automated

Table 2-10
Common Serology and Immunology Tests

Test	Examples of Clinical Significance
Bacterial Studies	
Antinuclear antibody (ANA)	Positive results in autoimmune disorders, specifically systemic lupus erythematosus.
Antistreptolysin O (ASO) titer	To demonstrate infection from streptococcus bacteria.
Cold agglutinins	Present in cases of atypical pneumonia.
Febrile agglutinins	Presence of antibodies to specific organisms indicates disease condition, *ie*, tularemia.
Rheumatoid factor (RF)	Presence of antibody indicates rheumatoid arthritis.
Rapid plasma reagin (RPR)	Positive screen indicates syphilis; positives need to be confirmed.
Viral Studies	
Anti-HIV	Human immunodeficiency virus is screened.
Cytomegalovirus antibody (CMV)	Confirmation test
Epstein-Barr virus (EBV)	Presence of this heterophil antibody indicates infectious mononucleosis.
Hepatitis B surface antigen (HBsAg)	Demonstrates the presence of hepatitis antigen on the surface of the red cells.
General Studies	
C-reactive protein (CRP)	Increased levels in inflammatory conditions.
Human chorionic gonadotropin (HCG)	Present in pregnancy (serum and urine).

instruments or manually. The UA is a routine test performed on urine involving physical, chemical, and microscopic evaluations (Table 2-11). The physical examination assesses the color, clarity, and specific gravity using a refractometer. The chemical evaluation, using chemical reagent strips, screens for substances such as sugar and protein. A microscopic examination identifies the presence or absence of blood cells, bacteria, crystals, and other substances. Urine culture, a very common test, is often delivered to the urinalysis area, but must be taken to the microbiology department first for culture and then returned to the urinalysis section for testing.

Table 2-11
Common Urinalysis Tests

Test	*Clinical Significance*
Physical Evaluation	
Color	Abnormal colors that are clinically significant result from blood, melanin, bilirubin, or urobilin in the sample.
Clarity	Turbidity may be due to chyle, fat, bacteria, RBCs, WBCs, or precipitated crystals.
Specific gravity	Variation in this indicator of dissolved solids in the urine is normal; inconsistencies suggest renal tubule involvement or ADH deficiency.
Chemical Evaluation	
Blood	Hematuria may be due to hemorrhage, infection, or trauma.
Bilirubin	Aids in differentiating obstructive jaundice from hemolytic jaundice, which will not cause increased bilirubin in the urine.
Glucose	Glucosuria could be due to diabetes mellitus, renal impairment, or ingestion of a large amount of carbohydrates.
Ketones	Occurs in uncontrolled diabetes mellitus.
Leukocyte esterase	Certain white cells (neutrophils) in abundance indicate urinary tract infection.
pH	Variations in pH indicate changes in acid–base balance which is normal; loss of ability to vary pH is indicative of tissue breakdown.
Protein	Proteinuria is indicator of renal disorders, such as injury and renal tube disfunction.
Nitrite	Positive result suggests bacterial infection but is only significant on first-morning specimen or urine incubated in bladder for at least 4 hours.
Urobilinogen	Occurs in increased amounts when patient has hepatic problems or hemolytic disorders.
Microscopic Evaluation	Analysis of urinary sediment reveals status of the urinary tract; hematuria, pyuria, and presence of casts and tissue cells are pathologic indicators.

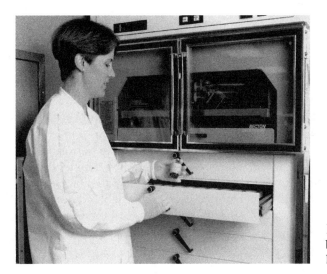

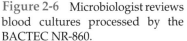

Figure 2-6   Microbiologist reviews blood cultures processed by the BACTEC NR-860.

Microbiology.   This department analyzes body fluids and tissues for the presence of microorganisms, primarily by means of culture and sensitivity (C & S) testing (Fig. 2-6). Results of a C & S tell the physician the type of organisms present as well as the particular antibiotic that would be most effective for treatment. Collecting and transporting microbiology specimens is very important in the identification of microorganisms. Subsections of microbiology are bacteriology (study of bacteria), parasitology (study of parasites), mycology (study of fungi), and virology (study of viruses). These subsections are growing rapidly in number of tests performed due to the increased number of contagious diseases (such as acquired immunodeficiency syndrome [AIDS]) and the increase in international travel, which exposes people to a wider range of microorganisms (Table 2-12).

Table 2-12
Common Microbiology Tests

Test	Clinical Significance
Acid fast bacilli	Positive stain means pulmonary tuberculosis; used to monitor the treatment for TB.
Blood culture	Positive culture results (bacterial growth in media) indicates bacteremia or septicemia.
Culture & sensitivity	Growth of a pathogenic microorganism indicates infection (culture); in vitro inhibition by an antibiotic (sensitivity) allows the physician to select the correct treatment.
Gram stain	Positive stain for specific types of pathogenic microorganisms permits antimicrobial therapy to begin before culture results are known.
Occult blood	Positive test indicates blood in the stool, which is associated with gastrointestinal bleeding from carcinoma.
Ova & parasites	Microscopic examination of stool sample showing ova and parasites solves many "etiology unknown" intestinal disorders.

Blood Bank or Immunohematology.   This department of the laboratory prepares blood products to be used for patient transfusions. Blood components dispensed include whole blood, platelets, packed cells, fresh frozen plasma, and cryoprecipitates. Blood samples from all donors and the recipient must be carefully tested before transfusions can be administered so that incompatibility and transfusion reactions can be avoided (Table 2-13). Antibody–antigen testing on red cells is routinely performed in this department on patient blood samples obtained in plain red top tubes. Correct patient identification and proper specimen labeling is the keystone of this department. The blood bank technologist relies on the person collecting the blood to perform identification of the patient without error. Transfusion services, offered by the blood bank department, collect, prepare, and store units of blood from donors or patients who wish to donate their own units for autologous transfusion, if necessary. All blood units from donors are tested for bloodborne pathogens, such as hepatitis and human immunodeficiency virus.

Anatomic and Surgical Pathology

Histology.   Histology is literally defined as the study of the microscopic structure of tissues. Before the pathologist studies the samples of tissue from autopsy or surgery, they must be processed and stained. This is the role of the histologist. Tissues can be evaluated by the anatomic pathologist as normal or pathological (diseased). Histological techniques include two of the most diagnostic tools found in the laboratory: (1) biopsy, obtaining samples by removal of a plug (small piece) of tissue from an organ and examining it microscopically; and (2) frozen sections, obtaining tissue from surgery and freezing and examining it immediately to determine whether more extensive surgery is needed.

Table 2-13
Common Bloodbank and Immunohematology Tests

Test	Clinical Significance
Antibody (Ab) screen	Agglutination indicates abnormal antibodies present in patient's blood.
Direct antihuman globulin test (DAT)	Positive results point to autoimmune hemolytic anemia, hemolytic disease of the newborn, and transfusion incompatibility.
Group and type	Determination of blood group (ABO) and type (Rh+) by identifying agglutinins present or absent.
Compatibility testing	Detection of unsuspected antibodies and antigens in recipient's and donor's blood that could cause severe reaction if transfused.
Human leukocyte antigens (HLA)	Determination of compatibility for tissue transplanting and donor platelets, determination of biologic parentage, and diagnoses of HLA-associated diseases.

Cytology.   Cytology and histology are often confused. In cytology, histologists process and prepare body fluids to study the structure, function, and pathology of the cells. A pathologist or cytotechnologist (CT) uses cytologic methods to screen carefully for signs of disease, such as cancer. The Pap smear, a test for early detection of cancer cells, primarily of the cervix and vagina, is one of the most common examinations performed by this department.

Cytogenetics.   An area found in larger labs is cytogenetics. In this section, samples are examined for chromosomal deficiencies that relate to genetic disease. Specimens used for chromosomal studies include tissue, blood, and amniotic fluid. Each day, new discoveries are being made in genetic research and the study of hereditary variations. The deoxyribonucleic acid (DNA) probe analysis is the latest in testing for infectious pathogens, genetic and malignant disorders, and DNA fingerprinting for forensic medicine. DNA probe technology can diagnose genetic disorders, such as HIV, Duchenne muscular dystrophy, sickle cell anemia, and cystic fibrosis.

Reference Accounts.   This newly emerging area has recently become important in many laboratories. Due to the changes in health care financing described in this chapter, hospitals are being forced to offer laboratory services to ambulatory care facilities. The purpose of this area is to market and handle accounts from doctors' offices and smaller laboratories that need laboratory testing services.

CLINICAL LABORATORY PERSONNEL

Laboratory Director/Pathologist

The pathologist is a physician who specializes in diagnosing disease, through the use of laboratory tests results, in tissues removed at operations and from postmortem examinations. It is his or her duty to direct laboratory services so they benefit the physician and patient. This includes establishing policies and protocols; providing consultation services to medical staff; teaching in educational programs; interpreting lab results, evaluating tissues from surgery and autopsies, and performing cytology evaluations and bone marrows examinations. The laboratory director may be a pathologist or a clinical laboratory scientist with a doctorate degree. The laboratory director and the laboratory administrator share responsibilities for managing the laboratory.

Laboratory Administrator/Laboratory Manager

The lab administrator is usually a technologist with an advanced degree and several years of experience. Duties of the administrator include overseeing all operations involving physician and patient services; establishing policies and procedures; hiring new personnel; developing and maintaining operational and capital budgets; ensuring that all standards are maintained; directing all inspections processes; providing continuing education for clinical and supervisory staff; and setting goals and objectives for the laboratory. Today, the laboratory administrator may supervise several ancillary services, such as radiology and respiratory therapy, or all the laboratory functions in a health care system consisting of separate lab facilities across a large geographic area.

Technical Supervisors

For each laboratory section or subsection, there is a technical supervisor who is responsible for the administration of the area and who reports to the laboratory administrator. The following responsibilities fall under this job description: ensuring adequate work coverage and the best use of personnel; evaluating technical procedures and specimen requirements; ensuring that procedures are followed by all section personnel; providing continuing education, instruction, and training for the section staff; maintaining and revising procedure manual; and contributing to the budgetary preparation.

Medical Technologist/Clinical Laboratory Scientist

The medical technologist (MT) or clinical laboratory scientist (CLS) generally has a bachelor's degree in chemistry or biology, with study in an MT program for 1 year or more. Some of the states require licensing for MTs but will often give reciprocity to those MTs who are nationally certified. The responsibilities of the MTs include performing all levels of testing, including chemical, hematologic, microbiological, and immunologic procedures pertaining to patient diagnosis; reporting results; performing quality control; and conducting preventive maintenance and troubleshooting on instruments.

Medical Laboratory Technicians/Clinical Laboratory Technicians

The medical laboratory technician (MLT) or clinical laboratory technician (CLT) is most often an individual with an associate degree from a 2-year program or certification from a military or proprietary (private) school. As with MTs, states requiring licensing for medical/clinical laboratory technicians may offer reciprocity to nationally certified technicians. The technician is responsible for performing routine testing; operating all equipment; performing basic instrument maintenance and recognizing instrument problems; and assisting in problem solving.

Clinical Laboratory Assistants

Before the arrival of computerized instrumentation in the laboratory, the clinical laboratory assistant was a recognized position. Today, due to reduction in the laboratory staff, this category of personnel has been revived. A clinical laboratory assistant is a person with phlebotomy experience who has skills in specimen processing and basic laboratory testing. Clinical laboratory assistants are generalists, responsible for assisting the MT or MLT with the workload in any area.

Phlebotomist

The phlebotomist is trained to collect blood for laboratory analysis which is necessary for diagnosis and care of the patient. A number of facilities use phlebotomists as laboratory assistants or specimen processors (see page 4 for duties). Formal phlebotomy programs in colleges and private schools usually require a high school diploma or the equivalent to enroll. After completing the program or acquiring 1 year of work experience, the phlebotomist can become certified by passing a national examination. A few states require licensing for this level of personnel and may offer reciprocity to nationally certified phlebotomists.

CLINICAL LABORATORY IMPROVEMENT ACT

The Clinical Laboratory Improvement Amendments of 1988 **(CLIA '88)** were signed into law on October 31, 1988, and became effective in 1992. This public law, administered by the Health Care Financing Administration (HCFA), mandates that all laboratories must be regulated using the same standards regardless of the location, type, or size. The law requires that every clinical laboratory facility in the country obtain a certificate from the federal government assuring the customers that laboratory testing performed at that facility is reliable and accurate. To maintain this certificate, labs must undergo a routine inspection by some government agency. Laboratories that perform tests such as pregnancy testing or urine dipsticks are considered "waived" from inspections because of the simplicity of the testing. Laboratories which fall under the CLIA regulations include those in hospitals, clinics, government facilities, independent laboratories, HMOs, and physician office laboratories (POLs). The regulations put into force by this law deal with, among other things, laboratory standards. The standards are designed for two types of laboratory facilities. The lab type is determined by the complexity of testing done at that facility, for example, moderately complex or highly complex. Personnel qualifications for each of the types are stated in the regulations.

Study & Review Questions

1. An institution that provides inpatient services is a
   a. clinic.
   b. doctor's office.
   c. hospital.
   d. day-surgery.

2. An example of a third-party payer is
   a. Medicare.
   b. DRGs.
   c. OSHA.
   d. none of the above.

3. When a provider does not bill the patient for costs exceeding those covered by insurance, it is called
   a. accepting assignment.
   b. ambulatory care.
   c. coinsurance.
   d. prospective payment system.

4. State and federally funded insurance is called
   a. OSHA.
   b. PPO.
   c. ASCP.
   d. Medicaid.

5. The specialty that treats disorders of old age is called
   a. cardiology.
   b. gerontology.
   c. pathology.
   d. psychiatry.

6. The department in the hospital that records brain waves for diagnosis is
   a. electroneurodiagnostics.
   b. occupational therapy.
   c. physical therapy.
   d. radiology.

7. The microbiology department in the laboratory performs
   a. compatibility.
   b. enzyme-linked immunoassay.
   c. electrolyte monitoring.
   d. blood culture testing.

8. The abbreviation for the routine hematology test that includes hemoglobin, hematocrit, red blood count, and white blood count determinations is called
   a. CDC.
   b. CRP.
   c. CBC.
   d. CPK.

Suggested Laboratory Activities

1. Tour a major hospital or other health care facility.

2. Summarize a news article concerning health issues.

3. Spend a day with a health care worker in a field other than phlebotomy.

4. Form class debate teams and discuss current hot topics in health care.

5. Tour a laboratory with a check-off list of terms related to departments and tests.

BIBLIOGRAPHY AND SUGGESTED READING

Byrne, C. J., Saxton, D. F., Pelikan, P. K., & Nugent, P. M. (1986). *Laboratory testing: Implications for nursing care* (2nd ed). Menlo Park, CA: Addison-Wesley Publishing.

CLIA '88. (1992). Final standard is published. *Clinical Chemistry News*, March.

Feldstein, P. J. (1993). *Health care economics* (4th ed.). New York: Delmar Publishers.

Illustrated guide to diagnostic tests (student version). (1994). Springhouse, PA: Springhouse.

Stanfield, P. S. (1990). *Introduction to the health professions.* Boston: Jones and Bartlett Publishers.

Watson, J., & Jaffe, M. (1995). *Nurse's manual of laboratory and diagnostic tests* (2nd ed.). Philadelphia, PA: F. A. Davis.

Williams, S., & Torrens, P. (1988). *Introduction to health services* (3rd ed.). New York: Delmar Publishers.

Williams, S. J. (1995). *Essentials of health services.* New York: Delmar Publishers.

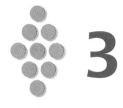

3

Medical Terminology

KEY TERMS

combining form   **combining vowel**   **prefix**   **suffix**   **word root**

OBJECTIVES

Upon successful completion of this chapter, the reader will be able to:

1. Describe how the meaning of a medical term is determined.
2. Define the terms *word root, prefix, suffix, combining vowel,* and *combining form.*
3. State the meanings of common word roots, prefixes, and suffixes, and identify unique plural endings.
4. State the meanings of common medical abbreviations and give their meanings.

All professions have a special vocabulary of scientific or technical terms necessary to speak or write effectively and precisely. **Medical terminology** is the special language of the health care professions. Medical terminology is based on an understanding of a few basic elements primarily derived from Greek and Latin words that form the foundation of nearly all medical terms. These elements are word roots, prefixes, suffixes, combining vowels, and combining forms.

WORD ROOTS

The foundation of all medical terms is a **word root**. A word root establishes the basic meaning of the term and usually signifies a tissue, organ, or body system involved. An example is the Greek root *nephr*, meaning "kidney." Sometimes there is both a Greek and Latin root with the same meaning. For example the Latin root *ren* also means "kidney." In a few cases, the same root will have very different meanings, such as the root *ped* which means both "foot" and "child." In these cases, it is necessary to consider the context in which the word is used. Some medical terms have more than one word root. An example is the word *cardiopulmonary*, which is made up of two word roots: *cardi*, meaning "heart," and *pulmo*, meaning "lung." See Table 3-1 for a list of common medical word roots.

PREFIXES

A **prefix** precedes a word root and modifies its meaning. A term is never made up of a prefix alone.

Table 3-1
Common Medical Word Roots

Root	Meaning	Example
aer	air	aerobic
angi	vessel	angiogram
arteri	artery	arteriosclerosis
arthr	joint	arthritis
bili	bile	bilirubin
bronch	bronchus	bronchitis
cardi	heart	electrocardiogram
cephal	head	cephalic
chondr	cartilage	osteochondritis
cry	cold	cryoglobulin
cyst	bladder	cystitis
cyt,cyte	cell	cytology
derm	skin	dermabrasion
encephal	brain	encephalitis
esophag	esophagus	esophagitis
gastr	stomach	gastrectomy
glyc	sugar	glycolysis
hem	blood	hematology
hepat	liver	hepatitis
lip	fat	liposuction
my	muscle	myalgia
nephr	kidney	nephritis
onc	tumor	oncologist
oste	bone	osteochondritis
path	disease	pathogen
phleb	vein	phlebotomy
pulmon	lung	pulmonary
ren	kidney	renal
scler	hard	sclerotic
thromb	clot	thrombosis
thorac	chest	thoracic
tox	poison	toxicology
vas	vessel	vasectomy
ven	vein	venipuncture

Example: A /   NUCLEAR
               prefix   root
               (without)   (nucleus)

The prefix "a" means "without." The word root "nuclear" means nucleus. The word "anuclear" means "without a nucleus." Table 3-2 lists common medical prefixes.

SUFFIXES

A **suffix**, often referred to as a word ending, follows a word root and either changes or adds to the meaning of the word root. A word meaning is best determined by starting with the suffix. As with a prefix, a suffix never stands alone.

Table 3-2
Common Medical Prefixes

Prefix	Meaning	Example
a-,an-,ar-	without	arrhythmia
aniso-	unequal	anisocytosis
anti-	against	antiseptic
bi-	two	bicuspid
brady-	slow	bradycardia
cyan-	blue	cyanotic
dys-	difficult	dyspnea
endo-	in, within	endothelium
epi-	on, over	epidermis
erythr-	red	erythrocyte
extra-	outside	extravascular
hetero-	different	heterosexual
homo-	same	homogeneous
hyper-	too much, high	hypertension
hypo-	low, under	hypoactive
intra-	within	intramuscular
inter-	between	intercellular
iso-	equal, same	isothermal
macro-	large, long	macrocyte
mal-	poor	malnutrition
micro-	small	microcyte
mono-	one	mononuclear
neo-	new	neonatal
poly-	many, much	polyuria
post-	after	postprandial
pre-	before	prenatal
per-	through	percutaneous
semi-	half	semilunar
tachy-	rapid	tachycardia
tri-	three	tricuspid

Example: GASTR /   IC
                 root   suffix
             (stomach)   (pertaining to)

The word root "gastr" means "stomach." The suffix "ic" means "pertaining to." The word gastric means "pertaining to the stomach." Table 3-3 lists common medical suffixes.

COMBINING VOWELS

A **combining vowel** (usually an "o") joins the word root to a suffix or another word root.

A combining vowel eases pronunciation.

Example: HEMAT   / O /   LOGY
                 root   combining vowel   suffix
             (blood)   (study of)

The word root "hemat," meaning "blood," is joined by the combining vowel "o" to "logy," meaning "the study of." Hematology thus means "the study of blood."

The combining vowel is usually dropped when the suffix begins with a vowel.

Table 3-3
Common Medical Suffixes

Suffix	Meaning	Example
ac,-al,	pertaining to	cardiac, neural
-algia	pain	neuralgia
-ar,-ary	pertaining to	muscular, urinary
-centesis	surgical puncture to remove a fluid	thoracentesis
-emia	blood condition	anemia
-gram	recording, writing	electrocardiogram
-ic	pertaining to	thoracic
-ism	condition	hypothyroidism
-itis	inflammation	tonsillitis
-logist	specialist in the study of	cardiologist
-lysis	breakdown, separation	hemolysis
-megaly	enlargement	acromegaly
-meter	instrument that measures or counts	thermometer
-oma	tumor	hepatoma
-osis	condition	necrosis
-oxia	oxygen level	hypoxia
-pathy	disease	cardiomyopathy
-penia	deficiency	leukopenia
-pnea	breathing	dyspnea
-stasis	stopping, controlling	hemostasis
-tomy	cutting, incision	phlebotomy

Example: PHLEB /   ITIS
          root   suffix
        (vein)   (inflammation)

Because the suffix "itis" begins with a vowel, a combining vowel is not used after the word root "phleb." Phlebitis means "inflammation of a vein."

In terms made up of two word roots, the combining vowel is kept between the word roots, even if the second root begins with a vowel.

Example: GASTR / O / ENTER / O / LOGY
        root   root   suffix
    (stomach)   (intestines)   (study of)

The combining vowel after "gastr" remains, even though the second root "enter" begins with a vowel. Gastroenterology means "study of the stomach and intestines."

COMBINING FORMS

A word root along with a combining vowel is called a **combining form**. A combining form can be attached to a suffix or another word root.

Example: LEUK   / O/   CYTE
               combining form
       root + combining vowel + root
      (white)   (cell)

The word "leuk," meaning "white," combined with the word "cyte," meaning "cell," combines to form leukocyte, meaning "white cell," or more commonly, "white blood cell."

PLURAL ENDINGS

Some medical terms have unique plural forms based on the ending of the word. Table 3-4 lists unique plural endings.

MEDICAL TERMINOLOGY REMINDERS

1. When defining a medical term, begin at the suffix and read back through the word to the beginning.
2. When a suffix starts with a vowel, drop the combining vowel before the suffix.
3. A combining vowel remains between word roots, even when the root begins with a vowel.

Table 3-4
Unique Plural Endings

Word Ending	Plural Ending	Singular Example	Plural Example
-a	-ae	vena cava	vena cavae (ka′ve)
-en	-ina	lumen	lumina (lu′min-a)
-ex,-ix	-ices	appendix	appendices (a-pen′di-sez)
-is	-es	crisis	crises (kri′sez)
-nx	-nges	phalanx	phalanges (fa-lan′-jez)
-on	-a	protozoon	protozoa (pro″to-zo′a)
-um	-a	ovum	ova (o′va)
-us	-i	nucleus	nuclei (nu′kle-i)

ABBREVIATIONS AND SYMBOLS

Some of the most common medical abbreviations and symbols are listed in Table 3-5.

Table 3-5
Common Medical Abbreviations and Symbols

ABGs	arterial blood gases
ABO	blood group system
a.c.	before meals
ACTH	adrenocorticotropic hormone
ADH	antidiuretic hormone
ad lib	as desired
AIDS	acquired immunodeficiency syndrome
ALL	acute lymphocytic leukemia
ALT	alanine transaminase (see SGPT)
AML	acute myelocytic leukemia
aq	water (aqua)
AST	aspartate aminotransferase (see SGOT)
ASO	antistreptolysin O
b.i.d.	twice a day (bis in die)
bili	bilirubin
BP	blood pressure
BUN	blood urea nitrogen
Bx	biopsy
$\bar{c}$	with (cum)
Ca	calcium
CAD	coronary artery disease
CBC	complete blood count
cc	cubic centimeter

(continued)

Table 3-5 (Continued)

CCU	coronary care unit
Chemo	chemotherapy
CK	creatine kinase
cm	centimeter
CML	chronic myelogenous leukemia
CNS	central nervous system
CO_2	carbon dioxide
COPD	chronic obstructive pulmonary disease
CPR	cardiopulmonary resuscitation
crit	hematocrit (see HCT)
C-section	cesarean section
CSF	cerebrospinal fluid
CT scan	computed tomography scan
CVA	cerebrovascular accident (stroke)
CXR	chest x-ray
DIC	disseminated intravascular coagulation
diff	differential count of white blood cells
dil	dilute
DNA	deoxyribonucleic acid
DOB	date of birth
Dx	diagnosis
EBV	Epstein-Barr virus
ECG	electrocardiogram
EEG	electroencephalogram
EKG	electrocardiogram
ENT	ear, nose, and throat
Eos	eosinophils
ER	emergency room
ESR	erythrocyte sedimentation rate (sed rate)
exc	excision
FBS	fasting blood sugar
Fe	iron
FSH	follicle stimulating hormone
FUO	fever of unknown origin
GI	gastrointestinal
Gm, gm, g	gram
GTT	glucose tolerance test
GYN	gynecology
h	hour
Hb, Hgb	hemoglobin
HbsAg	hepatitis B surface antigen
HCG	human chorionic gonadotropin
HCL	hydrochloric acid
Hct	hematocrit (see crit)
HDL	high density lipoprotein
Hg	mercury
HIV	human immunodeficiency virus

(continued)

Table 3-5 (Continued)

h/o	history of
H_2O	water
h.s.	at bedtime (hora somni)
hx	history
ICU	intensive care unit
IM	intramuscular
IV	intravenous
IVP	intravenous pyelogram
K^+	potassium
Kg	kilogram
L	liter
L	left
Lat	lateral
LD/LDH	lactic dehydrogenase
LDL	low density lipoprotein
LE	lupus erythematosus (lupus)
lymphs	lymphocytes
lytes	electrolytes
m	meter
MCH	mean corpuscular hemoglobin
MCHC	mean corpuscular hemoglobin concentration
MCV	mean corpuscular volume
mets	metastases
mg	milligram
Mg^{++}	magnesium
MI	myocardial infarction
mL	milliliter
mm	millimeter
mono	monocyte
MRI	magnetic resonance imaging
MS	multiple sclerosis
Na^+	sodium
neg	negative
NG	nasogastric
NPO	nothing by mouth (nulla per os)
O_2	oxygen
OB	obstetrics
O&P	ova and parasite
OR	operating room
P	pulse; phosphorus
Path	pathology
p.c.	after meals
PCO_2	pressure of carbon dioxide in the blood
Peds	pediatrics
pH	hydrogen ion concentration (measure of acidity or alkalinity)
PKU	phenylketonuria
PMNs	polymorphonuclear leukocytes

(continued)

Table 3-5 (Continued)

PO_2	pressure of oxygen in the blood
p/o	postoperative
p.o.	orally (per os)
polys	polymorphonuclear leukocytes
pos	positive
post-op	after operation
PP	after meals (postprandial)
pre-op	before operation
prep	prepare for
PRN, prn	as necessary (pro re nata)
PT	prothrombin time/protime
PTT	partial thromboplastin time
pt	patient
PVC	premature ventricular contraction
q.n.s.	quantity not sufficient
R	right
RA	rheumatoid arthritis
RBC	red blood cell (also rbc)
req	requisition
RIA	radioimmunoassay
R/O	rule out
RPR	rapid plasma reagin
RT	respiratory therapy
RR	recovery room
Rx	treatment
$\bar{s}$	without
Sed rate	erythrocyte sedimentation rate (ESR)
segs	segmented white blood cells
SGOT	serum glutamic-oxaloacetic transaminase (see AST)
SGPT	serum glutamic-pyruvic transaminase (see ALT)
SLE	systemic lupus erythematosus
SMAC	sequential multiple analyzer computerized
sol	solution
Staph	staphylococcus
STAT, stat	immediately
Strep	streptococcus
Sx	symptoms
T	temperature
T_3	triiodothyronine (a thyroid hormone)
T_4	thyroxine (a thyroid hormone)
TB	tuberculosis
T cells	lymphocytes from the thymus
T & C	type and crossmatch (type & x)
TIBC	total iron binding capacity
TPN	total parenteral nutrition (intravenous feeding)
TPR	temperature, pulse, and respiration
Trig	triglycerides

(continued)

Table 3-5 (Continued)

TSH	thyroid stimulating hormone
Tx	treatment
U	unit
UA, ua	urinalysis
URI	upper respiratory infection
UTI	urinary tract infection
UV	ultraviolet
VCU	voiding cystourethrogram
VD	venereal disease
VDRL	venereal disease research laboratory
W̸	water reactive
WBC, wbc	white blood cell
wd	wound
WT, wt	weight
y/o	years old

Study & Review Questions

1. What is the meaning of the term "dermatosis"?
   a. Abnormal condition of the skin
   b. Examination of the skin
   c. Inflammation of the skin
   d. Study of the skin

2. Which of the following terms means "inflammation of a vein"?
   a. Phlebitis
   b. Phlebology
   c. Phlebotomize
   d. Phlebotomy

3. To what part of the body does the word root "hepat" refer?
   a. Head
   b. Heart
   c. Liver
   d. Stomach

4. A hematologist specializes in the study of the
   a. blood.
   b. heart.
   c. liver.
   d. stomach.

5. Which part of gastr/o/enter/o/logy is the suffix?
   a. gastr
   b. enter
   c. o
   d. logy

6. Of the following word parts, which is a prefix?
   a. arthro
   b. hyper
   c. oste
   d. emia

7. What does the suffix "-algia" mean?
   a. Between
   b. Condition
   c. Disease
   d. Pain

8. Which of the following is the medical term for a red blood cell?
   a. Erythrocyte
   b. Hepatocyte
   c. Leukocyte
   d. Thrombocyte

Suggested Laboratory Activities

1. Make flash cards with word parts and meanings.

2. Have a spelling or "meaning of the term" bee.

3. Do matching exercises with medical terminology lists supplied by the instructor.

4. Write a fictional case study using a list of assigned terms.

BIBLIOGRAPHY AND SUGGESTED READINGS

Cohen, B. J. (1994). *Medical terminology: An illustrated guide.* Philadelphia: J. B. Lippincott.
Thomas, C. (1997). *Taber's cyclopedic medical dictionary* (18th ed.). Philadelphia: F. A. Davis.

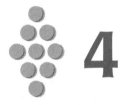

4

An Overview of the Anatomy and Physiology of the Human Body

KEY TERMS

anabolism	catabolism	inferior	superior
anatomic position	distal	metabolism	supine
anterior	dorsal cavities	prone	transverse
body cavities	frontal plane	proximal	plane
body plane	homeostasis	sagittal plane	ventral cavities

OBJECTIVES

Upon successful completion of this chapter, the reader will be able to:

1. Describe the anatomic, supine, and prone body positions.
2. Identify body planes and cavities, and use directional terms to describe the relationship of areas of the body with respect to the rest of the body.
3. Define homeostasis and the primary processes of metabolism.
4. Describe body organization; identify structural components of cells; and describe the four basic types of body tissue.
5. Describe the function, identify the components or major structures, and list disorders and diagnostic tests associated with each body system.

INTRODUCTION

The human body is a wonder, consisting of over 30 trillion cells, 206 bones, 700 muscles, 5 liters of blood, and 25 miles of blood vessels. To fully appreciate the workings of this wonder, it is necessary to have a basic understanding of the **anatomy** (structural composition) and **physiology** (functions) of the human body. Knowledge of human anatomy and physiology is also needed to understand fully the nature of the various disorders of the body and the rationale for the laboratory tests associated with them.

ANATOMIC POSITION

A person in the **anatomic position** is standing erect, arms at the side, with palms facing forward. When describing the direction or the location of a given point of the body, medical personnel always refer to the body as if the patient is in the anatomic position, regardless of actual body position.

OTHER BODY POSITIONS

Two other body positions of particular importance to a blood drawer are **supine**, in which the patient is lying on the back with the face up, and **prone**, in which the patient is lying face down. Prone also refers to the hand with the palm facing down. A way to equate supine with lying down is to think of the *ine* as in *recline*. An easy way to remember that a person who is supine is *face up* is to look for the word *up* in supine.

BODY PLANES

A **body plane** (Fig. 4-1) is a flat surface resulting from a real or imaginary cut through a body in the normal anatomic position. Areas of the body are often referred to according to their location with respect to one of the following body planes: frontal, sagittal, or transverse.

The **frontal** (or **coronal**) **plane** divides the body vertically into front and back portions.

The **sagittal plane** divides the body vertically into right and left portions. A vertical division resulting in equal right and left portions is called a **midsagittal** (or **medial**) **plane.**

The **transverse plane** divides the body horizontally into upper and lower portions.

A procedure called **computerized axial tomography (CT** or **CAT scan)** produces an x-ray in a transverse plane of the body. **Magnetic resonance imaging (MRI)** can produce images of the body in all three planes using magnetic waves instead of x-rays.

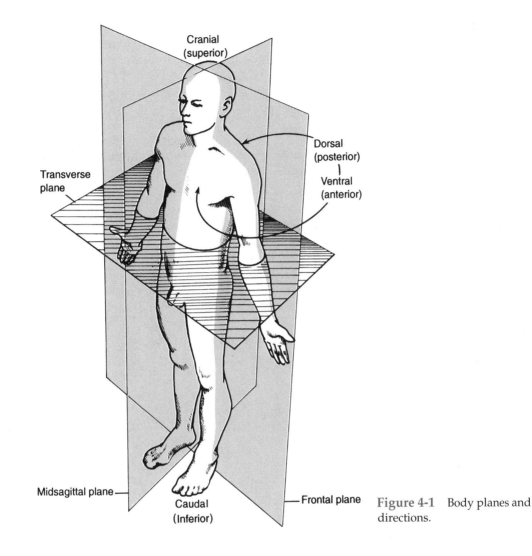

Cranial
(superior)

Dorsal
(posterior)

Ventral
(anterior)

Transverse
plane

Midsagittal plane

Caudal
(Inferior)

Frontal plane

Figure 4-1 Body planes and directions.

BODY DIRECTIONAL TERMS

Areas of the body are also identified using **directional terms**. Directional terms describe the relationship of an area or part of the body with respect to the rest of the body or body part. Directional terms are often paired with a term that means the opposite. The following are some of the more common paired directional terms:

Anterior (ventral) refers to the front. **Posterior (dorsal)** refers to the back.
External (superficial) means on or near the surface of the body. **Internal (deep)** means within or near the center of the body.
Medial means toward the midline or middle. **Lateral** means toward the side.

Proximal means nearest to the center of the body, origin, or point of attachment. **Distal** means farthest from the center of the body, origin, or point of attachment.

Superior (cranial) means higher, or above or toward the head. **Inferior (caudal)** means beneath, or lower or away from the head.

BODY CAVITIES

Various organs of the body are housed in large, hollow spaces called **body cavities** (Fig. 4-2). These body cavities are divided into two groups, according to their location within the body.

1. **Dorsal cavities** are located in the back of the body and include:
   The **cranial cavity**, which houses the brain.
   The **spinal cavity**, which encases the spinal cord.
2. **Ventral cavities** are located in the front of the body and include:
   The **thoracic cavity**, which houses primarily the heart and lungs.
   The **abdominal cavity**, which houses numerous organs including the stomach, liver, pancreas, gallbladder, spleen and kidneys. (It is separated from the thoracic cavity by a muscle called the **diaphragm**.)
   The **pelvic cavity**, which houses primarily the urinary bladder, and reproductive organs.

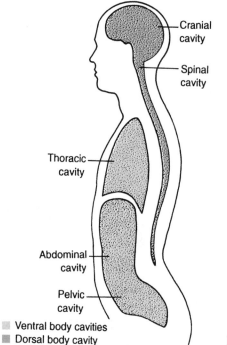

Figure 4-2   Side view of body cavities (Rosdahl C).

BODY FUNCTIONS

Homeostasis

The human body constantly strives to maintain its internal environment in a state of equilibrium or balance. This balanced or "steady state" condition is called **homeostasis** (ho'me-o-sta'sis), which literally translated means "staying the same." Homeostasis enables all the cells of the body to obtain the nutrients and oxygen necessary to maintain life.

Metabolism

Metabolism (me-tab'o-lizm) is the sum of all the physical and chemical reactions necessary to sustain life. There are two primary processes of metabolism: catabolism and anabolism.

Catabolism (kah-tab'o-lizm) is the process by which complex substances such as food are broken down into simple substances.

Anabolism (ah-nab'o-lizm) is the process by which the body converts simple compounds into complex substances needed to carry out the cellular activities of the body.

BODY ORGANIZATION

Cells

The cell (Fig. 4-3) is the basic structural unit of all life. The human body consists of trillions of cells, responsible for all the activities of the body. There are many categories of cells, each category specialized to perform a unique function. No matter what their function, all cells have the same basic structural components.

All cells have an outer covering called a **cell membrane** which has the selective capability of allowing certain substances in and out of the cell. The fluid that fills the cell is called **cytoplasm**. Within the cytoplasm are structures called organelles. These organelles are the **centrioles, endoplasmic reticulum, Golgi apparatus, lysosomes, mitochondria,** and **ribosomes**.

Also within the cell, surrounded by its own membrane, is the **nucleus** or command center of the cell. The nucleus contains the chromosomes or genetic material governing all the activities of the cell, including reproduction. The chromosomes contain DNA which is organized into separate units called genes. Most cells are able to replace themselves by a process called **mitosis** (mi-to'sis), which is also how the body grows.

Tissues

Tissues are groups of similar cells that work together to perform a special function. There are four basic tissue types:

1. **Connective** tissue supports and connects all parts of the body and includes adipose (fat) tissue, cartilage, bone, and blood.
2. **Epithelial** (ep-i-the'le-al) tissue covers and protects the body and lines organs, vessels, and cavities.

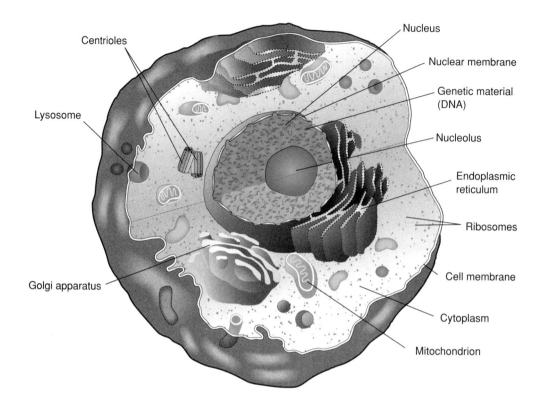

Centrioles

Nucleus

Nuclear membrane

Genetic material
(DNA)

Lysosome

Nucleolus

Endoplasmic
reticulum

Ribosomes

Cell membrane

Golgi apparatus

Cytoplasm

Mitochondrion

Figure 4-3   Diagram of a typical cell showing the main organelles.

3. **Muscle** tissue contracts to produce movement.
4. **Nerve** tissue has the ability to transmit electrical impulses.

Organs

Organs are structures composed of tissues functioning together for a common purpose.

BODY SYSTEMS

Body systems are structures and organs which are related to one another and function together. The following are 10 commonly recognized body systems.

Skeletal System
FUNCTIONS

The skeletal system (Fig. 4-4) is comprised of all the bones (206) and joints of the body. It is the framework that gives the body shape and support, protects internal organs, and, along with the muscular system, provides movement and leverage. In addition, the skeletal system is responsible for calcium storage and **hemopoiesis** (he'mo-

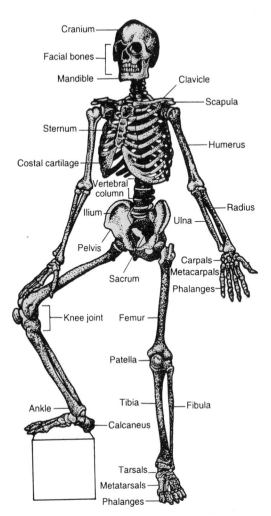

Figure 4-4   The human skeleton (Rosdahl C).

poy-e'sis), also called **hematopoiesis** (hem'a-to-poy-e'sis), the production of blood cells which normally occurs in the bone marrow.

TYPES OF BONES

The bones of the skeletal system are categorized by shape into four groups.

1. **Flat bones** such as rib and most skull (cranial) bones.
2. **Irregular bones** such as back bones (vertebrae) and some facial bones.
3. **Long bones** such as such as leg (femur, tibia, fibula), arm (humerus, radius, ulna), and hand bones (metacarpals and phalanges).
4. **Short bones** such as wrist (carpals) and ankle bones (tarsals).

Bones of particular importance in blood collection are the distal phalanx of the finger and the calcaneus or heel bone of the foot.

SKELETAL SYSTEM DISORDERS

- *Arthritis* (ar-thri'tis): a common joint disorder characterized by inflammation, usually accompanied by pain and swelling.
- *Bursitis* (bur-si'tis): inflammation of the fluid-filled sac (bursa) between muscle attachments and bone.
- *Gout* (gowt): a disorder of the joints (most commonly those of the feet), caused by faulty uric acid metabolism. It is a form of arthritis.
- *Osteomyelitis* (os'te-o-mi'el-i'tis): inflammation of the bone, especially the bone marrow, caused by bacterial infection.
- *Osteochondritis* (os'te-o-kon-dri'tis): inflammation of the bone and cartilage.
- *Osteoporosis* (os'te-o-por-o'sis): disorder involving loss of bone density.
- *Rickets* (rik'ets): abnormal bone formation indirectly resulting from lack of vitamin D which is necessary for calcium absorption.
- *Tumors:* abnormal bone growth.

DIAGNOSTIC TESTS

- Alkaline phosphatase (ALP)
- Calcium (Ca)
- Complete blood count (CBC)
- Erythrocyte sedimentation rate (ESR)
- Phosphorus (P)
- Synovial fluid analysis
- Uric acid
- Vitamin D

Muscular System

FUNCTIONS

The muscular system is comprised of all the muscles of the body. It includes not only those attached to the skeletal system, but also those that form the walls of the heart and those that line the walls of blood vessels and the digestive tract. Muscles give the body the ability to move, maintain posture, and produce heat.

TYPES OF MUSCLES

Muscles (Fig. 4-5) are classified according to their location, their **histologic** (microscopic) structure, and how they are controlled.

Skeletal muscle is attached to bone, has **striated** (stri'a-ted) or banded muscle fibers, and is under **voluntary** (conscious) control.

Visceral (vis'er-al) **muscle** lines the walls of blood vessels and most internal organs, is **non-striated**, and is under **involuntary** or unconscious control. Visceral muscle is often called **smooth** muscle.

Cardiac muscle forms the wall of the heart, is a special kind of **striated** muscle, and is under **involuntary** control.

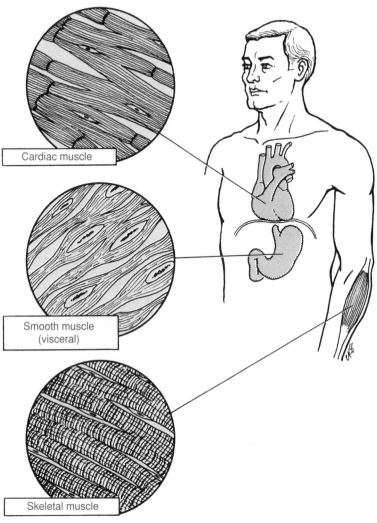

Figure 4-5 Types of muscle tissue.

MUSCULAR SYSTEM DISORDERS

- *Atrophy* (at'ro-fe): a decrease in size (wasting) of a muscle usually due to inactivity.
- *Muscular dystrophy* (dis'tro-fe): a genetic disease in which the muscles waste away or atrophy.
- *Myalgia* (mi-al'je-ah): painful muscle.
- *Tendinitis* (ten'di-ni'tis): inflammation of muscle tendons usually due to overexertion.

DIAGNOSTIC TESTS

- Autoimmune antibodies
- Creatine phosphokinase (CPK/CK)
- CPK/CK isoenzymes

- Lactic acid
- Lactic dehydrogenase (LD/LDH)
- Myoglobin
- Electromyography

Reproductive System

FUNCTIONS

The reproductive system (Fig. 4-6) produces the **gametes** (gam'eets), or **sex cells**, that are needed to form a new human being. In males, the gametes are called **spermatozoa** (sper'mat-o-zo'a), or sperm. In females, the gametes are called **ova** (o'va), or eggs. Reproduction occurs when an **ovum** (singular of ova) is fertilized by a sperm.

The reproductive system consists of glands called **gonads** (go'nads) and their associated structures and ducts. The gonads manufacture and store the gametes and produce the hormones (see Endocrine System) that regulate the reproductive process. The male gonads are the **testes**. The female gonads are the **ovaries**.

STRUCTURES

Structures of the female reproductive system include the ovaries, **fallopian** (fa-lo'pe-an) **tubes**, **uterus**, **cervix**, **vagina**, and **vulva**. Structures of the male reproductive system include the testes, **seminal vesicles**, **prostate**, **epididymis** (ep'i-did'i-mis), **vas deferens** (vas def'er-enz), **seminal ducts**, **urethra**, **penis**, **spermatic cords**, and **scrotum**.

REPRODUCTIVE SYSTEM DISORDERS

- *Cervical cancer:* cancer of the cervix.
- *Infertility:* a lower than normal ability to reproduce.
- *Ovarian cancer:* cancer of the ovaries.
- *Ovarian cyst:* a usually nonmalignant growth in an ovary.
- *Prostate cancer:* cancer of the prostate gland.
- *Sexually transmitted diseases (STDs):* diseases such as syphilis, gonorrhea, and genital herpes, which are usually transmitted by sexual contact.
- *Uterine cancer:* cancer of the uterus.

DIAGNOSTIC TESTS

- Acid phosphatase
- Estrogen
- Follicle stimulating hormone (FSH)
- Human chorionic gonadotropin (HCG)
- Luteinizing hormone (LH)
- Microbiological cultures
- PAP smear
- Prostate-specific antigen (PSA)
- Rapid plasmin reagin (RPR)
- Testosterone
- Viral tissue studies

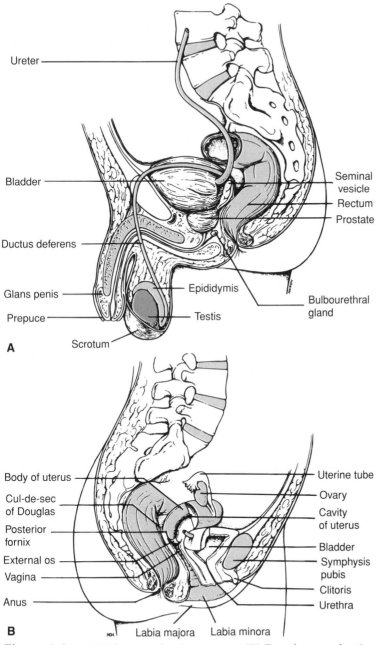

Figure 4-6 (**A**) Male reproductive system; (**B**) Female reproductive system (Rosdahl C).

Digestive System
FUNCTIONS

The digestive system (Fig. 4-7) provides the means by which the body takes in food, breaks it down into usable components for absorption, and eliminates waste products from this process.

STRUCTURES

The digestive system components form a continuous passageway called the **digestive tract**, which extends from the mouth to the anus. The digestive tract is often called the **gastrointestinal (GI) tract.** GI tract components include the **mouth, pharynx, throat, esophagus, stomach,** and **small** and **large intestines.**

The digestive system also includes and is assisted by a number of accessory organs and structures: **lips, teeth, tongue, salivary glands, liver, pancreas,** and **gallbladder.**

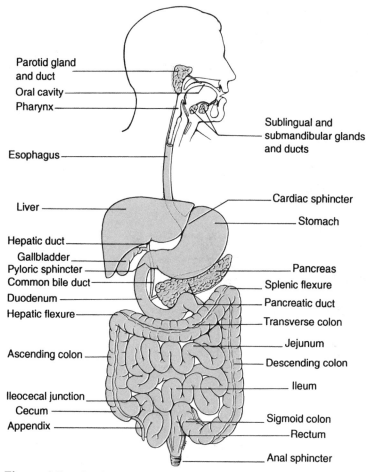

Figure 4-7   The digestive system (Rosdahl C).

Important digestive functions of the liver include glycogen storage, protein catabolism, the detoxification of harmful substances, and the secretion of bile necessary for the digestion of fat. Bile is concentrated and stored in the gallbladder. Digestive functions of the pancreas include the secretion of insulin and glucagon and the production of digestive enzymes, including amylase, lipase, and trypsin.

DIGESTIVE SYSTEM DISORDERS

- *Appendicitis* (a-pen'di-si'tis): inflammation of the appendix.
- *Cholecystitis* (ko'le-sis-ti'tis): inflammation of the gallbladder.
- *Colitis* (ko-li'tis): inflammation of the colon.
- *Diverticulosis* (di'ver-tik'u-lo'sis): pouches in the walls of the colon.
- *Gastritis* (gas-tri'tis): inflammation of the stomach lining.
- *Gastroenteritis* (gas'tro-en-ter-i'tis): inflammation of the stomach and intestinal tract.
- *Hepatitis* (hep'a-ti'tis): inflammation of the liver.
- *Pancreatitis* (pan'kre-a-ti'tis): inflammation of the pancreas.
- *Peritonitis* (per'i-to-ni'tis): inflammation of the abdominal cavity lining.
- *Ulcer:* open sore or lesion.

DIAGNOSTIC TESTS

- Amylase
- Bilirubin (bili)
- Carcinoembryonic antigen (CEA)
- Carotene
- Cholesterol
- Complete blood count (CBC)
- Glucose
- Glucose tolerance test (GTT)
- Lipase
- Occult blood
- Ova & parasite (O&P)
- Triglycerides

Endocrine System

FUNCTIONS

The word **endocrine** comes from the Greek words *endon,* meaning "within," and *krinein,* meaning "to secrete," and is used to describe a type of gland that secretes substances called hormones directly into the bloodstream. Glands of this type, also known as ductless glands, comprise the endocrine system (Fig. 4-8). The hormones secreted by these glands are powerful chemical substances that have a profound effect on metabolism, growth and development, reproduction, personality, and the ability of the body to react to stress and resist disease.

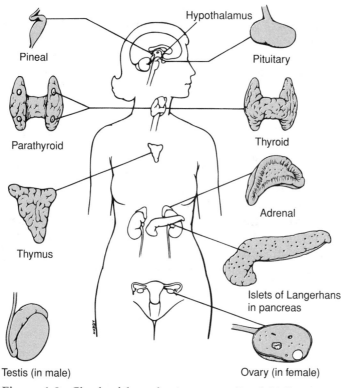

Figure 4-8   Glands of the endocrine system (Rosdahl C).

GLANDS OF THE ENDOCRINE SYSTEM

The **pituitary** (pi-tu′i-tar-ee) **gland**, located in the brain, is often called the master gland because it releases hormones that stimulate other glands. Examples of hormones released by the pituitary gland are **adrenocorticotropic** (ad-re′no-kor′ti-ko-trop′ik) **hormone (ACTH)**, which stimulates the **adrenal** (ad-re′nal) **glands**; **antidiuretic** (an′ti-di-u-ret′ik) **hormone (ADH)**, which decreases urine secretion; **follicle stimulating hormone (FSH)**, which affects the ovaries; **growth hormone (GH)**, which is important in regulating growth; and **thyroid** (thi′royd) **stimulating hormone (TSH)**, which controls thyroid activity.

The **pineal** (pin′e-al) **gland** is located posterior to the pituitary. The endocrine function of the pineal gland is not yet fully understood. A number of hormones have been isolated from this gland, but only **melatonin** (mel′a-to′nin) is known to be a major secretory product. Release of melatonin is inhibited by light and enhanced by darkness, causing melatonin levels in the blood to follow a **diurnal** (daily) **rhythm** with levels lowest around noon and peaking at night.

The **thyroid gland** is located in the throat near the larynx. The thyroid produces **calcitonin** (kal′si-to′nin), which regulates the amount of calcium in the blood, and **thyroxine** (thi-roks′in), or T_4, which increases the metabolic rate. Production of thyroid hormones requires the presence of iodine.

There are four **parathyroid** (par-a-thi′royd) **glands** located behind the thyroid gland, two on each side. The parathyroid glands produce **parathyroid hormone (PTH)**, which regulates calcium and phosphorous metabolism.

The **thymus** (thi′mus) is located in the chest behind the sternum (breastbone). The thymus produces the hormone **thymosin** (thi′mo-sin), which is necessary for the maturation of **T-lymphocytes** (specialized white blood cells) and the development of immunity. This gland is most active before birth and during childhood.

There are two **adrenal glands**, one located on top of each kidney. The inner portion of each adrenal gland produces the hormones **epinephrine** (ep-i-nef′rin) and **norepinephrine**, also called **adrenaline** (a-dren′a-lin) and **noradrenaline**. These hormones are known as the "fight-or-flight" hormones because of their effects when the body is under stress.

The outer portion of the adrenal glands produces numerous hormones. The major ones are **cortisol** (kor′ti-sol), which has the ability to suppress inflammation, and **aldosterone** (al-dos′ter-on), which is involved in regulating the amount of sodium and potassium in the bloodstream.

Special cells of the pancreas, known as **islets** (i′lets) **of Langerhans** (lahng′er-hanz), also perform endocrine activity. The islet cells secrete **insulin**, which is necessary for the normal movement of glucose from the blood into the cells, thus reducing the amount of glucose in the bloodstream. Islet cells also secrete **glucagon** (gloo′ka-gon), which stimulates the liver to release stored glucose into the bloodstream, counterbalancing the effect of insulin and increasing blood glucose levels.

The **testes** secrete the hormone **testosterone** (tes-tos′ter-on), which is responsible for the growth and functioning of the male reproductive system as well as the development of male sexual characteristics.

The **ovaries** secrete the hormones **estrogen** (es′tro-jen) and **progesterone** (pro′jester-on), which are responsible for the growth and functioning of the female reproductive system as well as the development of female sexual characteristics.

Other structures such as the **lining of the stomach,** the **placenta**, and the **kidneys** also have endocrine function. For example, the kidneys secrete **renin**, which increases blood pressure, and **erythropoietin** (e-rith′ro-poi′e-tin), which stimulates red blood cell formation.

ENDOCRINE SYSTEM DISORDERS

Endocrine disorders are most commonly caused by tumors, which can cause either **hypersecretion** (secreting too much) or **hyposecretion** (secreting too little) of the gland.

Pituitary disorders

- *Acromegaly* (ak′ro-meg′a-le): the overgrowth of the bones in the hands, feet, and face caused by excessive GH in adulthood.
- *Diabetes insipidus* (di′a-be′tez in-sip′id-us): a condition characterized by increased thirst and increased urine production caused by inadequate secretion of ADH, also called **vasopressin** (vas′o-pres′in).

- *Dwarfism:* the condition of being abnormally small, one cause of which is growth hormone (GH) deficiency in infancy.
- *Gigantism:* excessive development of the body or of a body part due to excessive GH.

Thyroid disorders

- *Congenital hypothyroidism:* insufficient thyroid activity in a newborn, either from a genetic deficiency or maternal factors such as lack of dietary iron during pregnancy.
- *Cretinism:* severe untreated congenital hypothyroidism in which the development of the child is impaired, resulting in a short, disproportionate body, thick tongue and neck, and mental handicap.
- *Goiter* (goy′ter): an enlargement of the thyroid gland.
- *Hyperthyroidism* (Graves′ disease): a condition characterized by weight loss, nervousness, and protruding eyeballs, due to an increased metabolic rate caused by excessive secretion of the thyroid gland.
- *Hypothyroidism:* a condition characterized weight gain and lethargy due to a decreased metabolic rate caused by decreased thyroid secretion.
- *Myxedema* (hypothyroid syndrome): a condition characterized by anemia, slow speech, mental apathy, drowsiness, and sensitivity to cold resulting from decreased functioning of the thyroid gland.

Parathyroid disorders

Hypersecretion of the parathyroids can lead to kidney stones and bone destruction. Hyposecretion can cause muscle spasms and convulsions.

Adrenal disorders

- *Addison′s disease:* a condition characterized by weight loss, dehydration, and hypotension (abnormally low blood pressure) caused by decreased glucose and sodium levels due to hyposecretion of the adrenal glands.
- *Aldosteronism:* a condition characterized by hypertension (high blood pressure) and edema caused by excessive sodium and water retention due to hypersecretion of aldosterone.
- *Cushing′s syndrome:* a condition characterized by a swollen, "moon-shaped" face and redistribution of fat to the abdomen and back of the neck caused by an excess of cortisone.

Pancreatic disorders

- *Diabetes mellitus:* a condition in which there is impaired carbohydrate, fat, and protein metabolism due to a deficiency of insulin.
- *Diabetes mellitus type I* or *insulin-dependent diabetes mellitus (IDDM):* a type of diabetes mellitus in which the body is totally unable to produce insulin. This type is often called juvenile-onset diabetes because it usually appears before 25 years of age.
- *Diabetes mellitus type II* or *non–insulin-dependent diabetes mellitus (NIDDM):* a type of diabetes mellitus in which the body is able to produce insulin, however either the amount produced is insufficient or there is impaired use of the insulin produced. This type of diabetes occurs predominantly in adults.

- *Hyperinsulinism:* a condition in which there is too much insulin in the blood due to excessive secretion of insulin or an overdose of insulin (insulin shock).
- *Hypoglycemia* (hi"po-gli-se'me-a): a condition in which the glucose (blood sugar) is abnormally low due to hyperinsulinism.

DIAGNOSTIC TESTS

- Adrenocorticotropic hormone (ACTH)
- Aldosterone
- Antidiuretic hormone (ADH)
- Cortisol
- Erythropoietin
- Glucagon
- Glucose tolerance test (GTT)
- Growth hormone (GH)
- Insulin level
- Renin
- Thyroid function studies (*eg*, T_3, T_4, TSH)

Nervous System

FUNCTIONS

The nervous system (Fig. 4-9, *left*) controls and coordinates activities of the various body systems by means of electrical impulses and chemical substances sent to and received from all parts of the body.

STRUCTURES

The fundamental unit of the nervous system is the **nerve cell** or **neuron** (see Fig. 4-9, *right*). Neurons are highly complex cells that are capable of conducting messages in the form of impulses that enable the body to interact with its internal and external environment.

There are two main structural divisions of the nervous system, the **central nervous system** and the **peripheral nervous system**.

Central nervous system

The **central nervous system (CNS)** consists of the **brain** and **spinal cord**, both of which are completely enclosed and protected by three layers of connective tissue called the **meninges** (me-nin'jez). The brain and spinal cord are surrounded, cushioned, and separated from the meninges by a space filled with a clear, plasma-like fluid called **cerebrospinal** (ser"e-bro-spi'nal) **fluid (CSF)**. A physician uses a procedure called **lumbar** (spinal) **puncture** to obtain CSF if needed for laboratory testing.

The CNS functions as command center of the nervous system by interpreting information and dictating responses. Every part of the body is in direct communication with the CNS by means of its own set of nerves. All of these nerves come together in one large trunk which forms the spinal cord.

(*text continues on page 76*)

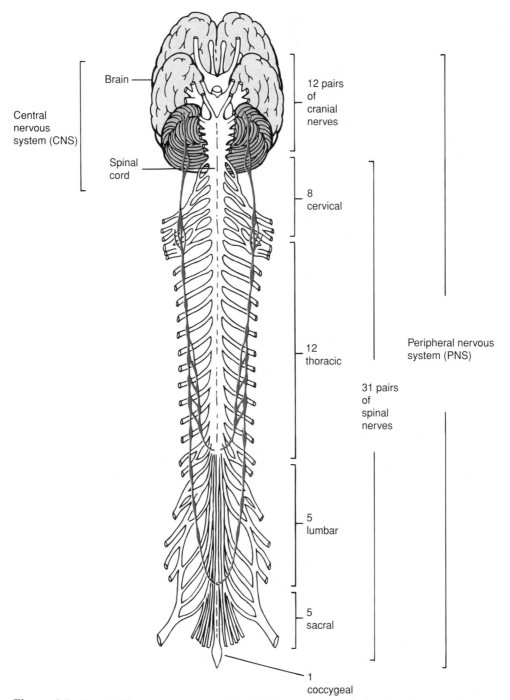

Figure 4-9   *Page 74*, The nervous system. *Page 75*, Motor neuron. The break in the axon denotes length; the arrows show the direction of the nerve impulse.

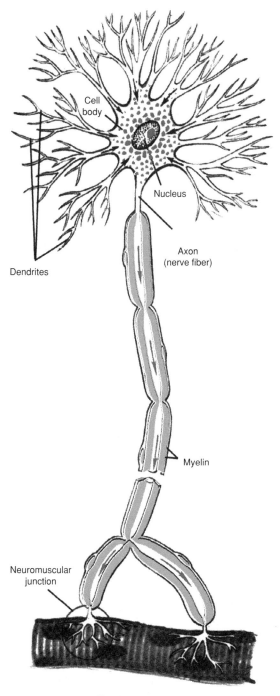

Figure 4-9 (Continued)

Peripheral nervous system

The **peripheral nervous system (PNS)** consists of all the nerves that connect the CNS to every part of the body. Two functional divisions of the PNS are the **sensory** or **afferent** (a'fer-ent) **division** and the **motor** or **efferent** (ef'fer-ent) **division**. **Sensory nerves** carry impulses *to* the CNS from sensory receptors in various parts of the body. **Motor nerves** carry impulses *from* the CNS to organs, glands, and muscles.

The motor division can be further subdivided into the **somatic** (so-mat'ik) or **voluntary nervous system** and the **autonomic** (aw-to-nom'ik) or **involuntary nervous system (ANS)**. The somatic nervous system conducts impulses from the CNS that allow an individual to consciously control skeletal muscles. The autonomic nervous system plays an important role in maintaining homeostasis by conducting impulses that affect involuntary activities of smooth muscle, cardiac muscle, and glands.

DISORDERS OF THE NERVOUS SYSTEM

- *Amyotrophic lateral sclerosis (ALS):* a disease involving muscle weakness and atrophy due to degeneration of portions of the brain and spinal cord.
- *Encephalitis:* inflammation of the brain.
- *Epilepsy:* recurrent pattern of seizures.
- *Hydrocephalus:* accumulation of cerebrospinal fluid in the brain.
- *Meningitis:* inflammation of the membranes of the spinal cord or brain.
- *Multiple sclerosis:* disease causing destruction of the myelin sheath (fat-like covering) of the nerves of the brain.
- *Neuralgia* (nu-ral'je-a): severe pain along a nerve.
- *Parkinson's disease:* chronic nervous disease characterized by fine muscle tremors and muscle weakness.
- *Shingles:* acute eruption of herpes blisters along the course of a peripheral nerve.

DIAGNOSTIC TESTS

- Acetylcholine receptor antibody
- Cerebral spinal fluid (CSF) analysis
  - Cell count
  - Glucose
  - Protein
  - Culture
- Cholinesterase
- Drug levels
- Serotonin

Urinary System
FUNCTIONS

The urinary system (Fig. 4-10) is responsible for filtering waste products of metabolism from the blood and eliminating them from the body. It also plays an important role in the regulation of body fluids. Activities of the urinary system result in the creation and elimination of urine.

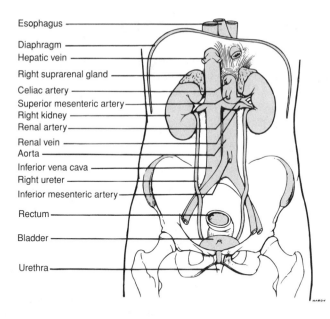

Esophagus

Diaphragm
Hepatic vein

Right suprarenal gland

Celiac artery
Superior mesenteric artery
Right kidney
Renal artery

Renal vein
Aorta
Inferior vena cava
Right ureter
Inferior mesenteric artery

Rectum

Bladder

Urethra

Figure 4-10 The urinary system (Rosdahl C).

STRUCTURES

The main structures of the urinary system are two kidneys, two ureters, a urinary bladder, and a urethra.

The **kidneys** are bean-shaped organs located at the back of the abdominal cavity, just above the waistline, one on each side of the body. The kidneys function to maintain water and electrolyte balance. **Electrolytes** include sodium, potassium, chloride, bicarbonate, and calcium ions and are essential to normal nerve, muscle, and heart activity. The kidneys also eliminate urea, a waste product of protein metabolism. In addition, the kidneys are responsible for the production of several hormones including erythropoietin.

The functional units of the kidneys are the **nephrons**, of which each kidney contains nearly a million. As blood travels through the nephrons, water and dissolved substances including wastes are filtered from the blood through a tuft of capillaries called the **glomerulus**. The resulting glomerular filtrate travels through other structures within the nephron, where water and essential amounts of substances such as sodium, potassium, and calcium are reabsorbed into the bloodstream. The remaining filtrate is called urine.

A narrow, muscular tube called a **ureter** transports the urine from the kidney to the **urinary bladder**. The urinary bladder, located in the anterior portion of the pelvic cavity, is a muscular sac that acts as a reservoir for the urine. Urine is voided (emptied) from the bladder to the outside of the body through a single tube called the **urethra**.

URINARY SYSTEM DISORDERS

- *Renal failure:* a sudden and severe impairment of renal function.
- *Nephritis:* inflammation of the kidneys.
- *Uremia:* impaired kidney function with a buildup of waste products in the blood.

- *Kidney stones:* uric acid, calcium phosphate, or oxalate stones in the kidneys, ureter, or bladder.
- *Cystitis:* Bladder inflammation.
- *Urinary tract infection (UTI):* an infection involving the organs or ducts of the urinary system.

DIAGNOSTIC TESTS
- Albumin
- Ammonia
- Blood urea nitrogen (BUN)
- Creatinine clearance
- Electrolytes
- Osmolality
- Urinalysis (UA)
- Urine C&S

Integumentary System
FUNCTIONS
Integument (in-teg'u-ment) means "covering" or "skin." The integumentary system is made up of the **skin** (Fig. 4-11) and its appendages: hair and nails. The skin, sometimes referred to as the largest organ of the body, is the cover that protects the body from bacterial invasion, dehydration, and the harmful rays of the sun. The skin also functions in the regulation of body temperature, the elimination of small amounts of waste (through sweat), the reception of environmental stimuli (sensation of heat, cold, touch, and pain), and the manufacture of vitamin D from sunlight.

LAYERS OF THE SKIN
There are two main layers of the skin, the **epidermis** (ep'i-der'mis) and the **dermis**. They are connected to a layer of **subcutaneous tissue** which connects the skin to surface muscles and bone.

The epidermis is the outermost and thinnest layer of the skin. It is primarily made up of **stratified** (layered), **squamous** (scale-like), **keratinized** (hardened) **epithelial** cells. The epidermis is avascular, meaning it contains no blood vessels. The only living cells of the epidermis are in its deepest layer, which is called the **stratum germinativum** (ger-mi-na-ti'vum). The stratum germinativum is the only layer of the skin where **mitosis** (cell division) occurs. It is also the layer where the skin pigment melanin is produced. The cells of the stratum germinativum are nourished by diffusion of nutrients from the dermis.

The **dermis**, also called **corium** or true skin, is the inner layer of the skin. It is much thicker than the epidermis and is composed of elastic and fibrous connective tissue.

Elevations called **papillae** (pa-pil'e) and resulting depressions in the dermis where it meets the epidermis give rise to the ridges and grooves that form fingerprints. This area is often referred to as the **papillary dermis**. The dermis contains blood and lymph vessels, nerves, sebaceous (se-ba'shus) and sudoriferous (su-dor-

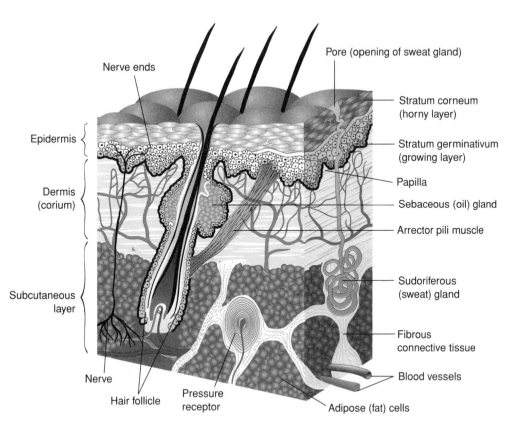

Figure 4-11 Cross section of the skin.

if′er-us) glands, and hair follicles. These structures can also extend into the subcutaneous layer.

The **subcutaneous** (under the skin) layer is composed of connective as well as adipose (fat) tissue that connects the skin to the surface of muscles.

MAJOR STRUCTURES OF THE SKIN

Hair follicles are the sheaths from which hair develops. Hair is nonliving and is primarily composed of **keratin** (ker′a-tin), a tough protein substance.

Nails are also nonliving and made of keratin. Nails grow continuously as new cells form from the nail root, located at the proximal end of the nail.

Sebaceous glands are connected to hair follicles. They are also referred to as oil glands because they secrete an oily substance called **sebum** (se′bum). Sebum helps lubricate the skin and hair and keeps it from drying out.

Sudoriferous glands, commonly called sweat glands, are coiled structures located in the dermis with ducts extending through the epidermis and ending in a pore on the surface of the skin. The sweat or perspiration produced by these glands is a mixture of water, salts, and waste.

Arrector pili are tiny, smooth muscles attached to hair follicles. These muscles are responsible for the formation of "goose bumps" as they react to pull the hair up straight when a person is cold or frightened.

INTEGUMENTARY SYSTEM DISORDERS

- *Acne:* inflammatory disease of the sebaceous gland and hair follicles.
- *Cancer:* basal cell, squamous, melanoma.
- *Dermatitis:* skin inflammation.
- *Fungal infections:* including tinea and ringworm.
- *Herpes:* including cold sore or viral infection.
- *Impetigo:* staph or strep infection.
- *Keloid:* fibrous tissue growth at scar area.
- *Pediculosis:* lice infestation.
- *Pruritus:* itching.
- *Psoriasis:* a chronic skin disease of unknown origin characterized by clearly defined red patches of scaly skin.

DIAGNOSTIC TESTS

- Biopsy
- Microbiology cultures
- Skin scrapings for fungal culture
- Tissue cultures

Respiratory System

The respiratory system (Fig. 4-12) functions along with the circulatory system to deliver a constant supply of oxygen (O_2) to all the cells of the body and to remove carbon dioxide (CO_2), a waste product of cell metabolism.

These functions are accomplished through **respiration**. Respiration permits the exchange of O_2 and CO_2 between the blood and the air and involves two processes, **external respiration** and **internal respiration**. External respiration is the process by which O_2 from the air enters the bloodstream in the lungs and CO_2 leaves the bloodstream and is breathed into the air from the lungs. Internal respiration involves the process by which O_2 leaves the bloodstream and enters the cells and CO_2 from the cells enters the bloodstream.

STRUCTURES

The major structures of the respiratory system form a continuous tract (pathway) for the flow of air to and from the lungs and include the nose, pharynx (throat), larynx (voice box), trachea, bronchi, and lungs.

The **nose** provides the main airway for respiration. (Some air enters and leaves through the mouth.) The nose also warms, moistens, and filters entering air. In addition, the nose provides a resonance chamber for the voice and contains receptors for the sense of smell.

From the nose the air moves into the **pharynx**, a funnel-shaped passageway for both food and air. The pharynx connects with the **larynx**, the enlarged upper end of the

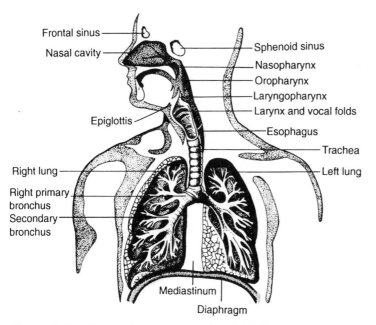

Frontal sinus
Nasal cavity
Sphenoid sinus
Nasopharynx
Oropharynx
Laryngopharynx
Larynx and vocal folds
Epiglottis
Esophagus
Trachea
Right lung
Left lung
Right primary bronchus
Secondary bronchus
Mediastinum
Diaphragm

Figure 4-12 The respiratory system (Rosdahl C).

trachea leading to the **lungs**, as well as the esophagus, which leads to the stomach. A thin, leaf-shaped cartilage structure called the **epiglottis** covers the entrance of the larynx during swallowing and acts as a switching mechanism, routing food and air into the proper pathway. Vocal chords within the larynx produce the sounds of the voice. The end of the vocal cords marks the division between the upper and lower respiratory tract.

Air from the larynx moves into the lower trachea, which branches into two main airways called **bronchi**, which lead into the lungs.

The human body has two lungs, a right with three lobes and a left with only two lobes because of the space needed for the heart. The lungs are encased in a thin membrane consisting of several layers called pleura. An infinitely small space between the layer that covers the lungs and one that lines the inner thoracic cavity is called the pleural cavity. Fluid within this cavity helps keep the lungs expanded by reducing surface tension. It also helps prevent friction as the lungs expand and contract.

Once the bronchi enter the lungs they divide into two branches which, in turn, divide many more times into smaller and smaller branches until they reach the **terminal bronchioles**. The terminal bronchioles branch into **respiratory bronchioles** which are attached to **alveolar** (al-ve'o-lar) **ducts**. The respiratory bronchioles, as well as the alveolar ducts, have cup-shaped outpouchings called **alveoli** (al-ve'o-li). The alveoli at the ends of the alveolar ducts are clustered together into **alveolar sacs**. Gas exchange between the air and the blood occurs across the walls of the alveoli.

The walls of the alveoli are composed of a singular layer of epithelium surrounded by a thin membrane. The thinness of the walls would ordinarily leave them prone to collapse. However, a coating of fluid called **surfactant** lowers the surface tension (or pull) on the walls and helps to stabilize them. (A deficiency of surfactant in premature babies allows their alveoli to collapse and is often involved in a condition called **infant respiratory distress syndrome** or **IRDS**.)

GAS EXCHANGE AND TRANSPORT

During normal external respiration (Fig. 4-13), oxygen and carbon dioxide are able to diffuse (go from an area of higher concentration to an area of lower concentration) through the walls of the alveoli and the tiny, one-cell thick blood vessels (capillaries) of the lungs. Because the blood in lung capillaries is low in O_2 and high in CO_2, O_2 from the alveoli diffuses into the blood in the capillaries while CO_2 diffuses from the capillaries into the alveoli to be **expired** (breathed out).

The amount of oxygen that can be carried dissolved in the blood plasma is not enough to meet the needs of the body. Fortunately, hemoglobin (a protein found in red blood cells) has the ability to bind oxygen, increasing the amount the blood can carry by over 70%. Most of the oxygen that diffuses into the capillaries in the lungs binds to the iron-containing heme portion of hemoglobin molecules in the red blood cells. Very little is dissolved in the blood plasma. Oxygen combined with hemoglobin is called **oxyhemoglobin**.

Hemoglobin also has the ability to bind with carbon dioxide. Hemoglobin combined with carbon dioxide is called **carbaminohemoglobin**. However, only around 20% of the carbon dioxide from the tissues is carried to the lungs in this manner. Approximately 10% is carried as gas dissolved in the blood plasma. The remaining 70% is carried as **bicarbonate ion** which was formed in the red blood cells and released into the blood plasma. In the lungs, the bicarbonate ion re-enters the red blood cells

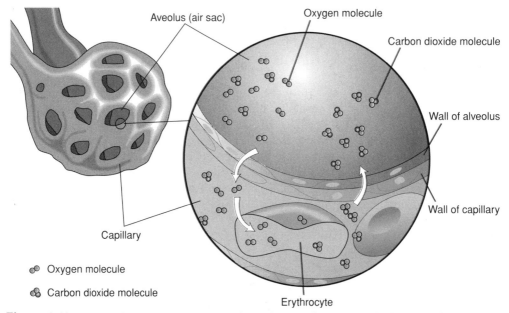

Figure 4-13   External respiration, showing the exchange of gas molecules between the air in the alveolus and the erythrocytes in a capillary.

and is released as carbon dioxide in order to diffuse through the alveoli and be exhaled by the body.

Carbon dioxide levels play a major role in acid–base (pH) balance of the blood. If CO_2 levels increase, blood pH decreases or becomes more acidic, which can lead to a dangerous condition called **acidosis**. The body responds by increasing the rate of respiration (hyperventilation) to increase oxygen levels. Prolonged hyperventilation causes a decrease in carbon dioxide, resulting in an increase in pH and a condition called **alkalosis.**

Whether oxygen or hemoglobin **associates** (combines) with or **disassociates** (releases) from hemoglobin depends upon the **partial pressure** of each gas. Partial pressure is defined as the pressure exerted by one gas in a mixture of gases. Oxygen associates with hemoglobin in the lungs, where the partial pressure of oxygen (PO_2) is increased, and disassociates from hemoglobin in the tissues, where the PO_2 is decreased. Carbon dioxide associates with hemoglobin in the tissues, where the partial pressure of carbon dioxide (PCO_2) is increased, and disassociates with hemoglobin in the lungs, where the PCO_2 is decreased.

RESPIRATORY SYSTEM DISORDERS

- *Apnea* (ap'ne-ah): a temporary cessation of breathing.
- *Asthma:* difficulty in breathing accompanied by wheezing caused by spasm or swelling of the bronchial tubes.
- *Bronchitis:* inflammation of the mucous membrane of the bronchial tubes.
- *Cystic fibrosis:* a genetic endocrine disease causing an excess production of mucus.
- *Dyspnea* (disp'ne-ah): difficult or labored breathing.
- *Emphysema:* chronic obstructive pulmonary disease (COPD).
- *Hypoxia* (hi-pok'se-ah): deficiency of oxygen.
- *Infant Respiratory Distress Syndrome (IRDS):* severe impairment of respiratory function in the newborn due to a lack of a substance called surfactant in the baby's lungs.
- *Pleurisy:* inflammation of the pleural membrane.
- *Pneumonia:* inflammation of the lungs.
- *Pulmonary edema:* accumulation of fluid in the lungs.
- *Tuberculosis (TB):* infectious disease affecting the respiratory system caused by the bacteria *Mycobacterium tuberculosis.*
- *Respiratory syncytial (sin-si'shal) virus:* a virus that is a major cause of respiratory distress in infants and children.
- *Rhinitis:* inflammation of the nasal mucous membranes.
- *Tonsillitis:* infection of the tonsils.
- *Upper respiratory infection (URI):* an infection of the nose, throat, larynx, or upper trachea such as caused by a cold virus.

DIAGNOSTIC TESTS

- Alkaline phosphatase (ALP)
- Arterial blood gases (ABG)
- Capillary blood gases (CBGs)
- Complete blood count (CBC)
- Drug levels

- Electrolytes (lytes)
- Microbiology cultures
- Pleuracentesis
- Skin tests: PPD (tuberculosis or TB test)

The Circulatory System

The circulatory system consists of the cardiovascular system (heart, blood, and blood vessels) along with the lymphatic system (lymph, lymph vessels, and nodes). The circulatory system is the means by which oxygen and food are carried to the cells of the body. It is also the means by which carbon dioxide and other wastes are carried away from the cells to the excretory organs: the kidneys, lungs, and skin. The circulatory system also aids in the coagulation process, assists in defending the body against disease, and plays an important role in the regulation of body temperature. The circulatory system is discussed in greater detail in Chapter 5.

Study & Review Questions

1. The transverse plane divides the body
   a. diagonally into upper and lower portions.
   b. horizontally into upper and lower portions.
   c. vertically into front and back portions.
   d. vertically into right and left portions.

2. Proximal is defined as
   a. away from the middle.
   b. farthest from the center.
   c. nearest to the point of attachment.
   d. closest to the middle.

3. The process by which the body maintains a state of equilibrium is
   a. anabolism.
   b. catabolism.
   c. homeostasis.
   d. venostasis.

4. Which of the following is *not* a function of the skeletal system?
   a. Protects internal organs
   b. Provides a framework for shape and support
   c. Produces red cells
   d. Transports oxygen to the cells

5. The type of muscle that lines the walls of blood vessels is called
   a. cardiac.
   b. skeletal.
   c. striated.
   d. visceral.

6. Which of the following is a test associated with the reproductive system?
   a. ABG
   b. BUN
   c. CK
   d. HCG

7. Which of the following is an accessory organ of the digestive system?
   a. Heart
   b. Lung
   c. Liver
   d. Ovary

8. Evaluation of the endocrine system involves
   a. blood gas studies.
   b. drug monitoring.
   c. spinal fluid analysis.
   d. hormone determinations.

9. The spinal cord and brain are covered by protective membranes called
   a. papillae.   c. neurons.
   b. meninges.   d. viscera.

10. The majority of gas exchange between blood and tissue takes place in the
    a. arterioles.   c. capillaries.
    b. pulmonary vein.   d. venules.

Suggested Laboratory Activities

1. Demonstrate anatomic position and identify body surfaces, planes, and directional terms on a fellow student.

2. Identify body cavities and organs using anatomic models.

3. Label diagrams of the various body systems.

4. Create a chart of diseases and diagnostic tests associated with each body system.

5. Watch a film such as *The Human Body: Systems Working Together* (Coronet Film and Video, Northbrook, IL).

BIBLIOGRAPHY AND SUGGESTED READINGS

Byrne, C. J., & Saxton, D. (1986). *Laboratory tests: Implications for nursing care*. San Francisco: Addison-Wesley.

Fischbach, F. (1996). *Laboratory diagnostic tests* (5th ed.). Philadelphia: Lippincott-Raven.

Marieb, E. (1989). *Human anatomy and physiology*. New York: Benjamin/Cummings.

Memmler, R. L., Cohen, B. J., & Wood, D. L. (1996). *The human body in health and disease* (8th ed.). Philadelphia: Lippincott-Raven.

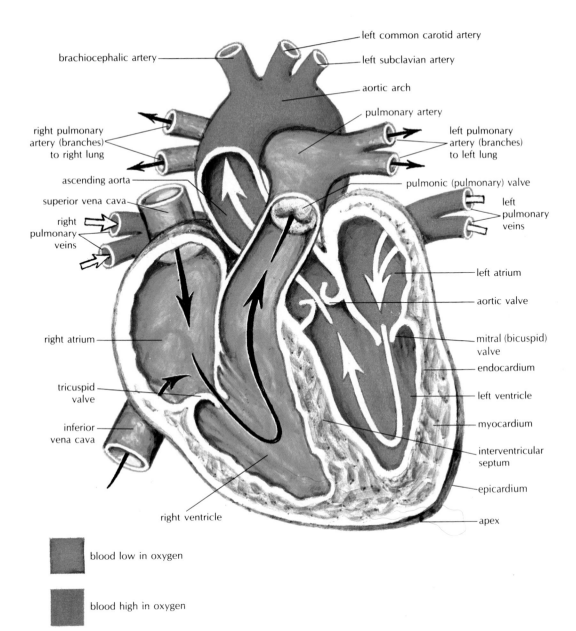

brachiocephalic artery

left common carotid artery

left subclavian artery

aortic arch

pulmonary artery

right pulmonary artery (branches) to right lung

left pulmonary artery (branches) to left lung

ascending aorta

pulmonic (pulmonary) valve

superior vena cava

left pulmonary veins

right pulmonary veins

left atrium

aortic valve

right atrium

mitral (bicuspid) valve

endocardium

tricuspid valve

left ventricle

inferior vena cava

myocardium

interventricular septum

epicardium

right ventricle

apex

blood low in oxygen

blood high in oxygen

Color Plate 1 Heart and great vessels.

HEMOGARD Closure	Conventional Stopper	Additive	Number of Inversions at Blood Collection (Invert gently, do not shake)	Laboratory Use
Gold		• Clot activator and gel for serum separation	5	SST Brand Tube for serum determinations in chemistry. Tube inversions ensure mixing of clot activator with blood and clotting within 30 minutes.
Light Green		• Lithium heparin and gel for plasma separation	8	PST Brand Tube for plasma determinations in chemistry. Tube inversions prevent clotting.
Red		• None	0	For serum determinations in chemistry, serology and blood banking.
Orange		• Thrombin	8	For stat serum determinations in chemistry. Tube inversions ensure complete clotting, usually in less than 5 minutes.
Royal Blue		• Sodium heparin • Na₂EDTA • None	8 8 0	For trace element, toxicology and nutrient determinations. Special stopper formulation offers the lowest verified levels of trace elements available (see package insert).
Green		• Sodium heparin • Lithium heparin • Ammonium heparin	8 8 8	For plasma determinations in chemistry. Tube inversions prevent clotting.

Color	Additive	Inversions	Use
Gray	• Potassium oxalate/ sodium fluoride • Sodium fluoride • Lithium iodoacetate • Lithium iodoacetate/ lithium heparin	8 8 8 8	For glucose determinations. Glycolytic inhibitors stabilize glucose values for up to 24 hours at room temperature with iodoacetate, and for at least 3 days with fluoride. Tube inversions ensure proper mixing of additive and blood. Oxalate and heparin, anticoagulants, will give plasma samples. Without them, samples are serum.
Brown	• Sodium heparin	8	For lead determinations. This tube is certified to contain less than .01 μg/mL (ppm) lead. Tube inversions prevent clotting.
Yellow	• Sodium polyanetholesulfonate (SPS)	8	For blood culture specimen collections in microbiology. Tube inversions prevent clotting.
Lavender	• Liquid K_3 EDTA • Freeze-dried Na_2 EDTA	8 8	For whole blood hematology determinations. Tube inversions prevent clotting.
Light Blue	• .105M sodium citrate (3.2%) • .129M sodium citrate (3.8%)	8 8	For coagulation determinations on plasma specimens. Tube inversions prevent clotting. NOTE: Certain tests require chilled specimens. Follow recommended procedures for collection and transport of specimen.

Color Plate 2 Common color-coded evacuated tube stoppers. (Courtesy Becton Dickinson, Franklin Lakes, NJ.)

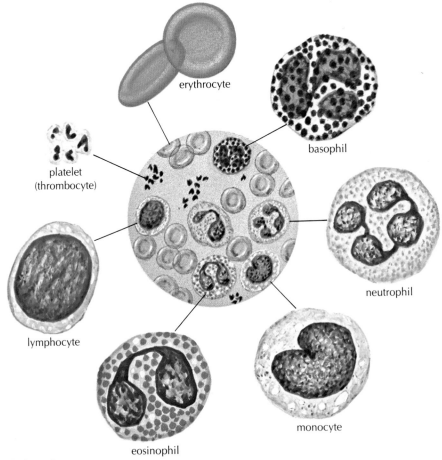

erythrocyte

basophil

platelet
(thrombocyte)

neutrophil

lymphocyte

monocyte

eosinophil

Color Plate 3 Formed elements of the blood.

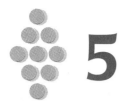

5

The Circulatory System

KEY TERMS

anticoagulant	crossmatch	median cubital vein
arrhythmia	diastole	pulmonary circulation
atria	electrocardiogram (ECG, EKG)	sphygmomanometer
basilic vein	extrinsic pathway	systemic circulation
blood pressure	fibrinolysis	systole
cardiac cycle	hemostasis	vasoconstriction
cephalic vein	intrinsic pathway	ventricles
coagulation		

OBJECTIVES

Upon successful completion of this chapter, the reader will be able to:

1. Identify the layers and structures of the heart.
2. Describe the cardiac cycle and how an ECG tracing relates to it; explain the origins of heart sounds and pulse rates.
3. Describe how to take blood pressure readings and what they represent.
4. Identify the two main divisions of the vascular system, describe the function of each, and trace the flow of blood throughout the system.
5. Identify the different types of blood vessels and describe the structure and function of each.
6. Name and locate the veins on which phlebotomy can be performed and describe the suitability of each.
7. List the major constituents of blood, differentiate between serum and plasma, and describe the function of each of the formed elements.
8. Describe how ABO and Rh blood types are determined, and the importance of compatibility testing prior to transfusion.
9. Define hemostasis and describe basic coagulation and fibrinolysis processes.
10. List the disorders and diagnostic tests of the circulatory system.
11. Identify the structures and vessels and describe the function of the lymphatic system.

THE HEART

The **heart** (Color Plate 1) is the major structure of the circulatory system. It is the "pump" that circulates blood throughout the body. It is located in the center of the thoracic cavity between the lungs with the apex (tip) pointing down and to the left of the body.

Heart Structure

The heart is a four-chambered, hollow, muscular organ, slightly larger than a man's closed fist. It has three layers and is surrounded by a thin, fluid-filled sac called the **pericardium** (per'i-kar'de-um). The heart has two sides, a right and a left, separated by a partition called the **septum**. Each side has two **chambers**, an upper and a lower. **Valves** between the chambers help prevent the back-flow of blood and keep it flowing through the heart in the right direction.

LAYERS OF THE HEART

The three layers of the heart are the epicardium, the myocardium, and the endocardium.

The **epicardium** (ep'-i-kar'de-um) is the thin outer layer of the heart, continuous with the lining of the pericardium. The **myocardium** (mi-o-kar'de-um) is the middle layer and is the thick, muscle layer of the heart. The **endocardium** (en"do-kar'de-um), the inner layer, is the thin membrane lining the heart. It is continuous with the lining of the blood vessels.

HEART CHAMBERS

The upper chambers on each side of the heart are called **atria** (a'tre-a), and the lower chambers are called **ventricles** (ven'trik-ls). The atria (singular is "atrium") are receiving chambers and the ventricles are pumping or delivering chambers.

The **right atrium** receives deoxygenated blood from the body via both the **superior (upper) vena cava** (ve'na ka'va) and **inferior (lower) vena cava** (plural is "vena cavae").

The **right ventricle** receives blood from the right atrium and pumps it to the lungs via the **pulmonary artery**.

The **left atrium** receives oxygenated blood from the lungs via the **pulmonary veins**.

The **left ventricle** receives blood from the left atrium and pumps it into the **aorta** (a-or'ta). The walls of the left ventricle are nearly three times as thick as the right ventricle owing to the force required to pump the blood into the arterial system.

VALVES

The valves at the entrance to the ventricles are called **atrioventricular** (a'tre-o-ven-trik'u-lar) **valves**. The valves that exit the ventricles are called **semilunar** (sem'e-lu'nar) **valves** because they are crescent-shaped, like the moon.

The right atrioventricular valve is called the **tricuspid** (tri-kus'pid) **valve** because it has three flaps or cusps. The left atrioventricular valve is called the **bicuspid** (bi-kus'pid) **valve** because it has two flaps. It is also called the **mitral** (mi'tral) **valve**.

Both of the atrioventricular valves are attached to the walls of the ventricles by thin threads of tissue called **chordae** (kor'de) **tendineae** (ten-din'e-e), which keep the valves from flipping back into the atria.

The right semilunar valve is called the **pulmonary** or **pulmonic semilunar valve** because blood passing through it goes into the pulmonary artery. The left semilunar valve is called the **aortic semilunar valve** because blood passing through it goes into the aorta.

CORONARY ARTERIES

The heart does not receive nourishment or oxygen from the blood passing through it. The heart receives its own blood supply via the right and left **coronary arteries** which are the first branches off of the aorta, just beyond the aortic semilunar valve. Obstruction of a coronary artery or one of its branches causes an insufficient supply of blood to meet oxygen needs of the heart muscle and results in a condition called **myocardial ischemia** (is-kee'me-ah). Complete obstruction or prolonged ischemia leads to **myocardial** (mi"o-kar'de-al) **infarction** (**MI**) or "heart attack" due to necrosis (ne-kro'sis) or death of the surrounding tissue from lack of oxygen.

Heart Function
CARDIAC CYCLE

One complete contraction and subsequent relaxation of the heart is called a **cardiac cycle.**

The contracting phase of the cardiac cycle is called **systole** (sis'to-le). It is followed by a relaxing phase called **diastole** (di-as'to-le).

ELECTRICAL CONDUCTION SYSTEM

Heart contraction is initiated by an electrical impulse generated from the **sinoatrial** (sin"o-a'tre-al) **node** or **SA node**, also called the **pacemaker**, located in the upper wall of the right atrium. The impulse causes both atria to contract simultaneously, pushing blood through the atrioventricular valves into the ventricles.

The impulse is then picked up by the **atrioventricular (AV) node** located in the lower right atrium. As the atria relax, the pulse is relayed through the **AV bundle (bundle of His)** and along the **Purkinje** (pur-kin'jee) **fibers** throughout the ventricular muscle. This causes the ventricles to contract, forcing blood through the semilunar valves. Both atria and ventricles relax briefly before the entire cycle starts again. Each cycle lasts approximately 0.8 seconds. (See Fig. 5-1 for diagram of the conduction system of the heart.)

ELECTROCARDIOGRAM

Because the electrical impulses are detectable on the surface of the body, the cardiac cycle can be recorded by means of an **electrocardiogram (ECG, EKG)**. The ECG is an actual record of the electrical currents that correspond to each event in the heart muscle contraction. These contractions can be recorded as waves when electrodes (leads or wires) are placed on the skin. This recording is called an ECG tracing (Fig. 5-2). The P wave of the tracing represents the activity of the atria and is usually the first wave seen. The QRS complex (a collection of three waves), along with the T wave, represents the activity of the ventricles. An ECG is useful in diagnosing heart muscle damage and abnormalities in heart rate. (See Chapter 11 for how to perform an ECG.)

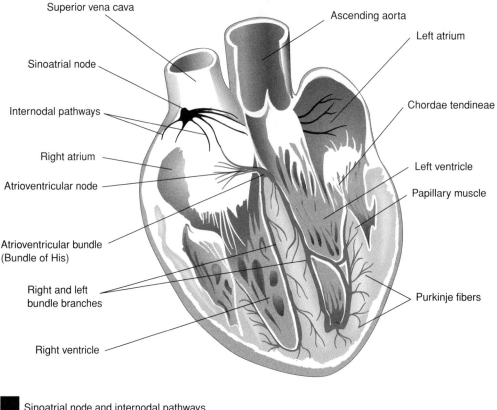

 Sinoatrial node and internodal pathways

Atrioventricular node and the bundle of His with its branches

Figure 5-1   Electrical conduction system of the heart.

ORIGIN OF THE HEART SOUNDS (HEART BEAT)

As the ventricles contract, the atrioventricular valves close, resulting in the first heart sound: a long, low-pitched sound commonly described as a "lubb." The second heart sound comes at the beginning of ventricular diastole and is due to the closing of the semilunar valves. It is shorter and sharper and described as a "dupp." Abnormal heart sounds, usually due to faulty valve action, are called **murmurs**.

HEART RATE AND CARDIAC OUTPUT

The number of heart beats per minute is called the **heart rate**. Normal adult heart rate is around 72 beats per minute. The volume of blood pumped by the heart in 1 minute is called the **cardiac output** and averages 5 liters per minute.

An irregularity in the heart rate, rhythm, or beat is called an **arrhythmia** (ah-rith'me-ah). A slow rate, less than 60 beats per minute, is called **bradycardia** (brad'e-kar'de-ah). A fast rate, over 100 beats per minute, is called **tachycardia** (tak'e-kar'de-ah). Extra beats before the normal beat are called **extrasystoles**. Rapid, uncoordinated contractions are called **fibrillations** and can result in lack of pumping action.

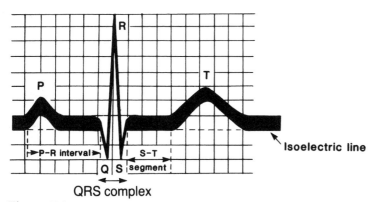

Figure 5-2   Normal ECG tracing showing one cardiac cycle (Jones SA, Weigel A, White RD, McSwain NE, Breiter M).

PULSE

The **pulse** is caused by a wave of increased pressure created as the ventricles contract and blood is forced out of the heart and through the arteries. In normal individuals, the **pulse rate** is the same as the heart rate. The pulse is most easily felt by compressing the radial artery on the thumb side of the wrist.

BLOOD PRESSURE

Blood pressure is a measure of the force (pressure) exerted by the blood on the walls of blood vessels. It is commonly measured in a large artery (such as the brachial artery in the upper arm). The pressure is measured using a **sphygmomanometer** (sfig'mo-mah-nom'e-ter), more commonly known as a "blood pressure cuff." Blood pressure results are expressed in millimeters of mercury (mm Hg) and are read from a manometer which is either a gauge or a mercury column, depending upon the type of blood pressure cuff used. Two components of the blood pressure are measured: the systolic (sis-tol'ik) and the diastolic (di-as-tol'ik).

Systolic pressure is the pressure in the arteries during contraction of the ventricles. It is the top number of a blood pressure reading and averages 120 mm Hg for adults.

Diastolic pressure is the pressure during relaxation of the ventricles. It is the lower reading and averages 80 mm Hg.

Taking a blood pressure reading involves placing a blood pressure cuff around the upper arm and a stethoscope over the brachial artery. The cuff is inflated until the brachial artery is compressed and the blood flow is cut off. Then the cuff is slowly deflated until the first heart sounds are heard with the stethoscope. The pressure reading at this time is equal to the systolic pressure. The cuff is then slowly deflated until a muffled sound is heard. The pressure at this time is equal to the diastolic pressure.

A blood pressure reading is expressed as the systolic pressure over the diastolic pressure. For example, normal blood pressure is verbally expressed as 120 over 80, and is written 120/80.

Heart Disorders

- *Angina pectoris* (an'-ji'na pek'to-ris): also called **ischemic heart disease (IHD)**; pain on exertion caused by decreased blood flow to the myocardium from the coronary artery.
- *Aortic stenosis* (a-or'tik ste-no'sis): narrowing of the aorta or its opening.
- *Bacterial endocarditis* (en'do-kar-di'tis): an infection of the lining of the heart, most commonly caused by streptococci.
- *Congestive heart failure (CHF):* impaired circulation caused by inadequate pumping of a diseased heart, resulting in fluid buildup (edema) in the lungs or other tissues.
- *Myocardial infarction (MI):* heart attack or death of heart muscle due to obstruction (occlusion) of a coronary artery.
- *Pericarditis* (per-i-kar-di'tis): inflammation of the pericardium.

Diagnostic Tests

- ABGs
- AST (SGOT)
- Cholesterol
- CK (CPK)
- CK isoenzymes
- ECG (EKG)
- Potassium (K)
- Triglycerides

THE VASCULAR SYSTEM

Functions

The vascular system is a closed system by which blood is circulated to all parts of the body. There are two divisions to this system, the pulmonary circulation and the systemic circulation.

THE PULMONARY CIRCULATION

The **pulmonary circulation** carries blood from the heart to the lungs to remove carbon dioxide and pick up oxygen. It then returns the oxygenated blood to the heart to be pumped throughout the body.

THE SYSTEMIC CIRCULATION

The **systemic circulation** carries oxygenated blood from the heart, along with nutrients from the digestive system, to all the cells of the body. The systemic circulation is also responsible for carrying carbon dioxide and other waste products of metabolism away from the cells for disposal.

Blood Vessels

Blood vessels are tube-like structures capable of expanding and contracting. Along with the heart, they form the closed system for the flow of blood.

TYPES OF BLOOD VESSELS
Arteries

Arteries (Fig. 5-3) carry blood away from the heart. They have thick walls because the blood is under pressure from the contraction of the ventricles. This pressure creates a pulse that can be felt and is one way arteries are distinguished from veins. When arterial blood is collected by syringe, this pressure usually causes the blood to "pump" or pulse into the syringe under its own power.

Except for the pulmonary artery, which is part of the pulmonary circulation and carries deoxygenated blood to the lungs, arteries carry blood that is oxygenated (full of oxygen). Because it is full of oxygen, normal systemic arterial blood is bright, cherry red in color.

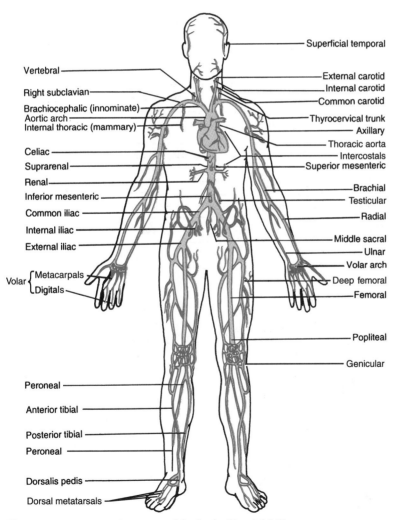

Figure 5-3   Principal arteries of the body (Rosdahl C).

The smallest branches of arteries are called **arterioles** (ar-te're-olz). The largest artery in the body is the aorta. It is approximately 1 inch (2.5 cm) in diameter.

Veins

Veins (Fig. 5-4) return blood to the heart. Veins carry blood that is low in oxygen (deoxygenated), except for the pulmonary vein which carries oxygenated blood from the lungs back to the heart. Because systemic venous blood is oxygen poor, it is much darker and more bluish-red in color than normal arterial blood. The walls of veins are thinner than arteries because the blood is under less pressure than arterial blood. Since the walls are thinner, veins can collapse more easily than arteries. Blood is kept moving through veins primarily due to skeletal muscle movement. In addition, most veins have

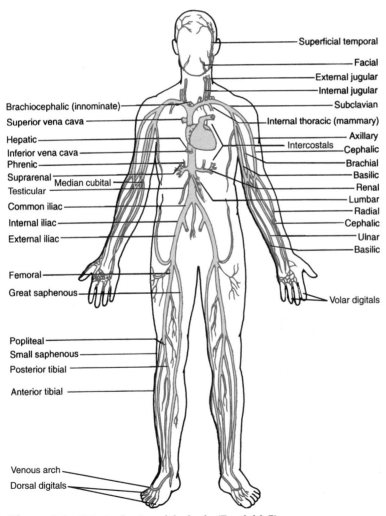

Figure 5-4   Principal veins of the body (Rosdahl C).

valves to prevent the backflow of blood and keep it moving along despite the fact that most of the venous system is flowing against the pull of gravity.

The smallest veins at the junction of the capillaries are called **venules** (ven'ulz). The largest vein in the body is the vena cava. The longest vein in the body is the **great saphenous** (sa-fe'nus) vein in the leg.

Capillaries

Capillaries are microscopic, one-cell thick vessels which connect the arterioles and venules. Blood in the capillaries is a mixture of both venous and arterial blood. In the systemic circulation, arterial blood delivers oxygen and nutrients to the capillaries. The thin capillary walls allow the exchange of oxygen for carbon dioxide and of nutrients for wastes to take place between the cells and the blood. Carbon dioxide and wastes are carried away in the venous blood. In the pulmonary circulation, carbon dioxide is delivered to the capillaries in the lungs and exchanged for oxygen.

BLOOD VESSEL STRUCTURE

Capillaries are composed of a single layer of endothelial cells enclosed in a basement membrane. Arteries and veins are composed of three layers. The thickness of the layers varies with the size and type of blood vessel. (See Fig. 5-5 for comparison diagram of arteries, veins, and capillaries.)

Blood vessel layers

- **Tunica** (tu'ni-ka) **adventitia** (ad'ven-tish'e-a): the outer layer of a blood vessel, sometimes called the tunica externa. It is made up of connective tissue and is thicker in arteries than veins.

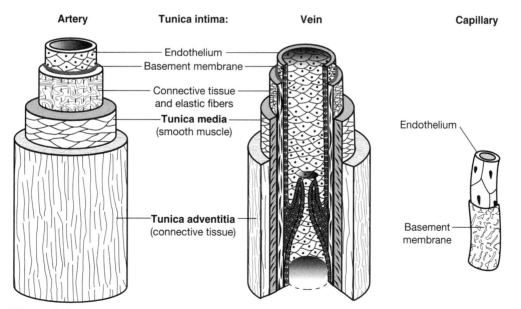

Figure 5-5   Artery, vein, and capillary structure.

- **Tunica media:** the middle layer of a blood vessel. It is made up of smooth muscle tissue and some elastic fibers. It is much thicker in arteries than in veins.
- **Tunica intima** (in'ti-ma): the inner layer or lining of a blood vessel, sometimes called the tunica interna. It is made up of a single layer of endothelial cells with an underlining basement membrane, a connective tissue layer, and an elastic internal membrane.

Lumen

The internal space of a blood vessel through which the blood flows is called the **lumen** (lu'men).

Valves

The presence of valves within veins is a major structural difference between arteries and veins. Venous blood is often flowing against gravity. As blood moves through veins, the valves, which are similar to the semilunar valves of the heart, open and close momentarily, helping to keep the blood flowing toward the heart.

The Flow of Blood

1. Oxygen-poor blood is returned to the heart via the superior and inferior (upper and lower) vena cavae and enters the right atrium of the heart.
2. Contraction of the right atrium forces the blood through the tricuspid valve into the right ventricle.
3. Contraction of the right ventricle forces the blood through the pulmonary semilunar valve into the pulmonary artery.
4. Blood flows through the pulmonary artery to the capillaries of the lungs where carbon dioxide is released from the red blood cells and exchanged for oxygen through the walls of the alveoli.

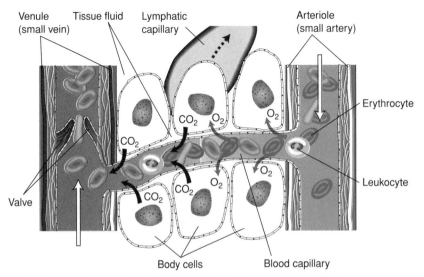

Figure 5-6 Oxygen and carbon dioxide exchange at the capillaries.

5. Oxygen-rich blood flows back to the heart by way of the pulmonary veins and enters the left atrium.
6. Contraction of the left atrium forces the blood through the bicuspid valve into the left ventricle.
7. Contraction of the left ventricle forces the blood through the aortic semilunar valve into the aorta.
8. The blood travels throughout the body by way of the arteries, which branch into smaller and smaller arteries, the smallest of which are the arterioles.
9. The arterioles connect with the capillaries where oxygen, water, and nutrients from the blood diffuse through the capillary walls to the cells. At the same time, carbon dioxide and other end products of metabolism enter the blood stream (Fig. 5-6).
10. The capillaries connect with the smallest branches of veins (venules).
11. The venules merge into larger and larger veins until the blood returns to the heart again by way of the superior or inferior vena cava and the cycle starts again (Fig. 5-7 and Color Plate 1).

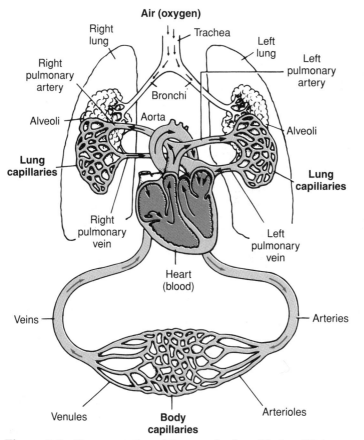

Figure 5-7   Representation of the vascular flow (National Tuberculosis and Respiratory Disease Association, New York, NY).

Vascular and Related Anatomy of the Arm and Leg
ANTECUBITAL FOSSA

The major veins for venipuncture are located in what is referred to as the **ante-cubital** (an'te-ku'bi-tal) **fossa.** This is the area of the arm that is anterior to (in front of) and below the bend of the elbow. Several major arm veins lie close to the surface in this area, making them easier to locate and penetrate with a needle. These major superficial veins are referred to as **antecubital veins** (Fig. 5-8*A*).

ANTECUBITAL VEINS SUBJECT TO VENIPUNCTURE

- **Median cubital vein:** the first-choice vein for venipuncture; it is usually large and well anchored, making it the easiest and least painful to puncture and also the least likely to bruise.
- **Cephalic vein:** the second-choice vein for venipuncture; it is often harder to palpate than the median cubital, but is fairly well anchored. It is often the only vein that can be palpated (felt) in obese patients.

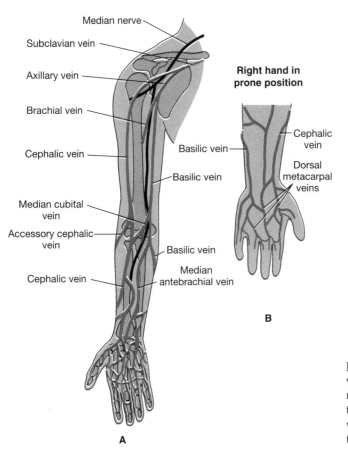

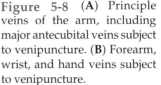

Figure 5-8 (A) Principle veins of the arm, including major antecubital veins subject to venipuncture. **(B)** Forearm, wrist, and hand veins subject to venipuncture.

- **Basilic vein:** The basilic vein is the third-choice vein for venipuncture. The basilic is generally easy to palpate, but it is not as well anchored and rolls and bruises more easily. Venipuncture of this vein tends to be more painful to the patient. There is also the possibility of accidental puncture of the median nerve, located in this area, or the brachial artery, which lies close to the skin surface in this area.

OTHER ARM AND HAND VEINS
SUBJECT TO VENIPUNCTURE

When antecubital veins are unsuitable or unavailable, other veins subject to venipuncture include veins of the forearm, the wrist, and the back of the hand (see Fig. 5-8*B*).

LEG, ANKLE, AND FOOT VEINS
SUBJECT TO VENIPUNCTURE

Leg, ankle, and foot veins (Fig. 5-9) should only be used for venipuncture when no other sites are available and with permission of the patient's physician. Puncture of the femoral vein is performed only by physicians or specially trained personnel.

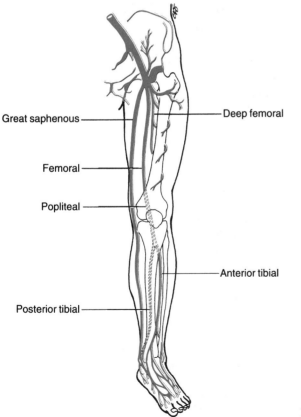

Figure 5-9   Major leg and foot veins.

ARTERIES SUBJECT TO PUNCTURE

Arterial puncture requires special training to perform, is more painful and hazardous to the patient, and is generally limited to the collection of arterial blood gas (ABG) specimens for evaluating respiratory function. Arteries of the arm subject to puncture are the **radial** and the **brachial arteries**. Puncture of the **femoral artery** of the leg may be performed during emergency situations or when no other arterial site is available. Puncture of the femoral artery is performed only by physicians and specially trained emergency room personnel. Arterial puncture is explained further in Chapter 13.

MEDIAN CUTANEOUS NERVE

Cutaneous nerves convey impulses for stimuli to the skin. The median cutaneous nerve is a major arm nerve that lies along the path of the brachial artery and in the vicinity of the basilic vein. Lawsuits have been filed over damage to major nerves as a result of venipuncture procedures.

Vascular System Disorders

- *Aneurysm* (an'u-rizm): a localized dilation or bulging in the wall of a blood vessel, usually an artery.
- *Arteriosclerosis* (ar-te're-o-skle-ro'sis): thickening, hardening, and loss of elasticity of artery walls.
- *Atherosclerosis* (ath'er-o'skle-ro'sis): a form of arteriosclerosis involving changes in the intima of the artery due to an accumulation of lipids and so on.
- *Embolism:* obstruction of a blood vessel by an embolus.
- *Embolus* (em'bo-lus): a blood clot, part of a blood clot, or other mass of undissolved matter circulating in the blood stream.
- *Hemorrhoids:* varicose veins in the rectal area.
- *Phlebitis* (fle-bi'tis): inflammation of a vein.
- *Thrombophlebitis* (throm'bo-fle-bi'tis): inflammation of a vein along with thrombus (blood clot) formation.
- *Thrombus:* a blood clot in a blood vessel.
- *Varicose veins* (varices): swollen, knotted superficial veins.

Diagnostic Tests

- Disseminated intravascular coagulation (DIC) screen
- lipoproteins
- Prothrombin Time (PT)
- Partial Thromboplastin Time (PTT/APTT)
- Triglycerides

THE BLOOD

Blood has been referred to as "the river of life." It flows throughout the circulatory system delivering nutrients, oxygen, and other substances to the cells and transporting waste products away from the cells for elimination.

Blood Composition

Blood is a mixture of fluid and cells that is about five times thicker than water, salty to the taste, and with a slightly alkaline pH of about 7.4 (pH is the degree of acidity or alkalinity on a scale of 1 to 14, with 7 being neutral). *In vivo* (in the living body) the fluid portion of the blood is called plasma and the cellular portion is referred to as the **formed elements** (Color Plate 3). The average adult weighing 70 kg (approximately 154 pounds) has a blood volume of about 5 liters (5.3 quarts), of which approximately 55% is plasma and 45% is formed elements.

PLASMA

Normal plasma is a clear, pale yellow fluid that is nearly 90% water (H_2O) and 10% solutes (dissolved substances). Composition of the solutes includes the following:

- Proteins, such as **albumin**, which is manufactured by the liver and functions to help regulate osmotic pressure or the tendency of blood to attract water; **antibodies**, which combat infection; and **fibrinogen**, which is also manufactured by the liver and functions in the clotting process.
- Nutrients, which supply energy. Plasma nutrients include **carbohydrates**, such as **glucose**, and **lipids (fats)** such as **triglycerides** and **cholesterol**.
- Minerals such as **sodium (Na)**, **potassium (K)**, **calcium (Ca)**, and **magnesium (Mg)**. Sodium helps maintain fluid balance, pH, and calcium and potassium balance necessary for normal heart action. Potassium is essential for normal muscle activity and the conduction of nerve impulses. Calcium is needed for proper bone and teeth formation, nerve conduction, and muscle contraction. In addition, calcium is essential to the clotting process.
- Gases, such as oxygen (O_2), carbon dioxide (CO_2), and nitrogen (N).
- Other substances, including vitamins, hormones, and waste products of metabolism such as urea (BUN), creatinine, and uric acid.

FORMED ELEMENTS
Erythrocytes

Erythrocytes (e-rith'ro-sites), better known as red blood cells (RBCs), are the most numerous cells in the blood, averaging 4.5 to 5 million per cubic millimeter of blood. Their main function is to carry oxygen from the lungs to the cells. They also carry carbon dioxide from the cells back to the lungs to be exhaled. RBCs are produced in the bone marrow. They are formed with a nucleus, which they lose as they mature and enter the blood stream. Immature RBCs in the blood stream that contain nuclear remnants are called **reticulocytes** (re-tik'u-lo-sits) or **retics**. Mature RBCs have a life span of approximately 120 days, after which they begin to disintegrate and are removed from the blood stream by the spleen and liver. The main component of RBCs is **hemoglobin (Hgb or Hb)**, which enables them to transport oxygen and carbon dioxide and also gives them their red color. RBCs are described as anuclear (no nucleus), biconcave (indented from both sides) disks approximately 7 to 8 microns in diameter. RBCs have **intravascular** function, which means that they do their job within the blood vessels. An old term for RBCs is red corpuscles.

Leukocytes

Leukocytes, or white blood cells (WBCs), are cells containing a nucleus. The average adult has from 5,000 to 10,000 WBCs per cubic millimeter of blood. WBCs are formed in the bone marrow and lymphatic tissue. They are said to have **extravascular** function because they are able to leave the blood stream and do their job in the tissues. The process by which WBCs are able to pass through the walls of the capillaries to enter the tissues is called **diapedesis** (di'a-ped-e'sis). WBCs may appear in the blood stream for only 6 to 8 hours but reside in the tissues for days, months, or even years. The life span of WBCs varies with the type.

The main function of WBCs is to destroy pathogens. They accomplish this by a method called **phagocytosis** (fag'o-si-to'sis), in which the pathogen is surrounded and engulfed by the WBC. Some WBCs produce antibodies that destroy pathogens indirectly or release substances that attack foreign matter. An old term for WBCs is white corpuscles.

There are different types of WBCs, each identified by their size, shape of the nucleus, and whether or not there are granules present in the cytoplasm when the cells are stained with a special blood stain called **Wright's** stain. WBCs containing easily visible granules are called **granulocytes** (gran'u-lo-sites"). WBCs lacking easily visible granules are called **agranulocytes.**

Granulocytes. Granulocytes can be differentiated by the color of their granules when stained with Wright's stain. There are three types of granulocytes: neutrophils, eosinophils, and basophils.

- **Neutrophils** (nu'tro-fils): Neutrophils are normally the most numerous of the WBCs, averaging 65% of the WBC total. The granules of neutrophils are fine in texture and stain lavender. Because a typical neutrophil is **polymorphonuclear (PMN)**, meaning its nucleus has several lobes or segments, neutrophils are sometimes referred to as **PMNs, polys**, or **segs**. Neutrophils are one of the main phagocytic cells. The presence of increased numbers of neutrophils is associated with bacterial infections. The life span of a neutrophil is from about 6 hours to a few days.
- **Eosinophils** (e'o-sin'o-fils): The granules of eosinophils **(Eos)** are bead-like and stain bright orange-red. The nucleus of an eosinophil has two lobes. Up to 3% of the WBCs of a normal adult are Eos. Eos ingest and detoxify foreign protein and help turn off immune reactions. Eos increase with allergies and parasitic infestations such as pinworms. The life span of an eosinophil is from 8 to 12 days.
- **Basophils** (ba'so-fils): Basophils **(basos)** are the least numerous of the WBCs, comprising less than 1% of the WBC population. The granules of basophils are large, stain dark blue, and often obscure the nucleus. Nuclei of basos are often in the shape of an "S." Basos release histamine and heparin, which enhance the inflammatory response. Basos are thought to live several days.

Agranulocytes. There are two types of agranulocytes: monocytes and lymphocytes.

- **Monocytes:** Monocytes **(monos)** are the largest of the WBCs. They comprise from 1% to 7% of the WBC population. Monos have fine, gray-blue cytoplasm and a large, dark-staining nucleus. Monos destroy pathogens by phagocytosis. They are sometimes referred to as macrophages after they leave the blood stream. The life span of a mono is several months.

- **Lymphocytes:** Lymphocytes are the second most numerous of the WBCs. They comprise approximately 15% to 30% of the WBC population. A typical lymphocyte has a large, round, dark purple nucleus that occupies the majority of the cell. The nucleus is surrounded by a thin rim of pale blue cytoplasm. The majority of lymphocytes stay in the lymph tissue, where they play an important role in immunity. Two main types of lymphocytes are **T-lymphocytes**, which directly attack infected cells, and **B-lymphocytes,** which give rise to plasma cells that produce immunoglobulins (antibodies) that are released into the blood stream, where they circulate and attack foreign cells. The life span of lymphocytes varies from only a few hours to a number of years.

Thrombocytes

Thrombocytes (throm'bo-sits), better known as **platelets**, are the smallest of the formed elements. Platelets are actually parts of a large cell called a **megakaryocyte** (meg'a-kar'e-o-sit'), which is formed in the bone marrow. The number of platelets in the blood (platelet count) of the average adult is from 150,000 to 400,000 per cubic millimeter. Platelets are essential to **coagulation** (the blood clotting process) and are the first cell on the scene when an injury occurs (see Hemostasis). The life span of a platelet is around 10 days.

Blood Type

An individual's blood type (also called blood group) is inherited and is determined by the type of antigen present on his or her red blood cells. Some blood type antigens cause formation of antibodies to the opposite blood type. If a person receives a blood transfusion of the wrong type, the person's antibodies may react with the donor RBCs and cause them to **agglutinate** (a-gloo'ti-nat) (clump together) and **lyse** (liz) (be destroyed). Such a reaction, which can be fatal, is called a **transfusion reaction**. A person will not normally produce antibodies against his or her own RBC antigens. The most commonly used method of blood typing recognizes two blood group systems: the ABO system and the Rh factor system.

ABO BLOOD GROUP SYSTEM

The **ABO blood group system** recognizes four blood types, A, B, AB, and O, based on the presence or absence of two antigens identified as A and B. An individual who is type A has the A antigen; type B has the B antigen; type AB has both antigens; and type O has neither A nor B. Type O is the most common type and type AB is the least common.

Unique to the ABO system are preformed antibodies (also called agglutinins) present in a person's blood that are directed against the opposite blood type. Type A blood will have an antibody (agglutinin) directed against type B called anti-B. A person with type B has anti-A; type O has both anti-A and anti-B; and type AB has neither. Table 5-1 shows the antigens and antibodies present in the four ABO group blood types.

Table 5-1
ABO Blood Group System

Blood Type	RBC Antigen	Plasma Antibodies (agglutinins)
A	A	Anti-B
B	B	Anti-A
AB	A and B	Neither anti-A nor anti-B
O	Neither	Anti-A and anti-B

Individuals with type AB blood were once referred to as **universal recipients** because they have neither A nor B antibody to the RBC antigens and can theoretically receive any ABO type blood. In the same manner, type O individuals were once called **universal donors** because they have neither A nor B antigen on their RBCs and in an emergency their type can theoretically be given to anyone. However, type O blood *does* contain plasma antibodies to both A and B antigens, and when given to an A or B type recipient, it can cause a mild transfusion reaction. To avoid reactions, patients are now given type-specific blood, even in emergencies.

RH BLOOD GROUP SYSTEM

The **Rh blood group system** is based upon the presence or absence of an RBC antigen called the D antigen, also known as Rh factor. An individual whose RBCs have the D antigen is said to be positive for the Rh factor, or **Rh positive (Rh+)**. An individual whose RBCs lack the D antigen is said to be **Rh negative (Rh−)**. It is important that a patient receive the correct Rh type blood as well as the correct ABO type. Approximately 85% of the population is Rh positive.

Unlike the ABO system, antibodies to the Rh factor (anti-Rh antibodies) are not preformed in the blood of Rh negative individuals. However, an Rh negative individual who receives Rh positive blood can become **sensitized**. This means that the individual may produce antibodies against the Rh factor. In addition, an Rh negative woman who is carrying an Rh positive fetus may become sensitized by the RBCs of the fetus, most commonly by leakage of the fetal cells into the mother's circulation during childbirth. This may lead to the destruction of the RBCs of a subsequent Rh positive fetus because Rh antibodies produced by the mother can cross the placenta into the fetal circulation. When this occurs, it is called **hemolytic disease of the newborn (HDN)**. A previously unsensitized Rh negative mother can be given **Rh immune globulin (RhIg)**, such as RhoGam, at certain times during her pregnancy as well as immediately after the baby's birth. RhIg will destroy any Rh positive fetal cells that may have entered her blood stream and prevent sensitization.

COMPATIBILITY TESTING/CROSSMATCH

Other factors in an individual's blood can cause adverse reactions during a blood transfusion, even with the correct ABO and Rh type blood. For this reason, a compatibility test or **crossmatch** is performed using the patient's serum and cells as well as the donor's serum and cells before a unit of blood is determined **compatible** for transfusion. Recently invented artificial blood, made by chemically altering donor blood, is being tested on humans. This blood is designed to be given to any blood type and poses no risk of transmitting disease.

Types of Blood Specimens

SERUM

Blood that has been removed from the body will coagulate or clot within 30 to 60 minutes. The clot consists of the blood cells enmeshed in a fibrin network (see Hemostasis). The remaining fluid portion is called **serum** and can be separated from the clot by centrifugation (spinning the clotted blood at high rpms in a machine called a centrifuge). Normal fasting serum is a clear, pale yellow fluid. Serum has the same composition as plasma *except* it *does not contain fibrinogen*, because the fibrinogen was used in the formation of the clot. Many laboratory tests, especially chemistry and immunology tests, are performed on serum.

PLASMA

Most coagulation tests cannot be performed on serum because the coagulation factors, particularly fibrinogen, have been used up in the process of clot formation. In addition, some chemistry test results are needed immediately (STAT) to respond to emergency situations; having to wait a minimum of 30 minutes for a specimen to clot would be unacceptable. If the blood is prevented from clotting, the coagulation factors are preserved and the specimen can be centrifuged immediately. Blood can be prevented from clotting by adding a substance called an **anticoagulant**. Most anticoagulants work by either binding calcium, which is critical to the coagulation process, or inhibiting the clotting component thrombin (see Anticoagulants, Chap. 7). When a blood specimen containing an anticoagulant is centrifuged, it will separate into three distinct layers (Fig. 5-10): a bottom layer of red blood cells; a thin, fluffy-looking, white-colored middle layer of WBCs and platelets referred to as the **buffy coat**; and a top layer of clear liquid called **plasma** that can be separated from the cells and used for testing. Normal fasting plasma is a clear, pale yellow fluid visually indistinguishable from serum. The major difference between plasma and serum is that *plasma contains fibrinogen.* Many laboratory tests can now be performed on either serum or plasma.

WHOLE BLOOD

Some tests, including most hematology tests and some chemistry tests such as ammonia and glycohemoglobin, cannot be performed on clotted blood. These tests need to be performed on **whole blood** or blood that is in the same form as when it circulated in the blood stream. This means the blood specimen must *not* be allowed to clot or separate. In order to obtain a whole blood specimen, it is necessary to add an anticoagulant. In addition, because the components will separate if the specimen is allowed to stand undisturbed, the specimen must be mixed for a minimum of 2 minutes prior to performing the test.

Blood Disorders

- *Anemia:* an abnormal reduction in the number of RBCs in the circulating blood.
- *Leukemia:* an increase in WBCs characterized by the presence of a large number of abnormal forms.

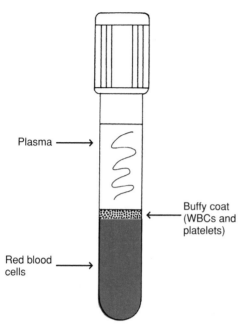

Figure 5-10   Centrifuged plasma specimen.

- *Leukocytosis:* an abnormal increase in WBCs in the circulating blood.
- *Leukopenia:* an abnormal decrease in WBCs.
- *Polycythemia:* an abnormal increase in RBCs.
- *Thrombocytosis:* increased platelets.
- *Thrombocytopenia:* decreased platelets.

Diagnostic Tests
- ABO and Rh type
- Bone marrow
- Complete blood count (CBC)
- Crossmatch
- Differential (diff.)
- Eosinophil (Eos) count
- Erythrocyte sedimentation rate (ESR)
- Ferritin
- Hematocrit (Hct)
- Hemoglobin (Hb or Hgb)
- Hemogram
- Indices (MCH, MCV, MCHC)
- Iron (Fe)
- Reticulocyte (retic) count
- Total iron binding capacity (TIBC)

HEMOSTASIS

Hemostasis (he'mo-sta'sis) is the process by which the body stops the leakage of blood from the vascular system after injury. It includes the process that leads to clot formation as well as clot dissolution. If an injury occurs to a blood vessel, the hemostatic process is set in motion to repair the injury. The process, also called the **coagulation** process, proceeds in four stages. Stages 1 and 2 are referred to as **primary hemostasis**, and stages 3 and 4 are referred to as **secondary hemostasis**.

Primary Hemostasis

- Stage 1: **Vasoconstriction.** The damaged vessel constricts (narrows) to decrease the flow of blood to the injured area.
- Stage 2: **Platelet plug formation.** Injury to the blood vessel exposes protein material in the basement membrane. Contact with this material causes the platelets to degranulate and stick to one another **(platelet aggregation)** and adhere to the injured area **(platelet adhesion)**, forming a "platelet plug." Normal platelet plug formation depends on an adequate concentration of platelets in the blood (determined by a platelet count), normal functioning of platelets, and blood vessel integrity. A bleeding time test assesses platelet plug formation.

For some injuries, such as a needle puncture of a vein, platelet plug formation is sufficient to seal the site and the hemostatic process goes no further. For larger injuries, the process continues to what is called **secondary hemostasis** involving formation of a tougher "fibrin" clot formed of RBCs, platelets, and fibrin.

Secondary Hemostasis

- Stage 3: **Fibrin clot formation.** Fibrin clot formation involves the complex interaction of a series of coagulation **factors** (also called procoagulants) designated by Roman numerals in the order of discovery. Once activated, each factor activates the next factor in sequence, somewhat like a cascade. This **coagulation cascade** (Fig. 5-11) can be initiated by two separate pathways, the intrinsic and the extrinsic, both of which eventually join to form a common pathway that ends in the formation of a fibrin clot. Both pathways require the presence of calcium and phospholipid from the platelets.
  - **Intrinsic pathway.** The intrinsic pathway involves coagulation factors circulating within the blood stream and is initiated with activation of factor XII. Functioning of the intrinsic pathway is measured by the **activated partial thromboplastin test (APTT or PTT)**, which is also useful in monitoring heparin therapy.
  - **Extrinsic pathway.** The extrinsic pathway is initiated by the release of thromboplastin (factor III) from injured tissue and the activation of factor VII. The prothrombin test (PT) measures the functioning of the extrinsic pathway and is used to monitor coumarin therapy.
  - **Common pathway.** Both pathways lead to the activation of factor X and the initiation of the factors of the common pathway. Ultimately, prothrombin (factor II) is converted into thrombin. Thrombin then splits fibrinogen (factor I) into the fibrin

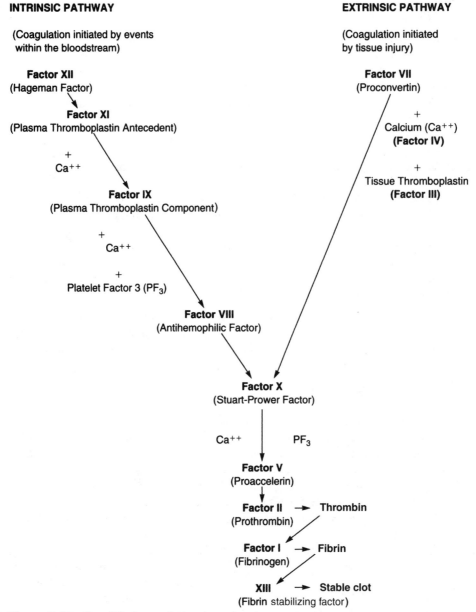

Figure 5-11   Simplified coagulation cascade.

necessary to form the fibrin clot, also known as the **hemostatic plug**. The fibrin clot is stabilized by factor XIII.

- Stage 4: **Fibrinolysis** (fi'brin-ol'i-sis). Fibrinolysis involves the ultimate removal or dissolution of the fibrin clot once healing has occurred. This process is possible because activation of the clotting process also releases substances that lead to the conversion of plasminogen to plasmin. Plasmin is an enzyme that breaks the fibrin into small fragments called **fibrin degradation products,** which are removed by reticuloendothelial cells (phagocytic cells).

The coagulation process is kept in check and limited to local sites by the action of natural inhibitors circulating in the plasma along with the coagulation factors. The inhibitors bind with coagulation factors that escape the clotting site and those remaining after clotting is complete.

The Role of the Liver in Hemostasis

The liver plays an important role in the hemostatic process. It is responsible for the synthesis (manufacture) of most of the coagulation factors, including fibrinogen, prothrombin, and heparin. In addition, it produces the bile salts necessary for the absorption of vitamin K, which is also necessary to the synthesis of the coagulation factors. When the liver is diseased, synthesis of coagulation factors is impaired and bleeding may result.

Hemostatic Disorders*

- *Disseminated intravascular coagulation (DIC):* a pathological form of diffuse coagulation in which coagulation factors are consumed to such an extent that bleeding occurs.
- *Hemophilia* (he'mo-fil'e-a): a hereditary condition characterized by bleeding due to increased coagulation time. The most common type of hemophilia is due to factor VIII deficiency.
- *Thrombocytopenia* (throm'bo-si'to-pe'ne-a): an abnormal decrease in platelets.

Diagnostic Tests

- Activated clotting time (ACT)
- Bleeding time (BT)
- Prothrombin time (PT)
- Partial thromboplastin time (PTT or APTT)
- Fibrin degradation products (FDP)
- D-dimer

THE LYMPHATIC SYSTEM

Functions

The lymphatic system returns tissue fluid to the blood stream, protects the body by removing microorganisms and impurities, processes lymphocytes, and delivers fats absorbed from the small intestine to the blood stream. Lymph vessels spread throughout the entire body much like blood vessels.

*See also Vascular Disorders.

Structures

The lymphatic system (Fig. 5-12) is made up of fluid called **lymph** and the **lymphatic vessels**, **ducts**, and **nodes** (masses of lymph tissue) through which the lymph flows.

Body cells are bathed in tissue fluid acquired from the blood stream. Water, oxygen, and nutrients continually diffuse through the capillary walls into the tissue spaces. Much of the fluid diffuses back into the capillaries along with waste products of metabolism. Excess tissue fluid filters into **lymphatic capillaries**, where it is called **lymph**. Lymph fluid is similar to plasma, but is 95% water.

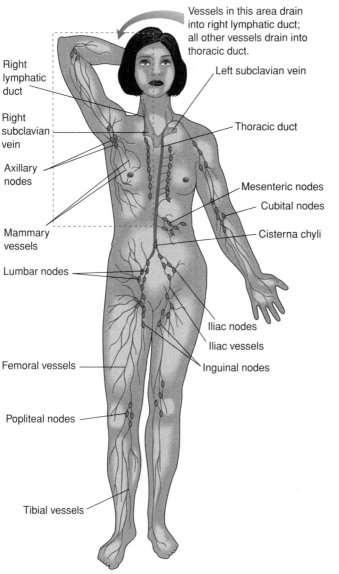

Vessels in this area drain into right lymphatic duct; all other vessels drain into thoracic duct.

Right lymphatic duct

Right subclavian vein

Axillary nodes

Mammary vessels

Lumbar nodes

Femoral vessels

Popliteal nodes

Tibial vessels

Left subclavian vein

Thoracic duct

Mesenteric nodes

Cubital nodes

Cisterna chyli

Iliac nodes

Iliac vessels

Inguinal nodes

Figure 5-12 Lymphatic system.

Lymphatic capillaries join with larger and larger lymphatic vessels until they empty into one of two terminal vessels, either the **right lymphatic duct** or the **thoracic duct**. These ducts then empty into large veins in the upper body. Lymph moves through the vessels primarily owing to skeletal muscle contraction, much like blood moves through the veins. Like veins, lymphatic vessels also have valves to keep the lymph flowing in the right direction.

Before reaching the ducts, the lymph passes through a series of structures called **lymph nodes**, which trap and destroy bacteria and foreign matter. The nodes also function in the production of lymphocytes. Lymph nodes are made of a special kind of tissue called **lymphoid tissue**. Lymphoid tissue has the ability to remove impurities and process lymphocytes. The tonsils, thymus, gastrointestinal tract, and spleen also contain lymphoid tissue.

Lymphatic System Disorders

- *Lymphangitis* (lim-fan-ji'tis): inflammation of the lymph vessels.
- *Lymphadenitis* (lim-fad'e-ni-tis): inflammation of lymph nodes. Inflamed lymph nodes may not be able to filter pathogens from the lymph before it returns to the blood stream. This could lead to **septicemia** (sep-ti-se'me-ah).
- *Lymphadenopathy* (lim-fad'e-nop'ah-the): disease of the lymph nodes, often associated with enlargement such as seen in mononucleosis.
- *Splenomegaly* (splen'no-meg'ah-le): spleen enlargement.
- *Hodgkin's disease:* a chronic, malignant disorder, common in males, characterized by lymph node enlargement.
- *Lymphosarcoma* (lim-fo-sar-ko'mah): a malignant lymphoid tumor.
- *Lymphoma:* the term for any lymphoid tumor, benign or malignant.

Diagnostic Tests

- Biopsy
- Complete blood count (CBC)
- Mononucleosis test (Monospot)
- Culture and sensitivity (C&S)
- Bone marrow biopsy

Study & Review Questions

1. The thin membrane lining the heart that is continuous with the lining of the blood vessels is the
   a. myocardium.
   b. epicardium.
   c. endocardium.
   d. pericardium.

2. The chamber of the heart that receives blood from the lungs is the
   a. left atrium.
   b. right atrium.
   c. left ventricle.
   d. right ventricle.

3. The mitral valve in the heart is also called the
   a. pulmonary semilunar valve.
   b. tricuspid valve.
   c. aortic valve.
   d. bicuspid valve.

4. The ECG shows P waves due to
   a. atrial contractions.
   b. delayed contractions.
   c. recovery of the electrical charge.
   d. ventricular contraction.

5. The relaxation phase of the heart is called the
   a. cardiac cycle.
   b. diastole.
   c. pulse.
   d. systole.

6. A heart disorder that is characterized by fluid buildup in the lungs is called
   a. aortic stenosis.
   b. bacterial endocarditis.
   c. congestive heart failure.
   d. myocardial infarction.

7. The internal space of a blood vessel is called the
   a. atrium.
   b. lumen.
   c. septum.
   d. valve.

8. The longest vein in the body is the
   a. cephalic.
   b. inferior vena cava.
   c. pulmonary vein.
   d. great saphenous.

9. An individual's blood type—A, B, AB, or O—is determined by the presence or absence of
   _____ on the red blood cells.
   a. antigens.
   b. chemicals.
   c. clotting factors.
   d. hormones.

10. Which is the correct sequence of events following vessel injury?
    a. Platelet aggregation, vasoconstriction, fibrin clot
    b. Vasoconstriction, platelet aggregation, fibrin clot
    c. Vasodilation, platelet adhesion, fibrin clot
    d. Fibrinolysis, platelet adhesion, vasoconstriction

Suggested Laboratory Activities

1. Identify structures of the heart using an anatomic model.

2. Demonstrate how to take the blood pressure of a fellow student.

3. Locate and take the pulse at several locations on a fellow student.

4. Examine and compare tubes of whole blood, serum, and plasma.

5. Locate the major antecubital veins, as well as other veins subject to venipuncture, on a fellow student.

6. Watch a film on the circulatory system.

7. Make a model of the pathways of the coagulation cascade.

BIBLIOGRAPHY AND SUGGESTED READINGS

Corriveau, D., & Fritsma, G. (1988). *Hemostasis and thrombosis in the clinical laboratory*. Philadelphia: J. B. Lippincott.

Memmler, R. L., Cohen, B. J., & Wood, D. L. (1996). *The human body in health and disease* (8th ed.). Philadelphia: Lippincott-Raven.

Quinley, E. (1993). *Immunohematology: Principles and practice*. Philadelphia: J. B. Lippincott.

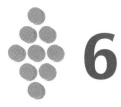

6

Infection Control, Safety, and First Aid

KEY TERMS

airborne precautions
biohazard
bloodborne pathogen
cardiopulmonary
   resuscitation (CPR)
Centers for Disease
   Control and
   Prevention (CDC)
contact precautions
causative agent
droplet precautions
engineering controls
Environmental
   Protection Agency
   (EPA)
fomites
hepatitis B virus (HBV)

Hospital Infection
   Control Practices
   Advisory Committee
   (HICPAC)
human
   immunodeficiency
   virus (HIV)
infection
   isolation procedures
material safety data
   sheets (MSDS)
microbes
nosocomial infection
occupational exposure
Occupational Safety and
Health Administration
   (OSHA)

OSHA bloodborne
   pathogen standard
parenteral
pathogenic
pathogens
percutaneous
personal protective
   equipment (PPE)
standard precautions
susceptible host
systemic
transmission-based
precautions
vector transmission
vehicle transmission
virulence

OBJECTIVES

Upon successful completion of this chapter, the reader will be able to:

1. Define infection and describe what is meant by the terms local, systemic, communicable, and nosocomial.

2. Identify the components of the chain of infection, give examples of each, and describe infection control procedures used to break the chain.

3. Identify organizations that regulate infection control, and name recent standards or guidelines.

(continued)

4. Define bloodborne pathogen, list examples, and describe the means of transmission of bloodborne pathogens in a health care setting.

5. Name four functions of infection control programs.

6. Describe proper procedures for handwashing, donning and removing protective clothing, and entering the nursery or neonatal ICU.

7. Describe standard precautions and transmission-based precautions outlined by the Centers for Disease Control and Prevention and the Hospital Infection Control Practices Advisory Committee, and compare them with traditional isolation systems.

8. State safety rules to follow when working in the laboratory or in patient areas.

9. Describe hazards, identify warning systems, list actions to take if incidents occur, and specify rules to follow for proper biological, electrical, fire, radiation, and chemical safety.

10. State first aid procedures for treating external hemorrhage and shock.

INFECTION CONTROL

Infection

Our environment is full of microorganisms (microscopic organisms) referred to as **microbes**. Microbes include bacteria, fungi, protozoa, and viruses. The majority of microbes are **nonpathogenic**, meaning they do not cause disease under normal conditions. Microbes that are capable of causing disease (*ie*, **pathogenic**) are called **pathogens**. If a pathogen invades the body and the conditions are favorable for it to multiply and cause injurious effects or disease, the resulting condition is called an **infection**. The pathogen responsible for causing the infection is referred to as the **infectious** or **causative agent**. Infection can be **local** (restricted to a small area of the body) or **systemic** (sistem'ik), in which the entire body is affected.

Communicable Infections

Some pathogenic microbes cause infections that can be spread from person to person. These infections are called **communicable infections** and the diseases that result are called **communicable diseases**. A division of the U.S. Public Health Service called the **Centers for Disease Control and Prevention (CDC)** is charged with the investigation and control of various diseases, especially those that are communicable and have epidemic potential. The CDC recommends safety precautions to protect health care workers and others from infection.

Nosocomial Infections

Approximately 5% of patients in the United States are exposed to and contract some sort of infection *after* admission to a hospital or other health care facility. These *hospital- or health care facility–acquired* infections are called **nosocomial infections**. Nosocomial infections can result from contact with infected personnel, other patients, visitors, or equipment. The most common nosocomial infection in the United States is urinary tract infection. The **Hospital Infection Control Practices Advisory Committee (HICPAC)**, established in 1991, advises the CDC on updating guidelines regarding prevention of nosocomial infection.

The Chain of Infection

Infection transmission requires the presence of three components which make up what is referred to as the **chain of infection** (Fig. 6-1). These components, or "links"

Chain of Infection

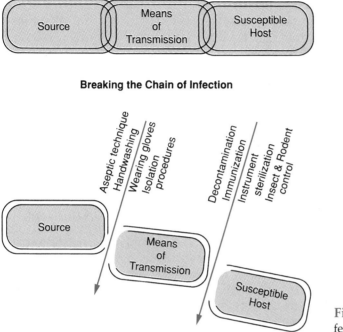

Breaking the Chain of Infection

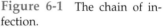

Figure 6-1 The chain of infection.

in the chain of infection, are a **source** of pathogenic or infectious microbes, a **means of transmission** for the microbe, and a **susceptible host**. For an infection to occur, this chain must be complete. If the process of infection is stopped at any component or link in the chain, an infection is prevented. Whenever a pathogen successfully enters a susceptible host, thus completing the chain, the host becomes a new source of infectious microorganisms and the process of infection continues. A phlebotomist, whose duties require coming in contact with many patients, must be fully aware of the infection process and take precautions to prevent the spread of infection.

Components of the Chain of Infection

SOURCE

Sources of infectious microbes include infected humans or animals and contaminated articles and equipment. In a health care setting, human sources of infectious microbes can be patients, personnel or visitors; and includes those with active disease, those whose disease is in the incubation period and those who are chronic carriers of a disease. Another potential source of infectious microbes is a person's own normal flora (microorganisms that normally live in the skin and other areas of the human body).

Contaminated articles and equipment can be a major source of infection in a health care setting. Whether or not an inanimate source is capable of transmitting infection depends upon the amount of contamination, the **viability** or ability of the organism to survive on the source, the **virulence** or degree to which an organism is capable of caus-ing disease, and the amount of time elapsed between when the source was contaminated and when it was contacted.

For example, the virus that causes hepatitis B is much more virulent, or capable of causing disease from a small amount of infective material, than the virus that causes acquired immunodeficiency syndrome (AIDS). It is also more viable, meaning it is capa-ble of surviving longer on surfaces than the AIDS virus. However, if a long enough time elapses from the time of contamination until contact by a susceptible host, the microbe is no longer alive and is not capable of transmitting disease.

MODES OF TRANSMISSION

There are five basic modes or routes of infection transmission: **contact**, **droplet**, **air-borne**, **vehicle**, and **vector**. The same microbe can be transmitted by more than one route.

Contact transmission

Contact transmission is the most frequent mode of infection transmission. There are two types of contact transmission, **direct transmission** and **indirect transmission**.

1. *Direct contact transmission* involves direct, physical transfer of a pathogenic microbe to a susceptible host through close or intimate contact such as touching or kissing.
2. *Indirect contact transmission* involves personal contact by a susceptible host with a conta-minated inanimate object, such as gloves, bed linens, dressings, instruments, eating uten-sils, needles, and clothing. Transfer of infectious microbes from contaminated hands is also considered contact transmission. Inanimate objects or substances that are capable of harboring infectious material and transmitting infection are called **fomites** (fo'mi-tez). Fomites in the laboratory include telephones, computer terminals, and countertops.

Droplet transmission

Droplet transmission involves the transfer of the infective microbe to the mucous membranes of the nose or mouth, or the conjunctiva (mucous membrane) of the eye, of a susceptible individual through sneezing, coughing, or talking by an infected person. Droplet transmission can also occur during procedures such as suctioning and throat swab collection. Droplet transmission is sometimes considered a type of contact transmission because droplets do not travel more than three feet. It differs from airborne transmission in that droplets do not remain suspended in air.

Airborne transmission

Airborne transmission involves dissemination of droplet nuclei. Droplet nuclei are the residue of evaporated droplets generated by sneezing, coughing, or talking. Infec-tious microbes within droplet nuclei can remain viable even though suspended in the air and in dust particles for long periods of time. Microbes carried in this manner can become widely dispersed before being inhaled by or deposited on a susceptible host. For this reason, special air handling and ventilation are required for rooms of patients having infections with airborne transmission. Persons entering the patient's room must wear a snug-fitting mask with a special filter. *Mycobacterium tuberculosis*, rubeola virus, and vari-cella virus are the most common microorganisms transmitted by the airborne route.

Vector transmission

Vector transmission involves the transfer of the microbe by an insect, arthropod, or animal. An example of vector transmission is the transmission of malaria by a mosquito or the plague by rodent fleas.

Vehicle transmission

Vehicle transmission involves the transmission of the infective microbe through contaminated food, water, or drugs. Examples of vehicle transmission are salmonella infection from handling contaminated chicken and shigella infection from drinking contaminated water. The transmission of hepatitis and human immunodeficiency virus (HIV) through blood transfusion is also considered vehicle transmission.

SUSCEPTIBLE HOST

A **susceptible host** can be anyone. Susceptibility is affected by age, health, and the immune status of the individual. For example, newborns whose immune systems are not yet developed and old people whose immune systems are no longer functioning properly are more susceptible to infections. A person's resistance may be compromised by disease, antibiotic treatment, and immunosuppressive drugs. Procedures such as surgery, anesthesia, and insertion of catheters can also leave a patient more susceptible to infection. A healthy person who has received a vaccination against a disease-causing virus, as well as someone who has recovered from a particular virus, has developed antibodies against that virus and is considered to be **immune**, or unlikely to develop the disease, and is therefore less susceptible.

Breaking the Chain of Infection

Breaking the chain of infection means stopping infections at the source, eliminating means of transmission, and reducing or eliminating the susceptibility of potential hosts. Ways to prevent transmission of infectious microbes are proper handwashing; use of gloves, gowns, masks, and other protective equipment when indicated; proper waste disposal; isolation procedures; insect and rodent control; and decontamination of surfaces and instruments. Susceptibility of potential hosts can be reduced through proper nutrition, reduction of stress, and immunization against common pathogens.

ORGANIZATIONS REGULATING INFECTION CONTROL

Organizations that establish or enforce regulations and guidelines for infection control include the following:

- Centers for Disease Control and Prevention (CDC)
- Hospital Infection Control Practices Advisory Committee (HICPAC)
- Joint Committee for Accrediting Healthcare Organizations (JCAHO)
- **Occupational Safety and Health Administration (OSHA)**
- State and local regulatory agencies

OSHA Regulations

OSHA regulations are federal standards or laws protecting employees that supersede all other regulatory agency requirements. The most current OSHA regulation affecting infection control in health care is the Occupational Exposure to Bloodborne Pathogens Standard, Final Rule (29CFR 1910.1030) (Federal Register Dec. 6:64004–64182, 1991).

Current CDC Guidelines Affecting Infection Control

- Guideline for Preventing the Transmission of Mycobacterium Tuberculosis in Healthcare Facilities, 1994
- Guideline for Isolation Precautions in Hospitals, 1995

Bloodborne Pathogens

Bloodborne pathogen is a term applied to any infectious microorganism present in blood and other body fluids and tissues. However, the term most commonly refers to hepatitis B virus and human immunodeficiency virus. Other bloodborne pathogens include other hepatitis viruses, cytomegalovirus (CMV), and the microorganisms that cause syphilis, malaria, relapsing fever, and Creutzfeldt-Jakob disease.

HEPATITIS B VIRUS

Hepatitis B (formerly called serum hepatitis) is the most frequently occurring laboratory-associated infection, making it the major infectious occupational health hazard in the health care industry. The virus that causes hepatitis B, **hepatitis B virus (HBV)**, is a potentially life-threatening bloodborne pathogen that targets the liver. (Hepatitis means "inflammation of the liver.") HBV can survive up to a week in dried blood on work surfaces, telephones, and other objects and surfaces. In a health care setting, HBV can be transmitted through needlesticks and other sharps injuries; contact with contaminated equipment, objects, and surfaces; and contact with infectious material through aerosols, spills, and splashing. In a nonmedical setting, it is transmitted primarily through sexual contact and sharing of dirty needles.

According to OSHA, every year approximately 8,700 health care workers contract hepatitis B and around 200 die as a result. Of those who recover, some become carriers with the ability to pass the disease on to others. Carriers are also at risk for developing cirrhosis of the liver and liver cancer. Presence of hepatitis B infection is commonly determined by the detecting of the presence of the hepatitis B surface antigen (HBsAg) in a patient's serum.

HUMAN IMMUNODEFICIENCY VIRUS

Human immunodeficiency virus (HIV) is the virus responsible for causing AIDS. The virus attacks the body's immune or "defense" system, leaving the host susceptible to opportunistic infections. Because HIV is a bloodborne pathogen and because infection with HIV has a poor prognosis at best, it is of great concern to health care workers. Although the incidence of work-related infection with HIV is relatively low, studies by the CDC have shown that phlebotomy procedures are dangerous work-related activities responsible for approximately 50% of the HIV exposures occurring so far in a health care setting.

Parenteral Transmission of Bloodborne Pathogens

The main **parenteral** (any route other than the digestive tract) means of transmission of bloodborne pathogens in a health care setting are as follows:

1. *Nonintact skin:* Direct contact of pathogen-containing material with both visible and invisible preexisting cuts and scratches (including those occurring with chapped hands), burns, lesions, and dermatitis.
2. *Percutaneous (through the skin):* Direct inoculation of blood or other body fluids by accidental needlesticks and injuries from other sharps such as broken glass and tubes. Human bites that break the skin and the transfusion of infected blood or blood products are also considered parenteral inoculation.
3. *Mucous membrane:* Contact of the oral, nasal, or conjunctival mucosa by droplets, aerosols, or splashes of infectious material; or touching the mouth, nose, or eyes with contaminated hands.

OSHA Bloodborne Pathogens Standard

OSHA has concluded that health care employees face a serious health risk as a result of occupational exposure to blood and other potentially infectious materials, including other body fluids and tissues, because they may contain pathogenic microorganisms. For this reason, OSHA promulgated (put into force) the **Occupational Exposure to Bloodborne Pathogens Standard**. Enforcement of this standard, which is mandated by federal law, is meant to minimize, if not eliminate, occupational exposure to the viruses that cause hepatitis B and AIDS, as well as other bloodborne pathogens. This standard outlines the necessary engineering and work practice controls that OSHA believes will help minimize or eliminate exposure of employees. In addition, the standard requires the availability and use of **personal protective equipment (PPE)** or clothing, special training, medical surveillance, and the availability of vaccination against HBV for all employees having contact with bloodborne pathogens.

Infection Control Programs

Every health care institution is required by the Joint Commission on the Accreditation of Healthcare Organizations (JCAHO) to have an infection control program responsible for implementing procedures designed to break the chain of infection. Such procedures are aimed at protecting not only patients, but also employees, visitors, and others. An infection control program is also responsible for monitoring and collecting data on all infections occurring within the health care institution and instituting special precautions in the event of outbreaks of particular infections.

EMPLOYEE SCREENING AND IMMUNIZATION

One way infection control programs help prevent infections is through employee health programs that screen employees for infectious diseases prior to or upon employment and on a regular basis throughout employment. Screening commonly includes tuberculosis (TB) testing, also called PPD (purified protein derivative) testing. Employees with positive TB tests receive chest x-ray evaluations to determine their TB status. Screening may also include RPR (rapid plasma reagin) testing for syphilis and screening for diarrheal and skin diseases. In addition, most health care employers require employees to have current HBV, MMR (measles, mumps, rubella), and tetanus vaccinations. Most employers provide vaccinations free of charge. Employers are required to offer HBV vaccine free of charge to employees with risk of exposure.

HEPATITIS B VACCINATION

The best defense against HBV infection is vaccination. Vaccination consists of a series of three equal intramuscular injections of vaccine: an initial dose, a second dose 1 month after the first, and a third dose 6 months following the initial dose. Success of immunization is confirmed by a blood test that detects the presence of the hepatitis B surface antibody (HBsAb) in the person's serum. One type of vaccine (*eg*, Recombivax B) is derived from yeast culture and poses no risk of transmitting HBV, HIV, or other bloodborne pathogens. Hepatitis B vaccine protects against HBV as well as delta hepatitis, which can only be contracted concurrently with HBV infection. Employers are required by OSHA to offer this vaccine free to employees within 10 days of being assigned to duties with possible exposure to bloodborne pathogens. Employees who decline the vaccination must sign a declination form.

EVALUATION AND TREATMENT

Infection control programs also provide evaluation and treatment for employees who are exposed to infections on the job. This includes OSHA-mandated confidential medical evaluation, treatment, counseling, and follow-up as a result of exposure to bloodborne pathogens (see Safety).

SURVEILLANCE

Surveillance or monitoring is a major function of an infection control program. This involves monitoring patients and employees at risk of acquiring infections, as well as collecting and evaluating data on infections in patients and employees. Infection control measures are updated and new policies are instituted based on this information.

Infection Control Methods
HANDWASHING

The most important means of preventing and controlling the spread of infection is proper handwashing. Handwashing by the phlebotomist should be performed:

- Before and after each patient contact.
- Between different procedures on the same patient.
- Before putting on gloves and after taking them off.
- Before leaving the laboratory.
- Before going to lunch or break.
- Before and after going to the restroom.
- Whenever hands become visibly or knowingly contaminated.

Routine handwash procedure
1. Remove rings and watch.
2. Stand back so that you do not touch the sink.

3. Wet hands under warm, running water.
4. Apply soap and work up a lather. Rub your hands together to create friction, which loosens dead skin, dirt, and other debris. Scrub everywhere, including between the fingers and around the knuckles. Wash for at least 15 seconds. Debris under fingernails should be removed with an orange stick or similar device.
5. Rinse your hands in a downward motion from wrists to fingertips.
6. Repeat steps 4 and 5.
7. Dry your hands with a clean paper towel.
8. Turn the faucet off with another clean paper towel.

PROTECTIVE CLOTHING
Masks, goggles, face shields, respirators

A mask is worn to provide protection from droplets generated by coughing or sneezing. To put on a mask, place it over the nose and mouth. Adjust the metal band (if applicable) to fit snugly over the nose. For masks with ties, fasten the top ties around the upper portion of the head, then tie the lower ones at the back of the neck. If the mask has elastic fasteners, slip them around the ears.

A mask and goggles, or a face shield, are worn to protect the eyes, nose, and mouth from splashes or sprays of body fluids. Blood-drawing activities that require goggles to be worn always require that a mask be worn also. Some masks have plastic eye shields attached.

Respirators are required when entering rooms of patients with pulmonary tuberculosis and other diseases with airborne transmission. Respirators must fit snugly with no air leaks. In addition, they must be N95 respirators (Fig. 6-2) approved by the National Institute for Occupational Safety and Health (NIOSH).

Gowns/Lab Coats

Clean, nonsterile, fluid-resistant gowns or lab coats are worn by health care workers to protect skin and prevent soiling of clothing during patient-care activities in which splashes or sprays of blood or body fluids are possible. In addition, sterile gowns are worn by health care workers to protect certain patients (*eg*, newborns and patients with compromised immune systems) from contaminants on health care worker clothing. Gowns are most often made of disposable cloth or paper, have long sleeves with knit cuffs, and are generous in size to adequately cover clothing. Gowns normally fasten in the back.

When putting on a gown, only inside surfaces of the gown should be touched. A properly worn gown has the sleeves pulled all the way to the wrist, the belt tied, and the gown overlapped, completely closed, and securely fastened. A gown is removed from the inside by sliding the arms out of the sleeves. The gown is then held away from the body and folded with the contaminated outside surface ending up inside.

Gloves

Clean, nonsterile gloves are to be worn when touching blood, other body fluids, or contaminated items and when touching nonintact skin or mucous membranes. To provide adequate protection, gloves should be worn pulled over the cuffs of gowns or lab coats. The three main reasons for wearing gloves are as follows:

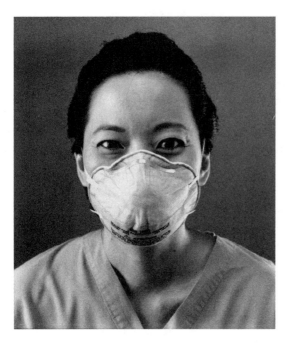

Figure 6-2 N95 respirator. (Courtesy 3M Health Care, St. Paul, MN)

1. To prevent contamination of the hands when handling blood or body fluids or when touching mucous membranes or nonintact skin. (Wearing gloves during most phlebotomy procedures is mandated by the OSHA Bloodborne Pathogens Standard.)
2. To reduce the chance of transmitting organisms on the hands of personnel to patients during invasive or other procedures that involve touching a patient's skin or mucous membranes.
3. To minimize the possibility of transmitting infectious microorganisms from one patient to another.

After use, gloves should be removed promptly in an aseptic manner and discarded (Fig. 6-3). To remove gloves aseptically, grasp one glove at the wrist and pull it inside out and off of the hand, ending up with it in the palm of the still-gloved hand. Slip fingers of the ungloved hand under the second glove at the wrist and pull it off of the hand, ending with one glove inside the other with the contaminated surfaces inside. Hands should be washed immediately after glove removal and before going to another patient.

Order to put on and remove protective clothing

When putting on complete protective clothing such as gown, mask, and gloves, the gown is put on first. The mask is next, making certain it covers the nose and mouth. Gloves are put on last and pulled over the cuffs of the gown (Fig. 6-4).

Protective clothing is removed in the opposite order from which it was put on. It must be removed carefully in an aseptic manner to prevent contamination of the health care worker. Gloves are removed first, being careful not to touch contaminated sur-

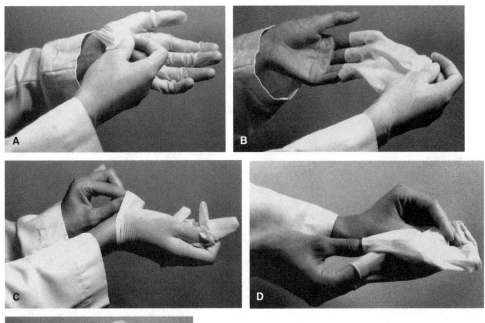

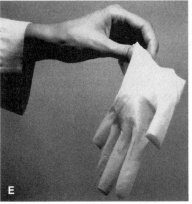

Figure 6-3   Glove removal. (**A**) The wrist of one glove is grasped with the opposite gloved hand; (**B**) the glove is pulled inside out over and off the hand; (**C**) with the first glove held in the gloved hand, the fingers of the non-gloved hand are slipped under the wrist of the remaining glove without touching the exterior surfaces; (**D**) the glove is then pulled inside out over the hand so that the first glove ends up inside of the second glove, no exterior glove surfaces are exposed; and (**E**) the contaminated gloves can then be dropped into the proper waste receptacle.

faces with ungloved hands. The mask is removed next, touching only the strings. The gown is removed last. Hands must be washed promptly after removal of protective clothing.

NURSERY AND NEONATAL ICU INFECTION CONTROL TECHNIQUE

Because their immune systems are not yet fully developed, newborns are more susceptible to infections than healthy older children and adults. For this reason, special infection control techniques should be used by the phlebotomist as well as all other personnel who enter the nursery. Most nurseries have a separate room just outside the nurs-

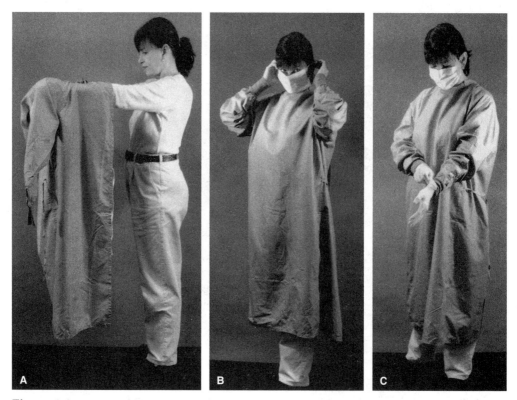

Figure 6-4   Protective clothing. (**A**) Phlebotomist slips arms into a protective gown; (**B**) A mask is applied by slipping the elastic band over the ears; (**C**) Gloves are put on last and pulled over the gown cuffs.

ery where handwashing, gowning, and so forth are performed before entering. Typical proper nursery infection control technique includes the following:

1. Washing hands thoroughly with an antiseptic hand cleaner
2. Putting on clean gloves, gown, and mask
3. Leaving the blood collection tray in the wash room outside the nursery and taking into the nursery only those items necessary to perform the specimen collection

Isolation Procedures

One way an infection control program minimizes spread of infection is through the establishment of **isolation procedures** designed to decrease the transmission of infectious microorganisms. Isolation procedures separate patients with certain transmissible infections or diseases from contact with other patients as well as limit their contact with hospital personnel and visitors. Isolating a patient requires a doctor's order and is implemented either to prevent the spread of infection from a patient with a contagious disease or to protect a patient whose immune system is compromised. Patients are most commonly isolated in a private room. The type of isolation, including a description of the precautions necessary, is generally posted on the patient's door. A cart containing all the supplies needed to enter the room and to care for the patient is placed outside the door.

PROTECTIVE OR REVERSE ISOLATION

A special kind of isolation called **protective** or **reverse** isolation is used for patients who are highly susceptible to infections. In this type of isolation, protective measures are used to keep health care workers and others from transmitting infection to the patient rather than vice versa. Examples of patients requiring protective isolation include patients with suppressed immune systems such as organ transplant patients, patients with AIDS, some chemotherapy patients, neutropenic patients (patients with low neutrophil counts), and patients with burns.

TRADITIONAL ISOLATION SYSTEMS

Traditionally, there were two basic types of isolation systems recommended by the CDC: the **category-specific** system and the **disease-specific** system. The diagnosis or suspicion of the presence of a transmissible disease was necessary before institution of either system.

Category-specific isolation

There were seven different categories in the category-specific system: strict, contact, respiratory, AFB (acid-fast bacillus or tuberculosis), enteric, drainage/secretion, and blood/body fluid precautions (Table 6-1). All categories required any article leaving an isolated patient's room to be double-bagged and labeled as biohazard prior to disposal or decontamination for reuse. Because categories covered many diseases, this system tended to result in overisolation of patients and needless increase in costs.

Disease-specific isolation

The disease-specific system employed specific isolation procedures based upon the mode of transmission for the most common diseases in the United States. Instead of categories, the system used a chart listing common diseases with check marks in columns identifying the specific precautions recommended for each disease.

UNIVERSAL PRECAUTIONS

Isolation practices in the United States were altered dramatically in 1985, when the CDC introduced a new strategy called **universal precautions (UP)** after reports of health care personnel becoming infected with HIV through needlesticks and other exposures to HIV-contaminated blood. UP replaced the blood/body fluid precautions, and these precautions were followed for all isolation categories. With the introduction of UP, the focus of infection control turned from prevention of patient-to-patient transmission to prevention of patient-to-personnel transmission. Under UP, the blood and certain body fluids of *all* individuals were considered potentially infectious for bloodborne pathogens. The CDC required that UP be part of an overall infection control plan, and OSHA mandated that they be part of a bloodborne pathogen exposure control plan.

BODY SUBSTANCE ISOLATION

Because, in some cases, transmission of infection can occur before a diagnosis is made, both the category-specific and the disease-specific systems were subject to error. Therefore, a new system called **body substance isolation (BSI)** (Fig. 6-5) gained acceptance.

Body substance isolation provided the equivalent of universal precautions for bloodborne pathogens while incorporating elements of disease-specific as well as category-specific precautions for all transmissible pathogens. BSI was followed for *every* patient without

Table 6-1
Category-Specific Isolation

Isolation Category	Description and Barrier Protection Required
Strict (complete)	Required for patients with highly contagious diseases, such as chicken pox, bubonic plague, and diphtheria, that can be spread by direct contact and through the air. Strict isolation requires the wearing of gowns, gloves, and masks by all persons entering the room.
Contact isolation	Indicated for highly transmittable diseases that are spread primarily by direct contact, but do not warrant strick isolation. These infections include influenza (flu) and infections with antibiotic-resistant bacteria. Contact isolation requirements include the use of gloves, gowns if soiling is likely, and masks if in close contact with the patient.
Respiratory	Used for patients with infections that can be spread via droplets or through the air, such as whooping cough (pertussis), *Haemophilus influenzae*, and meningococcal meningitis. Masks must be worn by those coming in close contact with the patient.
AFB (acid-fast bacillus)	Used for patients with active tuberculosis. Masks or particulate respirators, gowns, and gloves are indicated until there is clinical evidence that the infectiousness has substantially decreased and the patient is no longer coughing appreciably.
Drainage/secretion	Used for patients with skin infections, open wounds, or burns. It is sometimes used following surgery. Masks and gowns are indicated for procedures where splashing or soiling may occur.
Enteric	Used for patients with intestinal infections that can be transmitted by ingestion. Enteric infections include those caused by salmonella, shigella, campylobacter, and other organisms causing diarrhea or dysentery. Masks and gowns are indicated for procedures where soiling or splashing may occur.
Blood and body fluid	Patients with infections such as HIV and hepatitis B that can be transmitted through contact with the patient's blood and body fluids. Replaced by universal precautions.

the need of diagnosis or suspicion of a transmissible disease. Body substance isolation went beyond universal precautions by requiring the wearing of gloves when coming into contact with *any* moist body substance. Special "stop signs" (Fig. 6-6) alerted heath care workers when additional precautions were needed, such as for respiratory or strict isolation.

REVISED GUIDELINE FOR ISOLATION PRECAUTIONS IN HOSPITALS

In 1995, the CDC and HICPAC were prompted by a number of factors to issue a new Guideline for Isolation Precautions in Hospitals. The concerns that led to development of the new guideline included widespread variation in the use of UP or BSI; con-

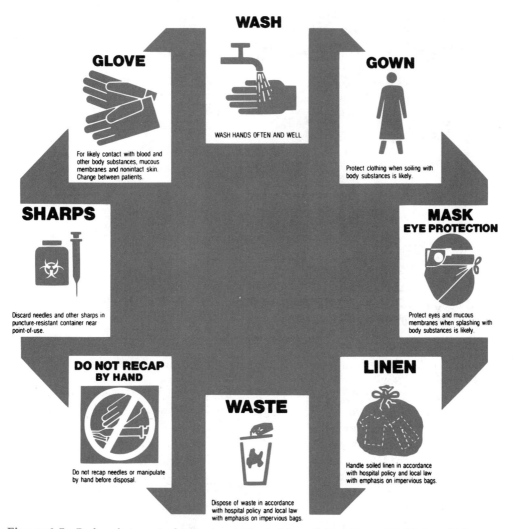

Figure 6-5   Body substance isolation sign. (Adapted from Briggs Corp., Des Moines, IA.)

fusion over which body fluids required precautions; and lack of agreement about the importance of handwashing when gloves were used and the need for additional precautions beyond BSI to prevent airborne, droplet, and contact transmission.

This guideline supersedes previous CDC recommendations for hospital isolation precautions. The guideline contains two tiers of precautions. The first tier, called **standard precautions**, contains precautions to be used in caring for all hospital patients regardless of their diagnosis or presumed infection status. The second tier, called **transmission-based precautions**, contains precautions to be used for patients suspected or known to be infected with certain pathogens transmitted by airborne, droplet, or contact transmission. The guideline also lists specific clinical syndromes or conditions that are highly suspicious for infection and identifies appropriate

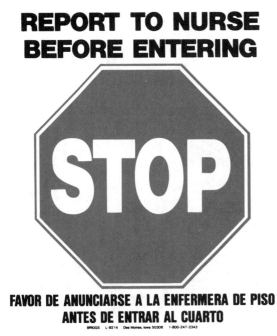

REPORT TO NURSE BEFORE ENTERING

FAVOR DE ANUNCIARSE A LA ENFERMERA DE PISO ANTES DE ENTRAR AL CUARTO

BRIGGS   L-9214   Des Moines, Iowa 50306   1-800-247-2343

Figure 6-6 Precaution "stop sign." (Adapted from Briggs Corp., Des Moines, IA.)

transmission-based precautions to use for each, in addition to standard precautions, until a diagnosis can be made.

Standard Precautions

[handwritten: All pts ; UP c̄ BSI   Apply to! mucous membranes blood, body fluids, non intact skin]

Standard precautions (Fig. 6-7) are intended to be the number-one strategy for successful **nosocomial infection** control. Standard precautions combine the major features of UP and BSI. The intent of standard precautions is to minimize the risk of infection transmission from both recognized and unrecognized sources. Standard precautions apply to blood, *all* body fluids (including all secretions and excretions except sweat, whether or not they contain visible blood), nonintact skin, and mucous membranes. They are to be used for the care of all patients.

Transmission-Based Precautions

Transmission-based precautions are to be used for patients known or suspected to be infected or colonized with highly transmissible or epidemiologically significant pathogens that require special precautions in addition to standard precautions. Table 6-2 lists clinical conditions that warrant transmission-based precautions pending diagnosis. Common diseases and conditions that require transmission-based precautions are listed in Table 6-3. Precautions may be combined for diseases that have more than one means of transmission. There are three types of transmission-based precautions:

1. *Airborne precautions:* Use **airborne precautions** (Fig. 6-8), or the equivalent, in addition to standard precautions for patients known or suspected to be infected with microorganisms transmitted by airborne droplet nuclei. Wear an N95 respirator (see Fig. 6-2) when entering rooms of patients with airborne precautions.

STANDARD PRECAUTIONS

FOR INFECTION CONTROL

Wash Hands (Plain soap)

Wash after touching **blood, body fluids, secretions, excretions,** and **contaminated items.** Wash immediately **after gloves are removed** and **between patient contacts.** Avoid transfer of microorganisms to other patients or environments.

Wear Gloves

Wear when touching **blood, body fluids, secretions, excretions,** and **contaminated items.** Put on **clean** gloves just **before touching mucous membranes** and **nonintact skin.** Change gloves between tasks and procedures on the same patient after contact with material that may contain high concentrations of microorganisms. Remove gloves promptly after use, before touching noncontaminated items and environmental surfaces, and before going to another patient, and wash hands immediately to avoid transfer of microorganisms to other patients or environments.

Wear Mask and Eye Protection or Face Shield

Protect mucous membranes of the eyes, nose and mouth during procedures and patient-care activities that are likely to generate **splashes** or **sprays** of **blood, body fluids, secretions,** or **excretions.**

Wear Gown

Protect skin and prevent soiling of clothing during procedures that are likely to generate **splashes** or **sprays** of **blood, body fluids, secretions,** or **excretions.** Remove a soiled gown as promptly as possible and wash hands to avoid transfer of microorganisms to other patients or environments.

Patient-Care Equipment

Handle used patient-care equipment soiled with **blood, body fluids, secretions,** or **excretions** in a manner that prevents skin and mucous membrane exposures, contamination of clothing, and transfer of microorganisms to other patients and environments. Ensure that reusable equipment is not used for the care of another patient until it has been appropriately cleaned and reprocessed and single use items are properly discarded.

Figure 6-7   Standard Precautions sign. (Courtesy Brevis Corp., Salt Lake City, UT.) *(continued)*

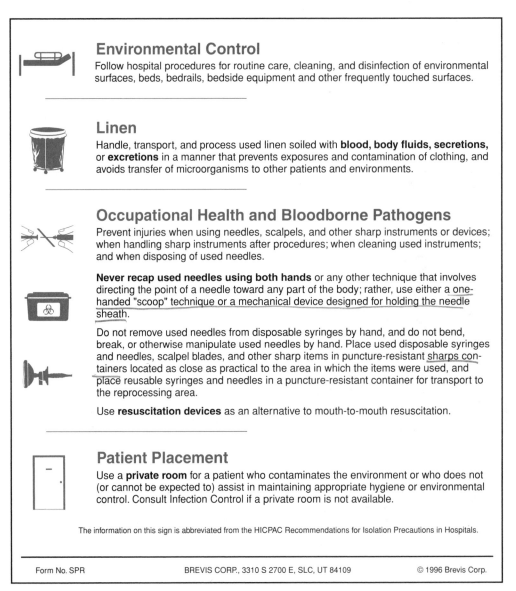

Environmental Control

Follow hospital procedures for routine care, cleaning, and disinfection of environmental surfaces, beds, bedrails, bedside equipment and other frequently touched surfaces.

Linen

Handle, transport, and process used linen soiled with **blood, body fluids, secretions, or excretions** in a manner that prevents exposures and contamination of clothing, and avoids transfer of microorganisms to other patients and environments.

Occupational Health and Bloodborne Pathogens

Prevent injuries when using needles, scalpels, and other sharp instruments or devices; when handling sharp instruments after procedures; when cleaning used instruments; and when disposing of used needles.

Never recap used needles using both hands or any other technique that involves directing the point of a needle toward any part of the body; rather, use either a one-handed "scoop" technique or a mechanical device designed for holding the needle sheath.

Do not remove used needles from disposable syringes by hand, and do not bend, break, or otherwise manipulate used needles by hand. Place used disposable syringes and needles, scalpel blades, and other sharp items in puncture-resistant sharps containers located as close as practical to the area in which the items were used, and place reusable syringes and needles in a puncture-resistant container for transport to the reprocessing area.

Use **resuscitation devices** as an alternative to mouth-to-mouth resuscitation.

Patient Placement

Use a **private room** for a patient who contaminates the environment or who does not (or cannot be expected to) assist in maintaining appropriate hygiene or environmental control. Consult Infection Control if a private room is not available.

The information on this sign is abbreviated from the HICPAC Recommendations for Isolation Precautions in Hospitals.

Form No. SPR   BREVIS CORP., 3310 S 2700 E, SLC, UT 84109   © 1996 Brevis Corp.

Figure 6-7 *(continued)*

2. *Droplet precautions:* **Droplet precautions** (Fig. 6-9), or the equivalent, are used in addition to standard precautions for patients known or suspected to be infected with microorganisms transmitted by droplets (particles larger than 5 micrometers in size), generated when a patient talks, coughs, or sneezes and during certain procedures.
3. *Contact precautions:* **Contact precautions** (Fig. 6-10), or the equivalent, are used in addition to standard precautions when a patient is known or suspected to be infected or colonized with epidemiologically important microorganisms that can be transmitted by direct contact with the patient or indirect contact with surfaces or patient-care items.

SAFETY

Providing quality care in an environment that is safe for employees as well as patients is a concern that is foremost in the minds of health care providers. Safe working conditions must be ensured by employers as mandated by the Occupational Safety and Health Act (OSHA) of 1970 and enforced by the Occupational Safety and Health Administration, also called OSHA. Even so, there are biological, electrical, radiation, and chemical hazards encountered in a health care setting, often on a daily basis. It is important for the phlebotomist to be aware of the existence of hazards and to have knowledge of the safety precautions and rules necessary to eliminate or minimize them.

General Laboratory Safety Rules

1. *Never* eat, drink, smoke, or chew gum in the laboratory. *Never* put pencils or pens in the mouth.
2. *Never* place food or beverages in a refrigerator used for storing reagents or specimens.
3. *Never* apply cosmetics, handle contact lenses, or rub eyes in the laboratory.
4. *Never* wear long chains, large or dangling earrings, or loose bracelets.
5. *Always* wear a fully buttoned lab coat when engaged in lab activities. *Never* wear a lab coat to lunch, on break, or when leaving the lab to go home. *Never* wear PPE outside the designated area for its use. ~Personal protective equipment~
6. *Always* tie back hair that is over shoulder length.
7. *Always* keep fingernails short and well manicured. *Do not* wear nail polish or artificial nails. *Never* bite nails.
8. *Always* wear a face shield when performing specimen processing or any activity that might generate splashes or aerosol of body fluids.
9. *Always* wear comfortable, sturdy shoes with nonslip soles. *Never* wear sandals, open-toed shoes, slippers, or high heels.
10. *Always* wear gloves for phlebotomy procedures and when specimen processing.

Safety Rules When in Patient Rooms and Other Patient Areas

1. Handle all specimens following standard precautions.
2. Properly dispose of used and contaminated specimen collection supplies and return all other equipment to the specimen collection tray before leaving the patient's room. *Do not* recap needles!
3. Replace bedrails that were let down during patient procedures.
4. *Do not* touch electrical equipment in patient rooms, especially when in the process of drawing blood. Electrical shock could pass through the phlebotomist and the needle and shock the patient.
5. Report infiltrated IVs or other IV problems to nursing personnel.
6. Report unresponsive patients to nursing personnel.
7. Watch out for and report food, liquid, and other items spilled or dropped on the floor to nursing or housekeeping personnel.
8. Report unusual odors to nursing personnel.
9. Be careful when entering and exiting patient rooms. Watch out for housekeeping equipment, dietary carts, x-ray machines, and other pieces of equipment which are often left in the halls outside patient rooms.
10. Avoid running. It is alarming to patients and visitors and may cause an accident.

Table 6-2
Clinical Conditions Warranting Transmission-Based Precautions Pending
Confirmation of Diagnosis

Condition	Potential Pathogen	Precaution
Diarrhea		
Acute diarrhea with a likely infectious cause in an incontinent or diapered patient	Enteric pathogen	Contact
Diarrhea in an adult with a history of broad-spectrum or long-term antibiotics	*Clostridium difficile*	Contact
Meningitis	*Neisseria meningitidis*	Droplet
Rash for inflamed skin eruptions		
Petechial/ecchymotic with fever	*Neisseria meningitidis*	Droplet
Vesicular	Varicella	Airborne & contact
Maculopapular	Rubeola (measles)	Airborne
Respiratory infections		
Cough/fever/upper lobe pulmonary infiltrate in an HIV-negative patient and a patient at low risk for HIV infection	*Mycobacterium tuberculosis*	Airborne
Cough/fever/pulmonary infiltrate in any lung location in an HIV-infected patient and at high risk for HIV infection	*Mycobacterium tuberculosis*	Airborne
Paroxysmal or severe persistent cough during periods of pertussis activity	*Bordetella pertussis*	Droplet
Respiratory infections, particularly bronchiolitis and croup, in infants and young children	Respiratory syncytial virus or para-influenza virus	Contact
Risk of multidrug-resistant microorganisms		
History of infection or colonization with multidrug-resistant organisms	Resistant bacteria	Contact
Skin, wound, or urinary tract infection in a patient with a recent hospital or nursing home stay in a facility where multidrug-resistant organisms are prevalent	Resistant bacteria	Contact
Skin or wound infection		
Abscess or draining wound that cannot be covered	*Staphylococcus aureus* Group A streptococcus	Contact

Table 6-3
Transmission-Based Precautions for Common Diseases and Conditions

Airborne Precautions	Droplet Precautions	Contact Precautions
Herpes zoster (shingles)**	Adenovirus infection*	Adenovirus infection*
Measles (rubeola)	Diphtheria (pharyngeal)	Cellulitis (uncontrolled drainage)
Pulmonary tuberculosis	*Haemophilus influenzae* meningitis	*Clostridium difficile*
Varicella (chickenpox)	Influenza	Conjunctivitis (acute viral)
	Meningococcal pneumonia	Decubitus ulcer (infected, major)
	Meningococcal sepsis	Diphtheria (cutaneous)
	Mumps (infectious parotitis)	Enteroviral infections*
	Mycoplasma pneumoniae	Herpes zoster (shingles)**
	Neisseria meningitidis	Impetigo
	Parvovirus B19	Parainfluenza virus
	Pertussis (whooping cough)	Pediculosis (lice)
	Pneumonic plague	Respiratory syncytial virus
	Rubella (German measles)	Rubella (congenital)
	Scarlet fever*	Scabies
		Varicella (chickenpox)

*Infants and children only

**Widely disseminated or in immunocompromised patients

Biological Hazards

A biological hazard or **biohazard** is any material or substance harmful to health. Biohazards are identified by a special symbol called a **biohazard symbol** (Fig. 6-11). Because the majority of laboratory specimens are blood and other body fluids and tissues with the potential to contain bloodborne pathogens and other infectious materials and agents that could be harmful to health, they are considered biohazards.

Common routes of entry for biohazards in a health care setting are as follows:

- *Airborne.* Biohazardous substances and microorganisms can be inhaled when splashes and aerosols are generated. Aerosols can be created during centrifugation of specimens and removal of stoppers, as well as when improperly aliquoting specimens. Dangerous fumes can be created when chemicals are improperly stored, mixed, or handled. Following proper procedures during handling and processing of specimens and when working with chemicals can minimize airborne exposure to biohazards. N95 respirators must be worn when entering rooms of patients with infections spread by airborne transmission.
- *Ingestion.* Biohazardous substances and microorganisms can be ingested when health care workers neglect to wash contaminated hands and subsequently handle food, gum, cigarettes, or drinks. Other activities such as covering the mouth with hands when coughing or sneezing, biting nails, chewing on pens or pencils, and licking fingers when turning pages in books or manuals can also lead to ingestion

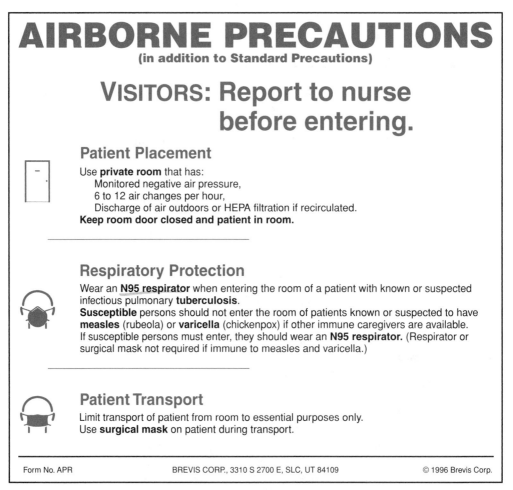

Figure 6-8   Airborne precautions sign. (Courtesy Brevis Corp., Salt Lake City, UT.)

of biohazardous substances. Frequent handwashing is the best defense against accidental ingestion of biohazardous substances.

- *Percutaneous inoculation.* Infection with biohazardous microorganisms can occur from needlesticks and injuries from other sharps including broken glass.
- *Skin contact.* Biohazardous substances and microorganisms can enter the body through abrasions, burns, cuts, sores, dermatitis, and chapped skin. Defects in the skin should be covered with waterproof or nonpermeable tape or bandages to prevent contamination, even when gloves are worn.
- *Permucosal (mucous membrane contact).* Infectious microorganisms can enter the body through the mucous membranes of the mouth and nose and the conjunctiva of the eyes through splashes, generation of aerosols, and rubbing the eyes with contaminated hands. Procedures should be followed to prevent or minimize the generation of splashes and aerosols. Rubbing the eyes should be avoided.

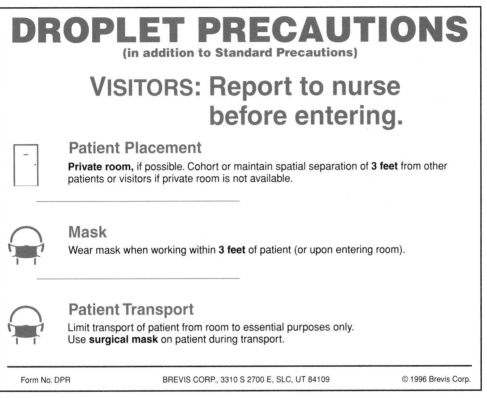

DROPLET PRECAUTIONS
(in addition to Standard Precautions)

VISITORS: Report to nurse before entering.

Patient Placement
Private room, if possible. Cohort or maintain spatial separation of **3 feet** from other patients or visitors if private room is not available.

Mask
Wear mask when working within **3 feet** of patient (or upon entering room).

Patient Transport
Limit transport of patient from room to essential purposes only.
Use **surgical mask** on patient during transport.

Form No. DPR   BREVIS CORP., 3310 S 2700 E, SLC, UT 84109   © 1996 Brevis Corp.

Figure 6-9   Droplet precautions sign. (Courtesy Brevis Corp., Salt Lake City, UT.)

OCCUPATIONAL EXPOSURE TO
BLOODBORNE PATHOGENS

Occupational exposure to bloodborne pathogens can occur if any of the following occurs while a health care worker is performing his or her duties.

- The skin is pierced by a contaminated needle or sharp object.
- Blood or other body fluid splashes into the eyes, nose, or mouth.
- Blood or other body fluid comes in contact with a cut, scratch, or abrasion.
- A human bite breaks the skin.

PROCEDURE FOR NEEDLESTICKS AND OTHER
EXPOSURE INCIDENTS

OSHA requires employers to provide free confidential medical evaluation and treatment to any employee in the event of an exposure incident. Initial response by the employee requires decontamination of a needlestick site with an appropriate antiseptic, such as povidone–iodine, for a minimum of 30 seconds. A mucous membrane exposure requires flushing the site with water for a minimum of 10 minutes. The employee must report the incident to his or her immediate supervisor. The employee is to then report

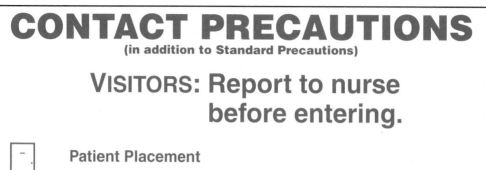

CONTACT PRECAUTIONS
(in addition to Standard Precautions)

VISITORS: Report to nurse before entering.

Patient Placement

Private room, if possible. Cohort if private room is not available.

Gloves

Wear gloves when entering patient room. **Change** gloves after having contact with infective material that may contain high concentrations of microorganisms (**fecal** material and **wound drainage**). **Remove** gloves before leaving patient room.

Wash

Wash hands with an **antimicrobial** agent immediately after glove removal. After glove removal and handwashing, ensure that hands do not touch potentially contaminated environmental surfaces or items in the patient's room to avoid transfer of microorganisms to other patients or environments.

Gown

Wear gown when **entering** patient room if you anticipate that your clothing will have substanital contact with the patient, environmental surfaces, or items in the patient's room, or if the patient is **incontinent**, or has **diarrhea**, an **ileostomy**, a **colostomy**, or **wound drainage** not contained by a dressing. **Remove** gown before leaving the patient's environment and ensure that clothing does not contact potentially contaminated environmental surfaces to avoid transfer of microorganisms to other patients or environments.

Patient Transport

Limit transport of patient to essential purposes only. During transport, ensure that precautions are maintained to minimize the risk of transmission of microorganisms to other patients and contamination of environmental surfaces and equipment.

Patient-Care Equipment

Dedicate the use of noncritical patient-care equipment to a single patient. If common equipment is used, clean and disinfect between patients.

Form No. CPR | BREVIS CORP., 3310 S 2700 E, SLC, UT 84109 | © 1996 Brevis Corp.

Figure 6-10   Contact precautions sign. (Courtesy Brevis Corp., Salt Lake City, UT.)

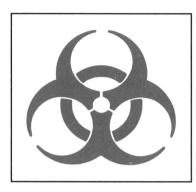

Figure 6-11   Biohazard symbol.

directly to a licensed health care provider for a medical evaluation and counseling, as well as any treatment required. Medical evaluation involves the following:

1. Testing the employees's blood for HIV in an accredited laboratory.
2. Testing the source patient for HIV and HBV, providing permission is granted by the patient.
3. If the source patient refuses testing or is HBV positive or in a high risk category, the employee may be given immune globulin or HBV vaccination.
4. If the source patient is HIV positive, the employee is counseled and tested for HIV infection immediately, and at periodic intervals, normally 6 weeks, 12 weeks, 6 months, and 1 year after exposure. The employee may be given azidothymidine (AZT) or other HIV therapy.
5. An exposed employee is counseled to be alert for acute retroviral syndrome (acute viral symptoms) within 12 weeks of exposure.

DECONTAMINATION OF SURFACES
Specimen collection and processing areas should be decontaminated at the end of each shift with a 1:10 bleach solution or other Environmental Protection Agency (EPA) approved disinfectant. Bleach solutions should be prepared daily. Gloves should be worn when cleaning.

BLOOD SPILL CLEAN-UP
Special EPA-approved chemical solutions are available for clean-up of blood and body fluid spills and for disinfecting surfaces. Gloves should always be worn during the cleaning process. Small spills of no more than a few drops can be absorbed carefully with a paper towel and the area cleaned with a disinfectant. Large blood or body fluid spills can be cleaned up using special clay- or chlorine-based powder that absorbs or gels the liquid and allows it to be scooped or swept up for disposal in a biohazard waste bag. The area is then wiped with a disinfectant. Dried spills should be moistened with disinfectant before clean-up to avoid scraping, which could disperse infectious organisms into the air. Clean-up procedures should concentrate on absorbing the material, while avoiding spread of the material over a wider area than that occupied by the original spill. Spills involving broken glass should be handled with heavy-duty utility gloves. Glass should

be scooped or swept up and not handled with the hands. Reusable materials used for clean-up should be disinfected after use.

BIOHAZARDOUS WASTE DISPOSAL

All discarded items contaminated with blood or body fluids are considered to be biohazardous waste and must be disposed of in special containers or bags marked with a biohazard symbol. Filled biohazardous waste containers require special handling in decontamination and disposal.

EXPOSURE CONTROL PLAN

In order to comply with the OSHA standard, employers must have a written exposure control plan which includes the following:

1. An exposure determination: A list of all job classifications in which employees have or may have occupational exposure to bloodborne pathogens, as well as a list of tasks and procedures in which exposure may occur.
2. Methods of implementation and compliance

   Universal precautions statement: Requires all employees to observe universal precautions.

   Engineering controls: Controls that isolate or remove the bloodborne pathogen hazard from the work place. Examples of **engineering controls** are readily accessible handwashing facilities, sharps disposal containers, and self-sheathing needles.

   Work practice controls: Practices that alter the manner in which a task is performed to reduce the likelihood of exposure. Examples of work practice controls are prohibiting needle bending, breaking, or recapping; requiring handwashing following glove removal; and prohibiting eating, drinking, smoking, or applying cosmetics in work areas of the laboratory.

   Personal protective equipment (PPE): PPE or barrier protection devices to minimize the risk of infection from bloodborne pathogens must be provided at no charge to all employees who have potential exposure. PPE includes gloves, gowns, lab coats, aprons, face shields, masks, and resuscitation mouthpieces. Laundry service for reusable protective outerwear such as gowns and lab coats must be provided by the employer.

   Housekeeping schedule and methods: Work surfaces must be cleaned at least once a day as well as after any contact with blood or other potentially infectious material. A 10% solution of household bleach (5.25% sodium hypochloride) is an acceptable disinfectant.
3. Hepatitis B vaccine and postexposure follow-up: Hepatitis B vaccine series must be offered free of charge to employees within 10 days of assignment to duties with potential exposure. Confidential medical evaluation and follow-up must be available immediately to employees with exposure incidents.
4. Communication of hazards to employees:

   Warning labels and signs must be affixed to containers of blood, contaminated waste containers, and other potentially infectious material. This includes refrigerators and freezers where infectious material may be stored. The labels should be predominantly fluorescent orange or orange-red, bearing the word "biohazard" and containing the biohazard symbol. Red bags or containers may be substituted for labels.

Training and information concerning bloodborne pathogens must be provided to employees at no cost and during working hours at the time of initial assignment to tasks involving occupational exposure. Employers should maintain an accessible copy of the Bloodborne Pathogen Standard as well as an explanation of its contents. Annual training is to be provided within 1 year of initial training.

5. Record keeping

Medical records: Employers are required to maintain confidential medical records on each employee with occupational exposure. These records must include the employee's name, social security number, and HBV vaccination status.

Training records: Employers are required to maintain records of training sessions that include the content, the qualifications of persons conducting the session, and the names and titles of persons attending.

Electrical Safety

There are potential hazards, such as fire and electrical shock, associated with the use of electrical equipment. Knowledge of the proper use, maintenance, and servicing of electrical equipment such as the centrifuge can minimize hazards associated with their use.

GUIDELINES FOR ELECTRICAL SAFETY

1. *Avoid* the use of extension cords.
2. *Do not* overload electrical circuits.
3. Inspect cords and plugs for breaks and fraying.
4. Unplug equipment when servicing, including when replacing a light bulb.
5. Unplug equipment that has had liquid spilled in it. Do not plug in again until the spill has been cleaned up and you are certain wiring is dry.
6. Unplug and do not use equipment that is malfunctioning.
7. *Do not* attempt to make repairs to equipment if you are not trained to do so.
8. *Do not* handle electrical equipment with wet hands or when standing on a wet floor.
9. Know the location of the circuit breaker box.
10. *Do not* touch electrical equipment in patient rooms, especially when in the process of drawing blood. Electrical shock could pass through the phlebotomist and the needle and shock the patient.

ACTIONS TO TAKE IF ELECTRICAL SHOCK OCCURS

1. Shut off the source of electricity.
2. If the source of electricity cannot be shut off, use nonconducting material (*eg,* hand inside a glass beaker) to remove the source of electricity from a victim.
3. Call for medical assistance.
4. Start cardiopulmonary resuscitation if indicated.
5. Keep the victim warm.

Fire Safety

All employees of any institution should be aware of procedures to follow in case of fire. They should know where fire extinguishers are located and be familiar with their use. They should also understand how to use fire blankets or heavy toweling to smother fires in clothing. In addition, they should be familiar with the location of emergency exits.

COMPONENTS OF FIRE

Three components, sometimes referred to as the fire triangle, are necessary for fire to occur. They are fuel, oxygen (or an oxidizing agent), and heat (or an ignition source).

CLASSES OF FIRE

Four classes of fire are recognized by the **National Fire Protection Association (NFPA)**. Classification depends on the fuel source of the fire. The four classes are as follows:

1. *Class A* fires occur with ordinary combustible materials such as wood, papers, or clothing. Class A fires require water or water-based solutions to cool or quench the fire in order to extinguish it.
2. *Class B* fires occur with flammable liquids and vapors such as paint, oil, grease, or gasoline. Class B fires require blocking the source of oxygen or smothering the fuel in order to extinguish the fire.
3. *Class C* fires occur with electrical equipment and require nonconducting agents to extinguish them.
4. *Class D* fires occur with combustible or reactive metals such as sodium, potassium, magnesium, and lithium. Class D fires require dry powder agents or sand to extinguish. They are the most difficult fires to control and frequently lead to explosions.

FIRE EXTINGUISHERS

There is a fire extinguisher class (Fig. 6-12) to correspond with each class of fire, except class D. Class D fires present unique problems and are best left to firefighting personnel to extinguish.

- *Class A extinguishers* use soda and acid or water to cool the fire.
- *Class B extinguishers* use foam, dry chemical, or carbon dioxide to smother the fire.
- *Class C extinguishers* use dry chemical, carbon dioxide, halon, or other nonconducting agents to smother the fire.
- *Class ABC (multipurpose) extinguishers* use dry chemical reagents to smother the fire. They can be used on Class A, B, and C fires and eliminate the confusion of having several different types of extinguishers. Multipurpose extinguishers are the type most frequently used in health care institutions.

DO'S AND DON'TS IF A FIRE OCCURS

- *Do* pull the nearest fire alarm.
- *Do* call the fire department.
- *Do* attempt to extinguish a small fire.
- *Do* close all doors and windows if leaving the area.
- *Do* smother a clothing fire with a fire blanket or have the person roll on the floor in an attempt to smother the fire.
- *Do* crawl to the nearest exit if there is heavy smoke present.
- *Don't* panic.
- *Don't* run.
- *Don't* use elevators.

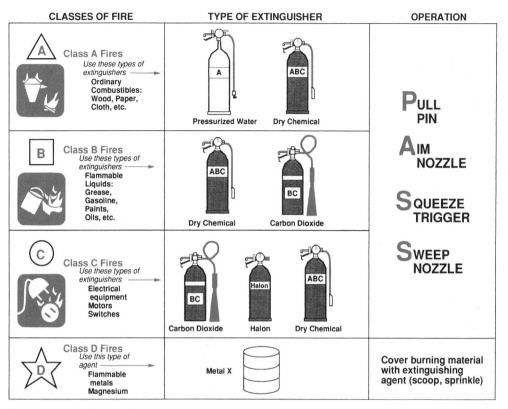

Figure 6-12   Classes of fire extinguishers. (Adapted with permission from the Environmental Health & Safety Department, The University of Texas, Houston, Health Science Center)

RACE

The NFPA code word for the order of action in the event of fire is RACE, where the letters stand for the following:

R = *Rescue* individuals in danger.
A = *Alarm:* sound the alarm.
C = *Confine* the fire by closing all doors and windows.
E = *Extinguish* the fire with the nearest suitable fire extinguisher.

Radiation Safety

The principles involved in radiation exposure are distance, shielding, and time. This means that the amount of radiation you are exposed to depends upon how far you are from the source of radioactivity, what protection you have from it, and how long you are exposed to it. Exposure time is important because radiation effects are cumulative.

A clearly posted **radiation hazard warning symbol** (Fig. 6-13) is required in areas where radioactive materials are used and on cabinet or refrigerator doors where radioactive materials are stored. In addition, radioactive reagents and specimens require

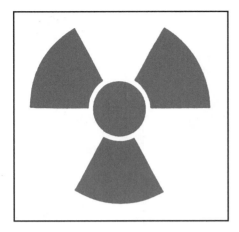

Figure 6-13   Radiation hazard symbol.

labeling with a radiation hazard symbol. A radiation hazard symbol on a patient's door signifies that a patient has been treated with radioactive isotopes.

The phlebotomist may encounter radiation hazards when collecting specimens from patients who have been injected with radioactive dyes, when collecting specimens from patients in the radiology department or nuclear medicine, and when delivering specimens to radioimmunoassay sections of the laboratory. The phlebotomist should be aware of institution radiation safety procedures. In addition, the phlebotomist should recognize the radiation hazard symbol and be cautious when entering areas displaying it. Because radiation is particularly hazardous to a fetus, pregnant employees should avoid areas displaying the radiation symbol and patients who have recently been injected with radioactive dyes.

Chemical Safety

The phlebotomist may come in contact with hazardous chemicals when using cleaning reagents, adding preservatives to 24-hour urine containers, or delivering specimens to the laboratory. Inappropriate use of chemicals can have dangerous consequences. For example, mixing bleach with other cleaning compounds can release dangerous gases. In addition, many chemicals are acids, such as the HCl used as a urine preservative, or alkalis, which can cause severe burns. Container labels provide important information regarding the nature of the contents and should always be read carefully before use.

GENERAL RULES FOR CHEMICAL SAFETY

1. *Always* wear proper protective clothing, including lab coat, apron, gloves, and safety goggles, when working with chemicals.
2. *Always* use proper chemical clean-up materials when cleaning up chemical spills.
3. *Never* store chemicals above eye level.
4. *Never* add water to acid.
5. *Never* indiscriminately mix chemicals together.
6. *Never* store chemicals in unlabeled containers.
7. *Never* pour chemicals into dirty containers, especially containers previously used to store other chemicals.
8. *Never* use chemicals in ways other than their intended use.

IDENTIFICATION OF CHEMICALS
OSHA Hazardous Communication (HazCom) Standard

Labeling of hazardous materials is required by the **OSHA Hazardous Communication (HazCom) Standard**. Labeling format may be different for each manufacturer; however, chemical manufacturers must comply with the labeling requirements set by the Manufacturers Chemical Association (MCA). Labels for hazardous chemicals must contain a statement of warning such as "danger" or "poison"; a statement of the hazard (*eg*, toxic, flammable, or combustible) and precautions to eliminate risk; and first aid measures in the event of a spill or other exposure.

Material Safety Data Sheets

In addition to labeling, the OSHA HazCom standard requires manufacturers to supply **material safety data sheets (MSDS)** for their products. An MSDS contains general information as well as precautionary and emergency information for the product. All products with a hazardous warning on the label require an MSDS to help assure that products will be used safely and as intended. Because the OSHA HazCom Standard includes this labeling requirement, it has become known as the "right to know" law.

Department of Transportation Labeling System

Hazardous materials may have additional labels of precaution, including a Department of Transportation (DOT) symbol incorporating a United Nations hazard classification number and symbol (Table 6-4). The DOT labeling system uses a diamond-shaped warning sign (Fig. 6-14) containing the United Nations hazard class number, the hazard class designation or four-digit identification number, and a symbol representing the hazard.

National Fire Protection Association Labeling System

Another hazardous material rating system was developed by the NFPA (Fig. 6-15) to label areas where hazardous chemicals and other materials are stored, thus alerting firefighters in the event of a fire. This system uses a diamond-shaped symbol divided into four quadrants. Health hazards are indicated in a blue diamond on the left; the level of fire hazard is indicated in the upper quadrant in a red diamond; stability or reactivity hazards are indicated in a yellow diamond on the right; and other specific hazards are indicated in a white quadrant on the bottom.

SAFETY SHOWERS AND EYE WASH STATIONS

The phlebotomist should know the location of and be instructed in the use of safety showers and eye wash stations (Fig. 6-16) in the event of a chemical spill or splash to the eyes or other body parts. The eyes or other body parts affected should be flushed with water for a minimum of 15 minutes, followed by a visit to the emergency room for evaluation.

CHEMICAL SPILL PROCEDURES

Chemical spills require clean-up using special kits (Fig. 6-17) containing absorbent and neutralizer materials. The type of materials used depends upon the type of chemical spilled. An indicator in the clean-up materials detects when the materials have been neutralized and are safe for disposal. Disposal of chemicals is regulated by the **Environmental Protection Agency (EPA)**.

Table 6-4
Placard Recognition Information

United Nations Hazard Class	Symbol	Background Color	Examples
Class 1 Explosives	Bursting ball	Orange	Fireworks Ammunition Dynamite
Class 2 Gases (compressed, liquified, or dissolved under pressure)	Flame	*Flammable* Red	Flammable: Butane Propane
	Cylinder	*Nonflammable* Green	Nonflammable: Ammonia Chlorine
Class 3 Flammable liquids	Flame	Red	Brake fluid Camphor oil Glycol ethers Gasoline
Class 4 Flammable solids or substances	Flame	*Flammable Solid* Red and white vertical stripes	Lithium Magnesium Phosphorus Titanium
	Slashed W	*Water-Reactive Materials* Red and white vertical stripes with blue top quadrant	
Class 5 Division 5.1: oxidizing substances	Circle with flame	Yellow	Ammonium nitrate Benzoyl peroxide Calcium chlorite
Division 5.2: organic peroxides			
Class 6 Poisonous and infectious substances	Skull with crossbones	White	Chemical mace Pesticides Cyanide AIDS specimens
Class 7 Radioactive materials	Propeller	Yellow over white	Cobalt 14 Plutonium Radioactive waste Uranium 235

(continued)

Table 6-4 (Continued)

United Nations Hazard Class	Symbol	Background Color	Examples
Class 8 Corrosives	Test tube over hand Test tube over metal	White over black	Caustic potash Caustic soda Hydrochloric acid Sulfuric acid
Class 9 Miscellaneous dangerous substances	ORM-A ORM-B ORM-C ORM-D ORM-E	White	ORM-A: dry ice ORM-B: quick lime ORM-C: sawdust ORM-D: hair spray ORM-E: hazardous waste

FIRST AID PROCEDURES

Ability to recognize and react quickly and skillfully to emergency situations may mean the difference between life and death for a victim.

External Hemorrhage

Control of hemorrhage (abnormal bleeding) from an obvious wound is most effectively accomplished by elevating the affected part above the level of the heart and applying direct pressure to the wound. However, do not attempt to elevate a broken

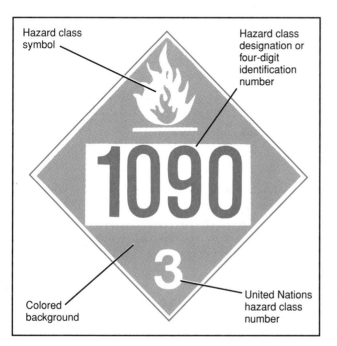

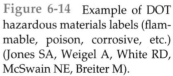

Figure 6-14 Example of DOT hazardous materials labels (flammable, poison, corrosive, etc.) (Jones SA, Weigel A, White RD, McSwain NE, Breiter M).

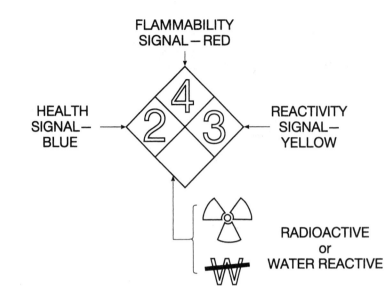

Identification of Health Hazard Color Code: BLUE		Identification of Flammability Color Code: RED		Identification of Reactivity (Stability) Color Code: YELLOW	
	Type of Possible Injury		Susceptibility of Materials to Burning		Susceptibility to Release of Energy
Signal		Signal		Signal	
4	Materials that on very short exposure could cause death or major residual injury even though prompt medical treatment was given.	**4**	Materials that will rapidly or completely vaporize at atmospheric pressure and normal ambient temperature, or that are readily dispersed in air and that will burn readily.	**4**	Materials that in themselves are readily capable of detonation or of explosive decomposition or reaction at normal temperatures and pressures.
3	Materials that on short exposure could cause serious temporary or residual injury even though prompt medical treatment was given.	**3**	Liquids and solids that can be ignited under almost all ambient temperature conditions.	**3**	Materials that in themselves are capable of detonation or explosive reaction but require a strong initiating source or that must be heated under confinement before initiation or that react explosively with water.
2	Materials that on intense or continued exposure could cause temporary incapacitation or possible residual injury unless prompt medical treatment is given.	**2**	Materials that must be moderately heated or exposed to relatively high ambient temperatures before ignition can occur.	**2**	Materials that in themselves are normally unstable and readily undergo violent chemical change but do not detonate. Also materials that may react violently with water or that may form potentially explosive mixtures with water.
1	Materials that on exposure would cause irritation but only minor residual injury even if no treatment is given.	**1**	Materials that must be preheated before ignition can occur.	**1**	Materials that in themselves are normally stable, but that can become unstable at elevated temperatures and pressures or that may react with water with some release of energy, but not violently.
0	Materials that on exposure under fire conditions would offer no hazard beyond that of ordinary combustible material.	**0**	Materials that will not burn.	**0**	Materials that in themselves are normally stable, even under fire exposure conditions, and that are not reactive with water.

Figure 6-15   National Fire Protection Association 704 marking system.

extremity. Pressure should be applied using a clean cloth or compress. If the compress should become soaked with blood, a new compress should be placed over the original. The original compress should not be removed as removal may disrupt the clotting process.

If applying pressure over the site is ineffective in controlling bleeding, such as may be the case with a very large injury, apply strong finger pressure over the pressure point of the main artery supplying the area. *Avoid* use of a tourniquet to control bleeding. A tourniquet should only be used as a last resort to save a patient's life after all other means to control bleeding are unsuccessful, such as may occur with an avulsion (amputation) or a severely mangled or crushed body part.

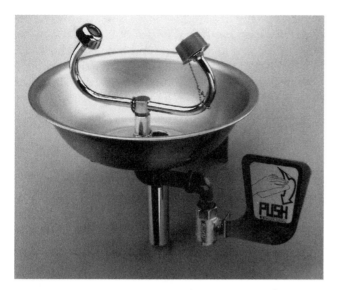

Figure 6-16 Eyewash station. (Courtesy Speakman Co., Wilmington, DE.)

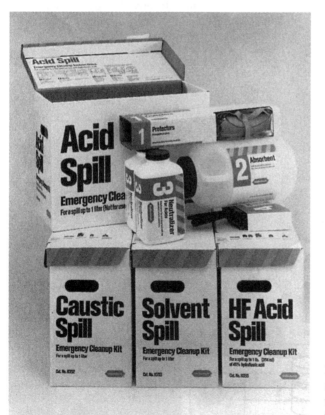

Figure 6-17 Spill cleanup kit. (Photo courtesy of Scientific Products Division, Baxter Healthcare Corporation.)

Shock

A state of shock results when there is insufficient return of blood flow to the heart, resulting in inadequate supply of oxygen to all organs and tissues of the body. Numerous conditions including hemorrhage, heart attack, trauma, and drug reactions can lead to some degree of shock. Because shock can be a life-threatening situation, it is important that the symptoms be recognized and dealt with immediately.

COMMON SYMPTOMS OF SHOCK

- Pale, cold, clammy skin
- Rapid, weak pulse
- Increased, shallow breathing rate
- Expressionless face and staring eyes

FIRST AID FOR SHOCK

1. Maintain an open airway for the victim.
2. Call for assistance.
3. Keep the victim lying down with the head lower than the rest of the body.
4. Attempt to control bleeding or other cause of shock if known.
5. Keep the victim warm.

Never give fluids if the patient is unconscious or semiconscious or has injuries likely to require surgery and anesthesia.

CARDIOPULMONARY RESUSCITATION

Most health care institutions require their personnel to be certified in **cardiopulmonary resuscitation (CPR)**. CPR instruction generally includes instruction in recognizing and treating foreign body airway obstruction (choking) and rescue breathing as well as CPR (Fig. 6-18). There are five different courses in CPR offered by the

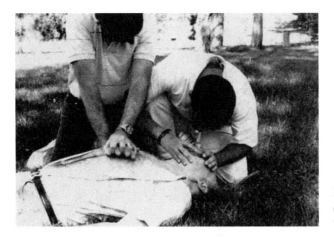

Figure 6-18 Two rescuers synchronize chest compression and ventilation.

American Heart Association. The "C" course is required for health care personnel. Certification must be renewed every 2 years. Most phlebotomy programs require CPR certification as a prerequisite or corequisite or include it as part of the course.

Study & Review Questions

1. Which of the following situations involves a nosocomial infection?
   a. A patient admitted to the hospital with a severe urinary tract infection
   b. An employee who contracts HBV infection from a needlestick
   c. A patient in ICU whose surgical wound is infected
   d. A baby in the nursery with congenital herpes

2. Reverse isolation may be used for
   a. a pediatric patient with measles.
   b. an adult patient with the flu.
   c. a patient with a urinary tract infection.
   d. a patient with severe burns.

3. The single most important means of preventing the spread of infection is
   a. proper handwashing.
   b. wearing a mask.
   c. wearing gloves.
   d. Nosocomial infections cannot be prevented.

4. Safe working conditions for employees are mandated by
   a. CDC.
   b. OSHA.
   c. CAP.
   d. ASCP.

5. The most frequently occurring lab-acquired infection is
   a. HBV infection.
   b. HIV infection.
   c. syphilis.
   d. tuberculosis.

6. Electrical safety involves
   a. distance, time, and shielding.
   b. knowing where the fire extinguishers are.
   c. knowing the circuit breaker box locations.
   d. none of the above.

7. In the event of a chemical splash in the eye, the first thing the victim should do is
   a. go to the emergency room.
   b. call the paramedics.
   c. wipe the eye with a tissue.
   d. immediately flush the eye with water for 15 minutes.

Suggested Laboratory Activities

1. Practice proper handwashing procedures.

2. Practice the proper way to put on and remove gloves.

3. Touch your hand to a blood agar plate after touching various surfaces or before and after handwashing. Incubate the plates overnight and observe growth of microorganisms.

4. Examine safety equipment such as face shields, goggles, and splash guards.

5. Determine the location of fire extinguishers and other safety equipment in your laboratory, as well as other areas of your facility.

6. Write an exposure control plan for the student laboratory.

BIBLIOGRAPHY AND SUGGESTED READINGS

Davis, B., Bishop, M. L., & Mass, D. (1989). *Clinical laboratory science: Strategies for practice.* Philadelphia: J. B. Lippincott.

Department of Health and Human Services, Centers for Disease Control and Prevention. (1994). *Guidelines for preventing transmission of Mycobacterium tuberculosis in health-care facilities.*

Grime, D., Grime, R., & Hamelink, M. (1991). *Infectious diseases.* St. Louis: Mosby Clinical Nursing Series.

National Committee for Clinical Laboratory Standards, M29-T2. (1992). *Protection of laboratory workers from infectious disease transmitted by blood, body fluids and tissue* (2nd ed.). Villanova, PA: NCCLS Tentative Guideline.

Occupational Safety and Health Administration (1991). *Occupational exposure to bloodborne pathogens: Final Rule.* 29CFR Part 1910.1030.

OSHA compliance encyclopedia. (Vol. III). (July 1992). Madison, CT: Business and Legal Reports.

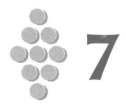

7

Blood Collection Equipment and Supplies

KEY TERMS

additive	bevel	gauge	thixotropic gel
anticoagulant	butterfly needle	glycolysis	separator
antiglycolytic	clot activator	lumen	tube additive
agent	disinfectants	order of draw	winged infusion
antiseptics	evacuated tubes	sharps container	set

OBJECTIVES

Upon successful completion of this chapter, the reader will be able to:

1. List the equipment and supplies needed to collect blood by venipuncture.
2. Contrast antiseptics and disinfectants.
3. Explain the purpose of using a tourniquet for venipuncture; name and describe the various types of tourniquets.
4. List and describe evacuated tube and syringe system components.
5. Identify types of additives used in blood collection and the color coding associated with each type of additive.
6. Describe the principle behind, and list the order of draw for the evacuated tube system and the syringe system.

GENERAL BLOOD COLLECTION EQUIPMENT

The primary duty of the phlebotomist is to collect blood specimens for laboratory analysis. Blood is collected by several means, including arterial puncture, skin puncture, and venipuncture. The following are general equipment and supplies commonly needed regardless of the method used to obtain the specimen.

Blood-Drawing Station

A blood-drawing station is a special area of the laboratory equipped for performing phlebotomy procedures on patients, primarily outpatients. (Outpatients are patients who are not hospitalized and who have been sent by their doctors to the laboratory to have blood tests performed.)

As a minimum, a blood-drawing station includes a table for supplies and a special phlebotomy chair (Fig. 7-1) for the patient. The table should be a convenient height for the phlebotomist to work from, with enough space to hold supplies for numerous phlebotomy procedures. The chair should be comfortable for the patient and have an adjustable armrest to achieve proper arm positioning. There should be a safety device to lock the armrest in place to prevent the patient from falling out should he or she become faint.

There should be a bed or reclining chair available for patients with a history of fainting, persons donating blood, and other special situations. A reclining chair does not require a locking armrest. A bed or padded table is also needed for performing heelsticks or other procedures on infants and small children.

Carts and Trays

The use of carts and trays makes blood-drawing equipment portable. This is especially important in a hospital setting and other instances where the patient cannot come to the lab.

Carts are made of stainless steel or strong synthetic material. They have swivel wheels, which glide the carts smoothly and quietly down hospital hallways and in and out of elevators. They normally have several shelves to carry adequate supplies for obtaining blood specimens from many patients. Carts are commonly used for early morning phlebotomy rounds when many patients need lab work and for scheduled "sweeps" (rounds which occur at regular intervals throughout the day). Because carts

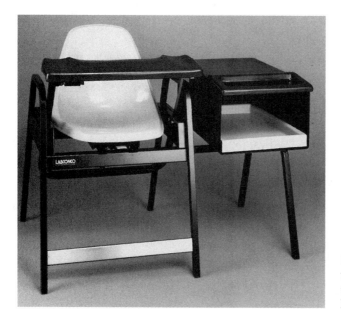

Figure 7-1 Phlebotomy chair with attached storage unit. (Courtesy Lab Conco, Kansas City, MO.)

can transmit nosocomial infections, they are not normally brought into patient rooms. Instead, they are parked outside in the hallway. In order to have extra supplies, as well as a container for needle disposal at the bedside as required by the Occupational Safety and Health Administration (OSHA), a tray of supplies to be taken into the room is often carried on the cart.

Phlebotomy trays (Fig. 7-2) come in a variety of styles and sizes designed to be easily carried by the phlebotomist and to contain enough equipment for numerous blood draws. They are convenient for "stat" or emergency situations or when relatively few patients need blood work. Trays are often part of the equipment on a phlebotomy cart.

Making certain carts and trays are adequately stocked is an important duty of the phlebotomist.

Gloves

Standard precautions guidelines by the Centers for Disease Control and Prevention (CDC) and the Hospital Infection Control Practices Advisory Committee (HICPAC), as well as regulations by OSHA, require the wearing of gloves when performing phlebotomy procedures (see Chap. 6). A new pair of gloves must be used for each patient and removed when the procedure is completed. Nonsterile, disposable latex, vinyl, or polyethylene examination gloves are acceptable for most phlebotomy procedures. A good fit is essential. Some gloves come lightly dusted with powder to make them more comfortable to wear and easier to slip on and off. However, the phlebotomist should be aware that glove powder can be a source of contamination for some tests, especially those collected by skin puncture. Cotton glove liners designed to be worn under latex or plastic gloves are available for persons who develop allergies or dermatitis from wearing gloves. The quality of gloves is regulated by the Food and Drug Administration (FDA).

Antiseptics and Disinfectants

Antiseptics are substances or solutions used to prevent **sepsis**, a disease state resulting from the presence of microorganisms or their toxic products in the bloodstream. Antiseptics are bacteriostatic, that is, they prevent or inhibit the growth of bacteria. They are safe for use on human skin and are used to clean the skin prior to

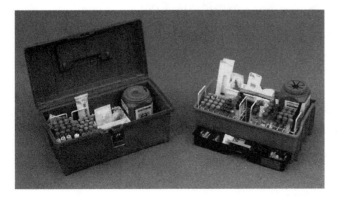

Figure 7-2 Two styles of phlebotomy trays: covered phlebotomy tray and phlebotomy tray with drawer. (Post Medical Inc., Atlanta, GA.)

venipuncture or skin puncture. Antiseptics used for blood collection include the following:

- 70% Isopropyl alcohol (isopropanol): the most common antiseptic used for routine blood collection, usually in the form of individually wrapped prep pads.
- Povidone–iodine: in several forms, including swab sticks and sponge pads for blood culture collection, and prep pads for blood gas collection.
- 0.5% Chlorhexidine gluconate: often used for those allergic to iodine.
- Benzalkonium chloride (*eg*, Zephiran Chloride): alternate antiseptic.

Disinfectants are bacteriocidal (kill bacteria). They are used on surfaces and instruments. They are not safe for use on human skin. Household bleach (5.25% sodium hypochlorite) in a 1:10 solution will kill the viruses causing AIDS and hepatitis and is commonly used to wipe surfaces and clean up blood spills.

Gauze Pads and Cotton Balls

Clean 2×2 inch gauze pads folded in fourths are used to hold pressure over the site following venipuncture or skin puncture. Special gauze pads with plastic backing are available to help prevent contamination of gloves from blood at the venipuncture site. Cotton (or synthetic, *eg*, Dacron) balls may be used to hold pressure, especially if the patient has dermatitis. A disadvantage of cotton balls is they have a tendency to stick to the site and re-initiate bleeding when removed.

Bandages

Adhesive bandages are used to cover the site once the bleeding has ceased. Paper, cloth, or knitted tape over a folded gauze square can also be used, especially for patients who are allergic to adhesive bandages. Two-inch-wide roll gauze or self adhesive gauze such as Coban (a special type of gauze that sticks to itself but not the skin) is occasionally used over a gauze pad or cotton ball to form a pressure bandage following arterial puncture or for patients with bleeding problems. Bandages are not to be used on babies younger than 2 years of age because of the danger of aspiration and suffocation.

Needle and Sharps Disposal Containers

Used needles, lancets, and other sharp objects must be disposed of immediately in special containers usually referred to as **"sharps" containers** (Fig. 7-3). A variety of styles and sizes are available from manufacturers. They are usually red or bright orange in color for easy identification and are also marked "biohazard." Containers must be rigid, puncture-resistant, leak-proof, disposable, and easily sealed when full. Those selected for phlebotomy use should contain a device to aid in removing needles from evacuated tube adapters. (See Evacuated Tube System for special needle disposal systems and containers.)

Slides

Precleaned 25×75 mm (1×3 inch) glass microscope slides are used to make blood films for hematology determinations. Slides are available either plain or with a frosted area at one end where the patient's name or other information can be written in pencil.

Pen

A phlebotomist should always carry a pen with indelible or nonsmear ink to label tubes and record other patient information.

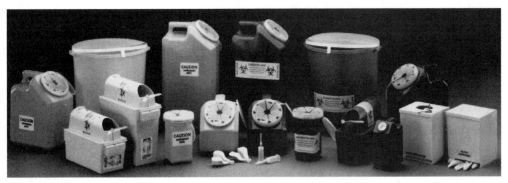

Figure 7-3 Several styles of sharps containers. (Courtesy of PRO TEC Containers, Inc., Irvine, CA.)

Watch

A watch, preferably with a sweep second hand or timer, is needed by the phlebotomist to determine specimen collection times accurately and time special tests.

ARTERIAL PUNCTURE EQUIPMENT

See Chapter 11.

SKIN PUNCTURE EQUIPMENT

See Chapter 10.

VENIPUNCTURE EQUIPMENT

In addition to the general blood collection supplies and equipment, venipuncture procedures require the use of the following special equipment.

Vein Locating Device

A transilluminator device such as the Venoscope (Fig. 7-4) is an optional but useful tool in locating veins that are difficult to see or feel. The Venoscope uses fiberoptic arms to deliver a halogen light source that illuminates the subcutaneous tissue of the venipuncture site. When the area is illuminated, veins stand out as dark lines between the fiberoptic arms. The Venoscope can be strapped to the patient's arm to illuminate the vein while venipuncture is performed. Pads or "skids" on the ends of the fiberoptic arms are disposable to minimize the possibility of infection transmission.

Tourniquet

A tourniquet (Fig. 7-5) is applied to a patient's arm prior to venipuncture. Tourniquet application causes the veins to enlarge, making them easier to find and penetrate with a needle. Tourniquets are available in adult and pediatric sizes.

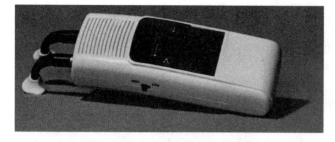

Figure 7-4 Venoscope® trans-illuminator. (Applied Biotech, Lafayette, LA.)

The most commonly used tourniquet is a flat strip of stretchable latex, 15 to 18 inches long. A length of latex Penrose drain tubing can also be used. Latex does not readily support bacterial growth and if soiled can easily be wiped clean with disinfectant. Inexpensive disposable latex tourniquets are available. These can be used more than once, but are normally thrown away if they become contaminated with blood.

A blood pressure cuff may be used in place of a tourniquet by those familiar with its operation. The patient's blood pressure is taken and the pressure is then maintained below the patient's diastolic pressure.

Velcro-closure tourniquets are also available. They usually are made of elastic material with a long band of Velcro to allow a wide range of adjustment capability. A disadvantage of Velcro tourniquets is that they may not fit around the arms of extremely obese patients. In addition, it is not easily cleaned when soiled with blood or otherwise contaminated.

Another type of tourniquet, called a Seraket tourniquet, is made of cloth webbing and has a buckle closure. This type stays on the patient's arm when released and can be tightened again if necessary. A disadvantage of this type, as with the Velcro tourniquet, is that it is not easily cleaned.

Needles

Needles used for phlebotomy include **multisample needles** (see Evacuated Tube System), **hypodermic needles** (see Syringe System), and **winged infusion**

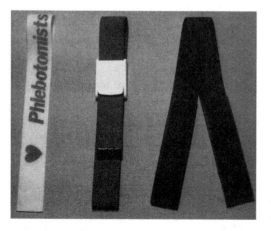

Figure 7-5 Several types of tourniquets (left to right): latex strap, Seraket®, and velcro closure.

(butterfly) needles (used with both the evacuated tube system and the syringe system). All blood-drawing needles are sterile, disposable, and for single use only. They are silicon coated, which enables them to penetrate the skin smoothly. The end of the needle that is inserted into the vein is called the **bevel** because it is "beveled" or cut on a slant to allow the needle to penetrate the vein easily and prevent coring (removal of a portion of the skin or vein). The long, cylindrical portion is called the **shaft**, and the end that connects to the blood-drawing apparatus is referred to as the **hub**.

The **gauge** of a needle indicates the size of the needle and refers to the diameter of the **lumen** (internal space) or "bore" of the needle. The diameter of the needle and the gauge number have an inverse (opposite) relationship, that is, the larger the gauge number, the smaller the actual diameter of the needle. Gauge selection depends upon the size and condition of the patient's vein.

Evacuated Tube System

The most common and preferred system for collecting blood samples is the **evacuated tube system** (Fig. 7-6). This system consists of a special blood-drawing needle attached to a plastic holder in which evacuated (vacuum) tubes are placed when collecting a blood specimen. It is a closed system in which the patient's blood goes directly from

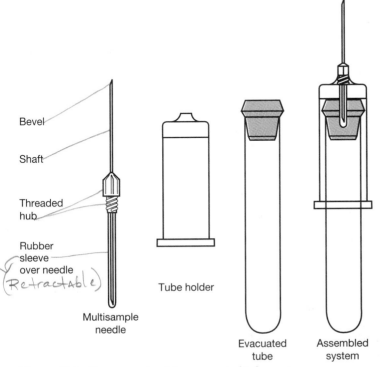

Bevel

Shaft

Threaded hub

Rubber sleeve over needle *(Retractable)*

Multisample needle

Tube holder

Evacuated tube

Assembled system

Figure 7-6 Components of the evacuated tube system.

the vein into a stoppered tube without being exposed to the air. The evacuated tube system allows numerous tubes to be collected using a single venipuncture. Evacuated tube collection systems are available from several manufacturers. Mixing components from different manufacturers may lead to problems, such as needles coming unscrewed and tubes popping off during venipuncture procedures. To avoid problems and ensure proper needle fit and smooth removal of tubes, it is necessary for all components of the system to be from the same manufacturer.

EVACUATED TUBE SYSTEM COMPONENTS

Needles.   Evacuated tube system needles (see Fig. 7-6) are threaded in the middle and have a beveled point on each end. One end is used to pierce the skin and enter the vein; the other end penetrates the rubber stopper of a collection tube. The threaded portion allows easy and secure attachment to a tube holder. The end of the needle that penetrates the vein is longer and has a longer bevel. The end of the needle that penetrates the stopper of the collecting tube has a retractable rubber sleeve or sheath, which covers it when the tube is removed. This feature prevents leakage of blood when changing tubes during a multiple-tube draw, as well as when the tube is removed prior to withdrawing the needle from the vein. Because multiple tubes of blood can be drawn during a single venipuncture using evacuated tube system needles, they are called **multisample needles**. Single-sample needles (needles without the retractable sleeve) are available, but are rarely used for phlebotomy, even for single-tube draws, because they allow blood to leak into the holder unless the needle is withdrawn from the vein while the tube is still attached.

Evacuated tube system needles come in two lengths: 1 inch and 1½ inches. Length selection depends primarily upon user preference and also the depth of the vein. Many phlebotomists prefer to use the 1-inch needle in routine situations because it is less intimidating to the patient. It is also less intimidating to a phlebotomy student. However, some phlebotomists feel that the 1½-inch needle allows for easier placement of the anchoring thumb. Evacuated tube system needles are available in sizes from 20 to 22 gauge, with 21 gauge most commonly used for routine venipuncture.

Needles come enclosed in sealed twist-apart shields to ensure sterility; they should *not* be used if the seal is already broken. The shields are color-coded by the manufacturer according to gauge for easy identification.

Needle and tube holders.   The needle and tube **holder** (Fig. 7-7A), sometimes referred to as an **adapter**, is a clear, plastic cylinder with a small opening at one end to receive the threaded needle. There is a large opening at the other end to receive the evacuated blood-drawing tube. There are flanges (extensions) on the sides of the tube end of the holder to aid in tube placement and removal.

Holders come in at least two sizes, one for regular-diameter tubes and a smaller one for small-diameter tubes used for pediatric patients or difficult draws. It is important to use the proper holder for the size of the tube. Some manufacturers supply tube adapter inserts so that small tubes may be used with the regular-sized holder. Special holders are available for drawing blood culture bottles (see Fig. 7-7B). Some have adapter inserts which allow collection of evacuated tubes after collecting blood culture specimens (see Fig. 7-7C).

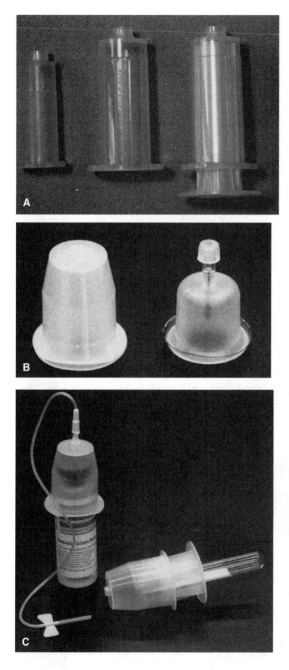

Figure 7-7 (**A**) Needle and tube holders (left to right): pediatric tube holder, regular size tube holder, and regular size tube holder with pediatric tube adapter insert; (**B**) Two styles of blood culture bottle holders: *Left*, blood culture holder from Organon Teknika Corp, Durham, NC; *Right*, the Angel Wing multiple-sample transfer set, Luer adapter holder from Sherwood Medical, St. Louis, MO; (**C**) Blood culture bottle holder and butterfly needle attached to blood culture bottles and the same style holder with adapter insert and evacuated tube.

Safety needle holders.   Special holders designed to reduce the risk of accidental needle sticks are available (Fig. 7-8). The PRO-JECT safety needle holder (PRO-TEC, Irvine, CA) (see Fig. 7-8A)has a special release mechanism that allows the user to release the needle into the needle container without unscrewing it from the holder. This prevents injuries associated with needle disposal caused by the needle slipping out of the holder while being unscrewed or the needle being stuck in the holder with the rubber guard end pointed up. It will not, however, protect the user from injuries associated with dropping the needle before disposal.

Two other holders, the Saf-T-Clik (Ryan Medical, Winfield Industries, San Diego, CA) (see Fig. 7-8B) and the Venipuncture Needle-Pro (SIMS, Inc., Keene, NH) (see Fig. 7-8C) have protective devices that cover the needle after use. The Saf-T-Clik has a locking shield that the user slides over the needle after use. The Venipuncture Needle-Pro has a locking shield that is pushed over the needle using the index finger. These holders, however, are not reusable and require a large needle disposal container to accommodate the increased bulk created by the holder, which produces much more waste than the needle by itself.

Needle disposal systems.   Several manufacturers have developed needle removal systems with safety in mind (Fig. 7-9). The Safety-Gard Phlebotomy System (Becton Dickinson Vacutainer Systems, Franklin Lakes, NJ) (see Fig. 7-9A and B) features a special reusable holder with a protective shield that the user can single-handedly slide over the needle and lock in place after the needle is withdrawn from the vein, providing immediate protection from accidental needle puncture. The needle holder is designed to be used with a Safety-Gard Needle Disposal Container (see Fig. 7-9C). When the shielded needle is safely inserted into a special mechanism in the disposal container, the protective sheath can be retracted and the needle removed with a twisting motion. Once the needle has been removed, the holder is ready to be used again.

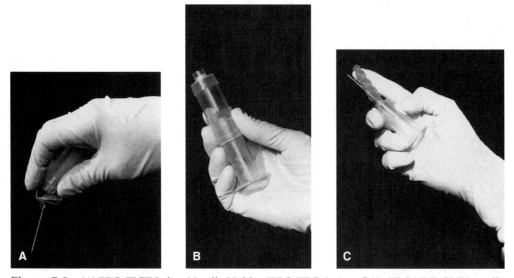

Figure 7-8   (**A**) PRO-JECT Safety Needle Holder (PRO-TEC, Irvine, CA); (**B**) SAF-T-CLIK needle holder (Ryan Medical, Winfield Industries, San Diego, CA); (**C**) Venipuncture Needle-Pro (SIMS, Inc., Keene, NH).

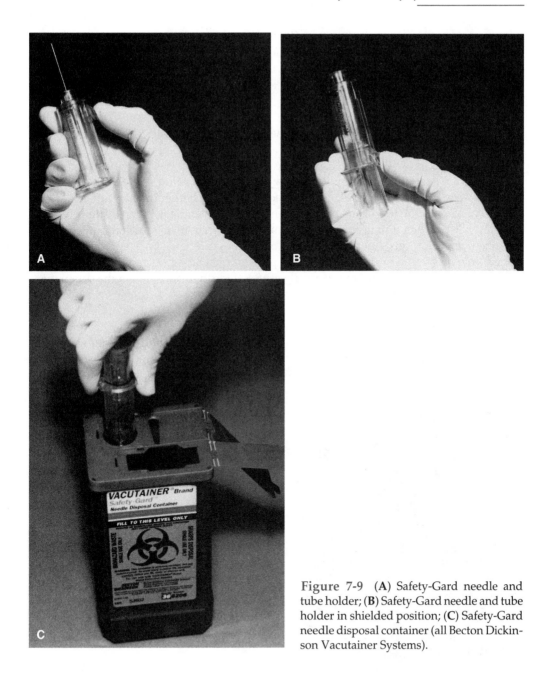

Figure 7-9 (**A**) Safety-Gard needle and tube holder; (**B**) Safety-Gard needle and tube holder in shielded position; (**C**) Safety-Gard needle disposal container (all Becton Dickinson Vacutainer Systems).

Another system, the Auto Drop needle holder and disposal container system (Sage Products, Crystal Lake, IL) (Fig. 7-10), has a special tube holder with a device that allows the user to eject the needle from the holder automatically. The needle can also be removed automatically by inserting the needle and holder into a special well in the top of the disposal container. Either method minimizes the chance of needle sticks associated with the needle removal process.

The A.N.D. (Automatic Needle Disconnect Containment System, Post Medical, Inc., Atlanta, GA) (Fig. 7-11) was designed to allow safe one-handed removal of evacuated tube system needles without the use of a special tube holder. Separate needle containment units are available for use with Becton Dickinson, Terumo, and Sherwood brand blood collection needles. A needle is removed from a tube holder by inserting it in a special mechanism in the top of the containment unit. The needle is given a slight twist to the left while pushing down, engaging the automatic mechanism which removes it from the tube holder. Lancets, Luer needles, and butterflies can be disposed of manually in a slotted hole on the top of the container. To prevent overfilling (a leading cause of accidental needle sticks), the automatic needle removal mechanism locks in the down position when the container reaches maximum safe capacity.

Evacuated Tubes

Evacuated tubes are used with both the evacuated tube system and the syringe method of obtaining blood specimens. With the evacuated tube system, the blood is collected directly into the tube during the venipuncture procedure. With the

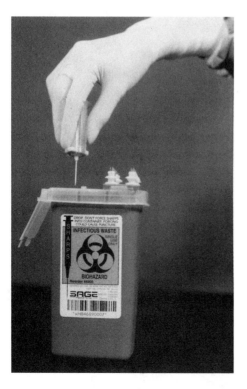

Figure 7-10 Auto Drop needle disposal system. (Sage Products, Inc., Crystal Lake, IL.)

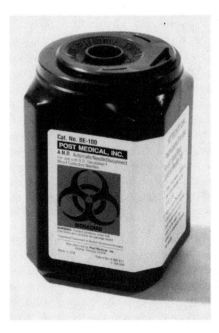

Figure 7-11   A.N.D. Automatic Needle Disconnect Containment System. (Courtesy Post Medical, Inc., Atlanta, GA.)

syringe method, the blood from the syringe must be transferred into the tubes after collection.

Evacuated tubes fill with blood automatically because of a vacuum that exists inside the tube. The amount of vacuum is premeasured so that the tube will draw a precise amount of blood. A tube that has lost its vacuum will not fill with blood. Tube vacuum is guaranteed by the manufacturer until the expiration date printed on the tube label; however, premature loss of vacuum can occur from opening the tube, dropping the tube, advancing the tube too far onto the needle holder prior to venipuncture, or pulling the needle bevel partially out of the skin during venipuncture.

Evacuated tubes are made of glass or plastic and come in sizes ranging from 2 to 15 mL. The size is selected according to the age of the patient, the amount of blood needed for the test, and the size and condition of the patient's vein. Some evacuated tubes, especially those for serum determinations, are coated on the inside with silicon to help prevent destruction of red blood cells and to keep the blood from sticking to the sides of the tube. Tubes for coagulation studies are coated with silicon to prevent activation of the clotting factors.

Evacuated tubes may or may not contain additives. Blood collected in tubes without additives will clot and yield serum on centrifugation. Tubes that contain additives may or may not clot, depending on the type of additive they contain.

TUBE ADDITIVES

A **tube additive** is any substance placed within a tube other than the coating of the tube or tube stopper (closure). The amount of additive in a tube is designed to function optimally with the amount of blood required to fill the tube. It is, therefore, important that additive tubes be filled until the vacuum is exhausted. They should also be inverted 5 to 8 times immediately after collection to ensure adequate mixing of the additive with the specimen. Tubes containing freeze-dried or powdered additive should be lightly tapped prior to use to settle the additive to the bottom of the tube. Additives have specific functions. The most common additives are categorized as follows.

Anticoagulants. An **anticoagulant** is a substance that prevents blood from coagulating or clotting. Anticoagulants prevent coagulation by either of two methods: chelating (binding) or precipitating calcium and making it unavailable for the coagulation process; or inhibiting formation of the thrombin needed to convert fibrinogen to fibrin.

Tubes containing anticoagulants yield whole blood specimens which are sometimes separated by centrifugation to yield plasma. The most common anticoagulants include the following:

- *Ethylenediaminetetraacetic acid (EDTA).* **EDTA** is commonly available in a dipotassium (K_2) or disodium (Na_2) freeze-dried powder, or a tripotassium (K_3) liquid base. EDTA prevents coagulation by binding or chelating calcium in the form of a potassium or sodium salt. EDTA is the anticoagulant of choice for whole blood hematology studies because it preserves cell morphology and inhibits platelet aggregation or clumping. Because the cells and plasma will separate if the specimen is allowed to stand undisturbed, the specimen must be mixed for a minimum of 2 minutes prior to performing the test. In addition, blood smears for hematology studies must be made within 1 hour of collection in EDTA because prolonged contact with the anticoagulant may change the staining characteristics of the formed elements. EDTA is contained in lavender stopper tubes and royal blue stopper tubes with lavender labels.
- *Heparin.* There are three **heparin** formulations: ammonium, lithium, and sodium heparin. Heparin prevents coagulation by inhibiting the conversion of prothrombin to thrombin. Heparin is the anticoagulant of choice for plasma chemistry determinations and is often used for stat chemistry determinations to save the time required for a serum specimen to clot. Heparin is contained in green stopper tubes and royal blue stopper tubes with green labels.
- *Sodium citrate.* **Sodium citrate** prevents coagulation by binding calcium. Sodium citrate is the anticoagulant of choice for coagulation studies because it best preserves the coagulation factors. Coagulation studies are performed on plasma. Sodium citrate tubes have light blue stoppers.
- *Potassium or ammonium oxalate.* **Potassium** and **ammonium oxalate** prevent coagulation by precipitating calcium. Oxalate along with an antiglycolytic agent (see below) is often used to collect plasma for glucose testing. Oxalate tubes have gray stoppers.

Special anticoagulants. Some anticoagulants have additional properties for special use situations. These anticoagulants include the following:

- *Acid citrate dextrose (ACD).* ACD solution prevents coagulation by binding calcium. The dextrose acts as both a red blood cell nutrient and a preservative by maintaining red cell viability. ACD solution is used for certain immunohematology tests such as paternity and transplant compatibility testing. ACD-containing tubes have yellow stoppers.

- *Sodium polyanethol sulfonate (SPS).* SPS prevents coagulation by binding calcium. It is used for blood culture collection because, in addition to being an anticoagulant, it inhibits complement (proteins in serum that destroy bacteria) and phagocytosis (ingestion of bacteria by leukocytes) and reduces activity of certain antibiotics. SPS tubes have a special yellow stopper.

Antiglycolytic agents.   An **antiglycolytic agent** is a substance that inhibits **glycolysis**, or metabolism of glucose by the cells of the blood. The most common antiglycolytic agents are **sodium fluoride** and **lithium iodoacetate**. Glucose stability is preserved for 24 hours in iodoacetate and for up to 3 days in sodium fluoride. A tube containing antiglycolytic agent alone will yield serum for testing. However, antiglycolytic agents are commonly used in combination with potassium oxalate to provide plasma specimens. Sodium fluoride and lithium iodoacetate tubes have gray stoppers.

Clot activators.   A **clot activator** is a substance that initiates or enhances coagulation. Clot activators include substances that provide increased surface for platelet activation, such as **glass** or **silica particles** and inert clays such as **siliceous earth** and **celite**, as well as clotting factors such as **thromboplastin** and **thrombin**. Glass and silica particles are the clot activators in serum separator tubes. Siliceous earth in a special gray stopper tube and celite in a special black stopper tube are used for two different methods of the activated clotting test. Thrombin is the additive in special light blue tubes for coagulation studies, as well as in Becton Dickinson orange Hemogard stopper tubes and mottled yellow and black rubber stopper tubes.

Thixotropic gel separators.   A **thixotropic gel separator** is an inert (nonreacting) synthetic substance that forms a physical barrier between the cellular portion of a specimen and the serum or plasma portion when the specimen is centrifuged. This physical separation prevents the cells from continuing to metabolize substances, particularly glucose, in the serum or plasma. The gel, which is initially contained in the bottom of the collection tube, has a density between that of the cells and serum or plasma. When the specimen is centrifuged, the gel undergoes a change in viscosity and moves to a position between the cellular and the serum or plasma portions of the specimen, forming the physical barrier. Gel separator serum tubes have yellow plastic or mottled red/gray rubber stoppers. Gel separator plasma tubes have light green plastic or mottled gray/green rubber stoppers.

TUBE STOPPERS

Tube stoppers (Color Plate 2) are commonly made of rubber and are color coded to indicate the presence and type of additive or the absence of additive in the tube. Stopper colors may vary slightly by manufacturer.

Becton Dickinson Hemogard Closure tubes (see Color Plate 2) have a rubber stopper covered by a plastic shield. The plastic shield is designed to protect lab personnel from blood remaining on the stopper after the tube is removed from the needle, as well as when the stopper is removed from the tube. The rigidity of the plastic also prevents a "thumb roll" technique and subsequent aerosol (misting) of contents when removing the stopper from the tube. The color coding of Hemogard stoppers varies slightly from that of regular stoppers.

Venoject II tubes (Fig. 7-12) (Terumo Medical Corp., Somerst, NJ) have a special peel-off stopper with a thin rubber seal.

The most common tube stopper colors and the type of additive they indicate are as follows:

Stopper Color	Additive
Red	None
Red/gray Gold Hemogard	Gel separator/glass or silica particles
Green/gray Light green Hemogard	Gel separator/lithium heparin
Green	Ammonium heparin Lithium heparin Sodium heparin
Lavender	Ethylenediaminetetraacetic acid (EDTA)
Royal blue (trace element–free tube)	None (red label) EDTA (lavender label) Sodium heparin (green label)
Light blue	Sodium citrate
Gray	Potassium oxalate/sodium fluoride Sodium fluoride Lithium iodoacetate Lithium iodoacetate/lithium heparin
Yellow	Sodium polyanetholesulfonate (SPS)
Yellow	Acid citrate dextrose (ACD)

Order of Draw

The order in which multiple specimen tubes are collected during a draw or filled from a syringe after a draw can affect test results. A special sequence of collection, referred to as the **order of draw**, was developed to minimize problems associated with multiple tube collections. Except for sterile specimens, which are collected first in either method to minimize the possibility of microbial contamination and the inhibiting effects of certain additives, the order of draw for the evacuated tube system of collection is different from the order in which tubes are filled when a syringe is used.

PRINCIPLE BEHIND THE EVACUATED TUBE SYSTEM
ORDER OF DRAW

The order of draw for the evacuated tube system of blood collection was designed to reduce interference in specimen testing caused by carryover of additives between tubes and to minimize the effects of tissue thromboplastin on coagulation specimens. Carryover or transfer of additive from one tube to the next can occur when blood

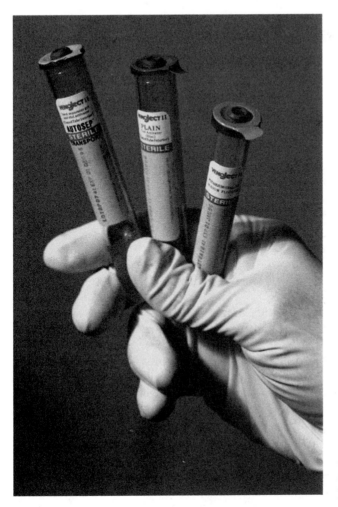

Figure 7-12 Venoject II plastic evacuated tubes with peel-off stoppers. (Terumo Medical Corporation, Somerset, NJ.)

in a tube that contains an additive is allowed to come in contact with the stopper puncturing needle during blood collection. Blood remaining on or within the needle may then be transferred to the next tube drawn, contaminating that tube and possibly affecting test results on that specimen. Table 7-1 shows some of the most common tests affected by additive contamination.

EDTA causes more carryover problems than any other additive. For example, EDTA (K_3) or EDTA (Na_2) contamination can have a major effect on sodium or potassium levels, respectively. Consequently, a tube for electrolytes or individual sodium or potassium tests should never be collected after an EDTA tube. In addition, because EDTA chelates calcium and iron, a calcium or serum iron specimen should never be collected immediately following an EDTA tube. Both EDTA and heparin can falsely increase values for coagulation tests, particularly prothrombin time and partial thromboplastin time tests. Tissue thromboplastin picked up by the needle during skin penetration can also interfere with coagulation testing.

Table 7-1
Common Tests Affected by Additive Contamination

Tests Affected by EDTA Contamination
Calcium
Partial thromboplastin
Potassium
Protime
Serum iron
Sodium

Tests Affected by Heparin Contamination
Activated clotting time
Partial thromboplastin
Protime

Tests Affected by Potassium Oxalate Contamination
Potassium
Red cell morphology

Potassium oxalate and sodium fluoride can falsely elevate potassium and sodium levels, respectively. In addition, oxalate damages cell membranes and may cause abnormal red blood cell morphology.

Remembering which tests are affected by the various additives can be difficult. The order of draw eliminates confusion by presenting a sequence of collection that results in the least amount of interference should carryover occur. Carryover can also be minimized by making certain that specimen tubes fill from the bottom up during collection and that the contents of the tube do not come in contact with the stopper puncturing needle during the draw. The order of draw for the evacuated tube system of collection follows:

EVACUATED TUBE SYSTEM ORDER OF DRAW

1. Sterile specimens (*ie*, blood culture tubes or bottles)
2. Red stopper: nonadditive
3. Light blue stopper: sodium citrate and other tubes for coagulation studies (*Note:* If a light blue stoppered tube or other coagulation tube is the first or only tube to be drawn, a 5-mL red stopper tube should be drawn first and discarded to eliminate contamination from tissue thromboplastin picked up during needle penetration.)
4. Green stopper: heparin
5. Lavender stopper: EDTA (K_3 or Na_2)
6. Gray stopper: oxalate/fluoride

An easy way to remember the evacuated tube order of draw is to remember the phrase "stop, red light, green light, go." The first letter of each word in the phrase stands for a tube in the evacuated tube system order of draw: S = sterile, R = red, L = light blue, G = green, L = lavender, and G = gray.

PRINCIPLE BEHIND THE SYRINGE SYSTEM
ORDER OF DRAW

The order of draw for the syringe method was designed to deliver blood first to those tubes most affected by microclot formation. This method assumes that the blood that enters the syringe last is the freshest and that this blood will be the first blood out of the syringe during the transfer process. Because the clotting process is activated the minute that the blood starts to fill the syringe, it is important to transfer the blood quickly and to fill anticoagulant tubes before serum tubes. Carryover of additive can occur using this method. To prevent carryover, the phlebotomist *must* keep the transfer needle above the fill level of the tube so that the needle does not come in contact with the blood in the tube.

SYRINGE SYSTEM ORDER OF DRAW

1. Sterile specimens (*ie*, blood culture tubes or bottles)
2. Light blue stopper: sodium citrate or other citrate-containing tubes or tubes for coagulation studies
3. Lavender stopper: EDTA (K_3 or Na_2)
4. Green stopper: heparin
5. Gray stopper: oxalate/fluoride
6. Red stopper or red/gray stopper: nonadditive and gel separator, respectively

---

An easy way to remember the order of draw for the syringe method is to think of the nonsense jingle "Silly ladies love green and gray roses," where the first letter in each word stands for a tube in the syringe order of draw: S = sterile, L = light blue, L = lavender, G = green, and G = gray.

Syringe System

Although the evacuated tube system is the preferred method of blood collection, a syringe system (Fig. 7-13) is sometimes used for patients with difficult veins. The syringe system consists of a sterile hypodermic, Luer-Lok needle attached to a disposable plastic (occasionally nondisposable glass) syringe.

SYRINGE NEEDLES

Syringe needles (see Fig. 7-13) are sterile, prepackaged, and come in a wide range of gauges for many different uses. Only those gauges appropriate for phlebotomy procedures should be used, generally 21 to 23 gauge for blood drawing. Syringe needles also come in different lengths, with 1-inch and 1½-inch lengths most commonly used for blood drawing.

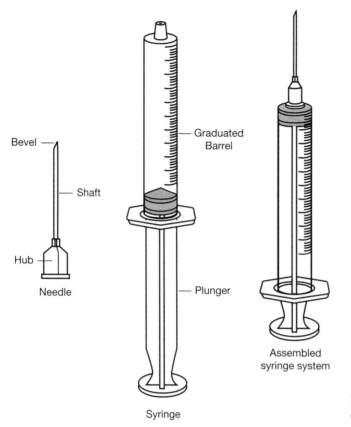

Bevel

Shaft

Hub

Needle

Graduated
Barrel

Plunger

Syringe

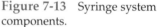

Assembled
syringe system

Figure 7-13   Syringe system
components.

SYRINGES

Syringes (see Fig. 7-13) come in various sizes, with 2 to 10 mL most commonly used for phlebotomy procedures. Syringes have two parts, a **barrel** with graduated markings in either milliliters (mL) or cubic centimeters (cc), and a **plunger** which fits into the barrel of the syringe. When drawing blood with a syringe, the plunger is slowly retracted by the phlebotomist, allowing the barrel to fill with blood. Blood specimens collected by syringe must be transferred to evacuated tubes following the proper order of draw for the syringe method. Safety syringes with shields that slide over the needle prior to disposal are available.

Winged Infusion Set

A **winged infusion set** (butterfly) consists of a ½- to ¾-inch stainless steel needle connected to a 5- to 12-inch length of tubing. It is called a butterfly because of its wing-shaped plastic extensions, which are used for gripping the needle.

Butterflies generally come with attachments that allow them to be used with syringes. There are, however, butterflies that come with special multiple sample Luer adapters that allow them to be used with an evacuated tube system. Multiple sample Luer adapters are also available separately to convert a syringe attachment butterfly for use with the evacuated tube system. See Figure 7-14 for several styles of winged infusion sets.

The **butterfly needle** is an indispensable tool for collecting blood from small or difficult veins such as hand veins or veins of elderly or pediatric patients. It allows much more flexibility and precision than a needle and syringe. Butterfly needles come in various sizes, with a 23 gauge being the one most commonly used in difficult phlebotomy situations. Using a needle with a bore smaller than a 23 gauge increases the chance of hemolyzing the specimen.

Several types of safety butterfly needles (Fig. 7-15) are now available. These needles contain a shield, which covers the needle upon withdrawal from the patient's vein, reducing the possibility of accidental needle sticks. Examples are the Becton Dickinson Luer-Lok safety winged infusion set (Becton Dickinson Vacutainer Systems, Franklin Lakes, NJ), the Angel Wing Safety Needle System (Sherwood Medical, St. Louis, MO), the Shamrock safety winged set (Ryan Medical, Winfield Industries, San Diego, CA), and the Puncture-Guard wing set (Bio-Plexus, Tolland, CT).

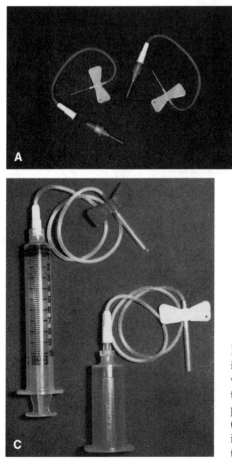

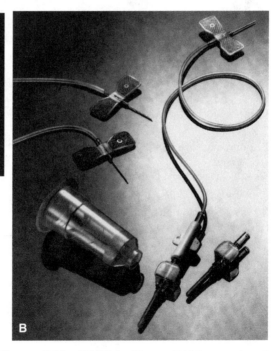

Figure 7-14 (**A**) *Right*, Becton Dickinson winged infusion set and Luer adapter; *left*, winged infusion set with Luer adapter attached (Becton Dickinson Vacutainer Systems, Franklin Lakes, NJ); (**B**) Multiple-sample Luer Adapter with winged needle collection set (Courtesy Kawasumi Medical, Tampa, FL); (**C**) Winged infusion sets: *Left*, attached to a syringe; *right*, attached to evacuated tube holder by means of a Luer adapter.

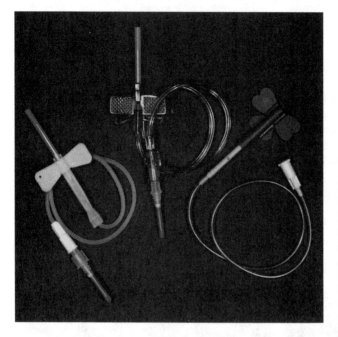

Figure 7-15   Safety winged infusion sets (from left to right): Luer-Lok safety winged infusion set (Becton Dickinson Vacutainer Systems, Franklin Lakes, NJ); Angel Wing Safety Needle System (Sherwood Medical, St. Louis, MO); and the Shamrock safety winged set (Ryan Medical, Winfield Industries, San Diego, CA).

Study & Review Questions

1. Containers used for disposing of needles and other sharp objects must be all of the following *except*
   a. clearly marked "biohazard."
   b. disposable.
   c. puncture resistant.
   d. recyclable.

2. The most common antiseptic for routine blood collection is
   a. antibacterial soap and water.
   b. povidone–iodine.
   c. 70% isopropyl alcohol.
   d. 5.25% sodium hypochlorite.

3. Needles are color coded according to their
   a. brand.
   b. gauge.
   c. length.
   d. expiration date.

4. The needle gauge with the smallest diameter is
   a. 19.
   b. 20.
   c. 21.
   d. 23.

5. In the recommended order of draw for the evacuated tube method, which tube should be filled last?
   a. Red top
   b. Lavender top
   c. Light blue top
   d. Blood culture

6. The color-coded tube that is most often associated with hematology tests is
   a. green.
   b. light blue.
   c. lavender.
   d. red.

Suggested Laboratory Activities

1. Identify, handle, and describe the uses of various pieces of blood collection equipment. Practice equipment assembly, if applicable.

2. Properly stock a laboratory blood collection tray.

3. Make 8 × 10 cards with different collection tubes attached and write a thought-provoking question on each concerning its use.

4. Arrange blood collecting tubes in the proper order of draw for both the evacuated tube and the syringe methods.

BIBLIOGRAPHY AND SUGGESTED READINGS

National Committee for Clinical Laboratory Standards, H3-A3. (July 1991). *Procedures for the collection of diagnostic blood specimens by venipuncture* (3rd ed.). Villanova, PA: NCCLS.

National Committee for Clinical Laboratory Standards, H4-A3. (July 1991). *Procedures for the collection of diagnostic blood specimens by skin puncture* (3rd ed.). Villanova, PA: NCCLS.

National Committee for Clinical Laboratory Standards, H14-A2. (July 1990). *Devices for collection of skin puncture blood specimens* (2nd ed.). Villanova, PA: NCCLS.

National Committee for Clinical Laboratory Standards, M29-T2. (September 1992). *Protection of laboratory workers from infectious disease transmitted by blood, body fluids and tissue* (Tentative guideline) (2nd ed.). Villanova, PA: NCCLS.

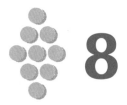

8

Factors to Consider Prior to Blood Collection

KEY TERMS

basal state	hematoma	patency	syncope
cannula	hemoconcentration	petechiae	vascular access
diurnal variations	hemolysis	reflux	device (VAD)
edema	heparin lock	STAT (stat)	venous stasis
fistula	lipemic		

OBJECTIVES

Upon successful completion of this chapter, the reader will be able to:

1. Define basal state and list factors influencing this state.
2. List and define test status designations and describe the procedure to follow for each.
3. List factors to consider in site selection; describe causes for concern and procedures to follow when encountering each.
4. Identify various vascular access devices.
5. List complications associated with blood collection and describe how they may affect the patient or the integrity of the specimen.
6. Describe how to avoid complications and how to handle those that occur.

PHYSIOLOGIC FACTORS

Basal State

Because constituents of the blood are affected by diet, exercise, and other factors, the ideal time for collecting blood specimens is early in the morning while the body is still at rest and **fasting,** or approximately 12 hours after the last intake of food. This condition is known as **basal state. Reference (normal)** values for lab tests on hospital patients are usually established using basal state specimens. Outpatient specimens are not basal state specimens and may have slightly different normal values.

Factors Influencing Basal State

AGE

Values for numerous blood components vary considerably with the age of the patient. For example, red blood cell (RBC) and white blood cell (WBC) values are higher in newborns than adults.

Some physiologic functions decrease with age in adults. For example, creatinine clearance, a kidney function test, is directly related to the age of the patient, which must be used in calculating test results.

ALTITUDE

Decreased oxygen content of the air at higher altitudes causes the body to produce more red blood cells to fulfill the body's oxygen requirements. The higher the altitude, the greater the increase. RBC counts and related determinations such as hemoglobin (Hgb) and hematocrit (Hct) will have higher normal ranges at higher elevations.

DEHYDRATION

Dehydration (a decrease in total body fluid) that occurs with persistent vomiting or diarrhea, for example, causes **hemoconcentration**, which can falsely increase some blood components such as RBCs, enzymes, iron (Fe), calcium (Ca), and sodium (Na). In addition, it is often much more difficult to obtain a blood specimen from a dehydrated patient.

DIET

Blood composition is significantly altered by ingestion of food. Glucose levels increase dramatically with the ingestion of sugar-laden substances but should return to normal within 2 hours.

Ingestion of fatty substances, including many fast food items, butter, and cheese, increases lipid content in the blood for anywhere from 1 to 10 hours or more, causing the serum or plasma to appear **lipemic** (cloudy or turbid). In fact, accurate testing of triglycerides (a type of lipid) requires a 12-hour fast. In addition, some chemistry tests cannot be performed on lipemic specimens because the cloudiness interferes with the testing procedure.

Some laboratory tests are affected by ingestion of certain foods, which must be eliminated from the diet for several days before the test specimen is collected.

Excessive fluid intake may cause decreased Hgb levels and alter electrolyte balance. Consumption of caffeine has been demonstrated to affect cortisol levels. Recent alcohol ingestion may also affect test values, especially glucose values. Most dietary influences on blood as well as urine specimens can be eliminated by requesting a fasting specimen.

DIURNAL (DAILY) VARIATIONS

Many blood constituents show **diurnal variations** or normal fluctuations throughout the day. White blood counts, eosinophil counts, and iron levels are lower in the morning than in the afternoon. Cortisol and testosterone levels are highest in the morning.

DRUGS

Many drugs alter physiologic functions. In most instances, the effect is desired. In some individuals, however, there are also unwanted physiologic effects called side effects or sensitivities. For example, thiazide diuretics often cause increased calcium levels and may cause low potassium levels. Chemotherapy drugs often cause a decrease in the cells of the blood, especially WBCs and platelets. Numerous drugs are toxic to the liver, causing an increase in liver enzymes such as serum glutamic-oxaloacetic transaminase (SGOT) (aspartate transaminase; AST), alkaline phosphatase, and lactate dehydrogenase (LDH). Steroids and diuretics can cause pancreatitis and an increase in serum amylase and lipase values. To check for side effects, it is not uncommon for physicians to monitor levels of certain blood components while a person is receiving drug therapy.

Drugs may also interfere with the performance of the test in the laboratory, causing false increases or decreases in test results. Many lab test procedures are based on fluorescent, chromogenic (color producing), peroxide-generating, or reagent-binding reactions. A drug may compete with the test reagents for the substance being tested, causing a false-negative or falsely low result, or the drug may enhance the reaction, causing a false-positive or falsely high result. An acronym used for substances that interfere with the testing process is *CRUD*, which stands for *compounds reacting unfortunately* as the *desired*.

The **College of American Pathologists (CAP)** has developed guideline for drugs known to interfere with testing procedures. According to CAP, drugs known to interfere with blood tests should be stopped or avoided 4 to 24 hours prior to obtaining the blood sample for testing. Drugs known to interfere with urine testing should be avoided for 48 to 72 hours prior to urine sample collection.

It is up to the physician to recognize or eliminate drug interferences; however, it is helpful to the technician or technologist performing the test in the laboratory if the phlebotomist notes on the lab slip when he or she observes medication being administered just prior to blood collection.

ENVIRONMENT

Environmental factors such as temperature and humidity are known to affect test values. Environmental factors associated with geographic location are accounted for when establishing normal or reference values. Temperature and humidity in the laboratory are closely monitored to ensure proper functioning of equipment as well as to maintain specimen integrity.

EXERCISE

Muscular activity, however moderate, will elevate the blood levels of a number of blood components, such as lactic acid, creatinine, protein, and certain enzymes. Levels of these substances return to normal soon after the activity is stopped, with the exception of enzymes such as creatine kinase (CK) and LDH, which may remain elevated 24 hours or more.

GENDER

A patient's gender or sex has a determining effect on the concentration of numerous blood components. Most differences are apparent only after sexual maturity. These differences are reflected in separate normal values for male and female patients. For example, RBC, Hgb, and Hct normal values are higher for males.

POSITION

The position of a patient both before and during venipuncture influences blood composition. Going from a supine (lying down) position to standing causes the water or plasma portion of the blood to filter into the tissues, resulting in a decrease in plasma volume and an increase in nonfilterable elements, or substances such as proteins, iron, calcium, and blood cells, that cannot easily pass through the walls of the blood vessels. For example, the RBC count on a patient who has been standing for approximately 15 minutes will be higher than the basal state RBC on the same patient.

PREGNANCY

Pregnancy causes physiologic changes in many body systems. As a result of these changes, a number of laboratory test results will differ from regular normal values and must be compared to normal ranges established for pregnant populations. For example, body fluid increases, which are normal during pregnancy, have a diluting effect on the red blood cells, leading to lower red blood counts.

SMOKING

Patients who smoke prior to specimen collection may have increased cortisol levels and white blood counts. Chronic smoking often leads to decreased pulmonary function and increased hemoglobin levels. In addition, skin puncture specimens may be more difficult to obtain from smokers because of impaired circulation in the fingertips.

STRESS

Emotional stress in the form of fear or anxiety has been shown to cause short-lived elevations in WBC counts, decreases in serum iron, and increases in adrenal hormone values. For example, studies on crying infants demonstrated marked increases in WBC counts. Counts returned to normal within 1 hour after crying stopped. For this reason, complete blood cell (CBC) or WBC specimens should not be obtained unless the baby has been sleeping or resting quietly for approximately 1 hour.

A new field called **psychoneuroimmunology (PNI)** deals with the study of interactions between the brain, the endocrine system, and the immune system. Studies in this field have demonstrated that receptors on the cell membrane of WBCs can sense stress in a person and react by stimulating an increase in cell numbers.

TEST STATUS

Some tests require specimens collected at specific times or under specific conditions. Certain test requests take priority over others. The "status" of the test request should be clearly noted on the test request form. It is up to the phlebotomist to assess each test request and determine the priority and conditions involved in obtaining the specimen. Test status designations, priorities, and response times are determined by individual laboratories and may differ somewhat from one lab to another. The following are common test status designations.

STAT

STAT (stat) comes from the Latin word *statim*, meaning immediately. Stat tests should only be ordered on patients whose condition is or has become critical and test results are urgently needed to respond to the situation. Stat requests have the highest priority and should not only be drawn expeditiously, but processed with results reported immediately. The phlebotomist who draws and delivers a stat specimen to the lab should alert lab personnel to its presence.

Medical Emergency

Due to misuse of the term stat, such as using the designation for requesting tests when there is not a medical emergency, some institutions have started using the designation **Med Emerg** to identify specimens that are needed in critical or life-or-death situations. This designation replaces the stat designation, consequently the same procedure is followed.

Timed Specimens

Some tests are requested to be collected at a particular time. It is important that the specimen be collected as near to the time requested as possible with the actual time of collection recorded on the request form as well as on the specimen container.

Commonly ordered timed tests include 2-hour postprandial glucose levels, glucose tolerance tests, cortisol levels, cardiac enzymes, and specimens for therapeutic drug monitoring (TDM) peaks and troughs.

ASAP

ASAP stands for "as soon as possible." This means that test results are needed soon for the physician to respond to a serious situation, but the patient's condition is not critical. Most laboratories have specific protocol for how quickly ASAP tests are collected, depending upon the type of test ordered and how close the order comes to a regular sweep (scheduled collection time for other tests.)

Fasting

Some tests such as glucose, cholesterol, and triglycerides require that the patient abstain from eating or drinking (except water) for approximately 12 hours prior to collection of the specimen. It is up to the phlebotomist to ascertain if the patient is fasting. If the test has been ordered fasting and the phlebotomist determines that the patient has eaten, the phlebotomist must check with the patient's nurse (or the phlebotomy supervisor in the case of outpatients) to find out whether the test should still be performed. If the test is still wanted, the phlebotomist should draw the specimen and write "nonfasting" on the lab slip.

Fasting should not be confused with NPO, which comes from Latin *nulla per os* which means "nothing by mouth." NPO differs from fasting in that the patient is not allowed food or water. Patients are NPO prior to surgery or other procedures requiring anesthesia. A phlebotomist will not always know if a patient is NPO and should therefore refer all patient requests for food or water to the patient's nurse.

Pre-op/Post-op

"Pre-op" means before an operation or surgery, and "post-op" means after. Pre-op tests are needed to determine whether the patient's condition is suitable for surgery. Examples of pre-op tests include CBC, partial thromboplastin time, and bleeding time tests. Post-op tests evaluate the patient's condition following surgery. A hemoglobin and hematocrit (H & H) is a common post-op test.

Routine

Routine tests are those tests commonly ordered by the physician in the course of establishing a diagnosis or monitoring a patient's progress. Specimens should be collected in a timely fashion; however, there is no immediate urgency involved. Most routine tests are ordered for early morning rounds. Routine tests ordered after morning rounds are collected during the next scheduled rounds or sweeps.

Routine Admission

Routine admission tests may be required of all patients by the health care facility on admission. For example, many hospitals require all patients to have a CBC, chemistry profile, and urinalysis (UA) upon admission. This procedure is changing, however, because many reimbursement policies now require physicians to base their choice of tests on medical necessity and not on traditional tests or admission panels that are available.

FACTORS TO CONSIDER IN SITE SELECTION

Burns and Scars

Avoid burned, scarred, or tattooed areas. Veins are difficult to palpate as well as penetrate in scarred areas. Healed burn sites with extensive scarring may have impaired circulation and yield erroneous test results. Newly burned areas are painful and also susceptible to infection.

Cutdown

A cutdown is a surgical procedure used to locate a vein or artery in which to insert an intravenous (IV) or arterial line to deliver drugs or fluids. It is performed in patients whose blood vessels have collapsed owing to shock or other causes. Tourniquet application may disrupt the healing of a recent cutdown. Veins may be hard to palpate or feel near older cutdown sites and the possibility of impaired circulation to the site may lead to erroneous (inaccurate) test results. If no other site is available, check with the patient's nurse to find out whether it is acceptable either to apply the tourniquet and draw the specimen well below the cutdown site or to collect the specimen by finger puncture.

Damaged Veins

Some patient's veins feel hard and cord-like and lack resiliency. These veins are said to be hardened or sclerosed. This may be due to inflammation, disease, or the irritation of chemotherapy drugs. Sometimes it is due to the scarring caused by numerous venipunctures, as in the case of regular blood donors and people with chronic illnesses. Damaged veins are difficult to penetrate, often yield erroneous test results owing to impaired blood flow, and should be avoided. Draw below (or distal to) the damaged area or choose another site.

Edema

Edema is the result of an accumulation of fluid in the tissues. Drawing blood specimens from edematous areas may result in inaccurate test results. Edematous tissue may also be fragile and easily injured by tourniquet and antiseptic application. Choose another site if possible.

Hematoma

A venipuncture should not be made in the area of a **hematoma**. A hematoma is a swelling or mass of blood (usually clotted) caused by blood leaking from a blood vessel during or following venipuncture. A slowdown of blood flow to the area (hemostasis) due to obstruction by the hematoma may lead to inaccurate test results. The area may also be painful to the patient. If there is no alternative site, it is acceptable to perform the venipuncture distal to the hematoma.

Mastectomy

The patient's physician should be consulted before drawing blood from an arm on the same side as a mastectomy (breast removal). Due to lymphostasis (a stoppage of lymph flow) caused by lymph node removal, blood specimens obtained from the arm on the same side as a mastectomy may yield erroneous test results. These patients are also more susceptible to infection. In addition, application of a tourniquet to that arm may cause injury. If the patient has had a mastectomy on both sides, the most recent site should be avoided.

Obesity

Obese patients often present a challenge to the phlebotomist. Veins on obese patients may be deep and difficult to find. In addition, conventional latex tourniquets may be too short to fit around the arm without rolling and twisting. A long length of Penrose drain tubing or a long Velcro closure strap often works better than a latex strap. Proper tourniquet selection and application is the first step to a successful venipuncture.

Obese patients who have a double crease in the antecubital area often have an easily palpable median cubital vein between the two creases. If this is not the case, another site to try is the cephalic vein. To locate the cephalic vein, the patient's arm is rotated so that the hand is prone. In this position, the weight of excess tissue often pulls downward, making the cephalic vein easy to feel and penetrate with a needle.

Intravenous Therapy

It is preferred that blood specimens not be drawn from an arm with an IV line. Drawing a specimen from an arm with an IV may result in dilution of the blood with the IV fluid, causing erroneous results, especially if the specimen is drawn above the IV. However, if no other site is available, the specimen may be collected *below* the IV (*never above*) using the following NCCLS recommended procedure:

1. Have the nurse turn off the IV for a minimum of 2 minutes prior to collection.
2. Apply the tourniquet distal to the IV.

3. Perform the venipuncture in a different vein than the one with the IV.
4. Collect a 5-mL tube of blood (10 mL for coagulation tests) and discard before collecting test specimens.
5. Have the nurse restart the IV.
6. State on the requisition form that the specimen was collected from an arm with an IV. It is also helpful to indicate the type of IV fluid.

VASCULAR ACCESS DEVICES

A **vascular access device (VAD)**, also called an **indwelling line**, consists of tubing inserted into a main vein or artery. It is used primarily for administering fluids and medications, monitoring pressures, and drawing blood. VADs that are to be used for drawing blood should only be accessed by specially trained personnel. However, the phlebotomist may be asked to assist in transferring the specimen to the appropriate tubes. Because most lines are routinely flushed with heparin, a minimum of 5 mL of blood must be discarded before a test specimen is collected. Because of possible interference due to heparin, line draws are not recommended for collection of coagulation specimens. However, some health care institution policies allow the sample to be drawn after discarding the first 10 mL of blood.

Central Venous Catheter (CVC)

The most common type of VAD is a **central venous catheter (CVC)**, also called a **central venous line**. A CVC (Fig. 8-1) is inserted into a large vein such as the subclavian and advanced into the superior vena cava, proximal to the right atrium. The exit end is surgically tunneled under the skin to a site several inches away in the chest. Several inches of tubing protrude from the exit site, which is normally covered with a transparent dressing. There are a number of different types of CVCs, including Broviac, Groshong, and Hickman (Fig. 8-2).

Implanted Port

Another type of VAD, an **implanted port** (Fig. 8-3), is a small chamber that is attached to an indwelling line. The chamber is surgically implanted under the skin. The device is located by palpating the skin. Access is gained by inserting a special noncoring needle through the skin into the self-sealing septum (wall) of the chamber. The site is not normally covered with a bandage when not in use.

Peripherally Inserted Central Catheter

A **peripherally inserted central catheter (PICC)** (Fig. 8-4) is inserted into the peripheral venous system (veins of the extremities) and threaded into the central venous system (main veins leading to the heart). It does not require surgical insertion. PICCs are commonly placed in either the basilic or cephalic vein with the exit in the antecubital area. Because a PICC tends to collapse on aspiration, drawing blood from a PICC is not recommended.

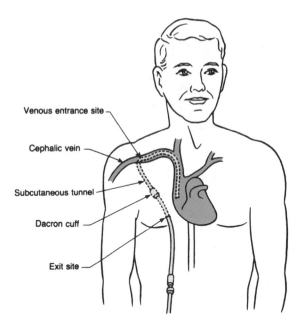

Venous entrance site

Cephalic vein

Subcutaneous tunnel

Dacron cuff

Exit site

Figure 8-1 Central venous catheter (CVC) (Metheny NM).

Arterial Line

An intraarterial line or catheter is most commonly located in the radial artery and is used to provide continuous measurement of a patient's blood pressure. It is also used for collection of blood gas specimens.

Heparin or Saline Lock

A **heparin** or **saline lock** (Fig. 8-5) is a special winged needle set or **cannula** that can be left in a patient's vein for up to 48 hours. It is commonly located in the lower arm

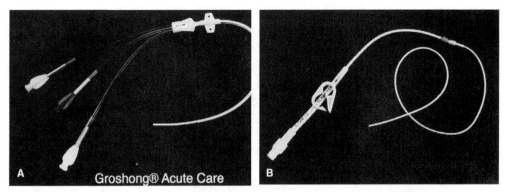

Figure 8-2 Central venous catheters. (Courtesy Bard Access Systems, Inc., Salt Lake City, UT.) (**A**) Groshong®. (**B**) Hickman®.

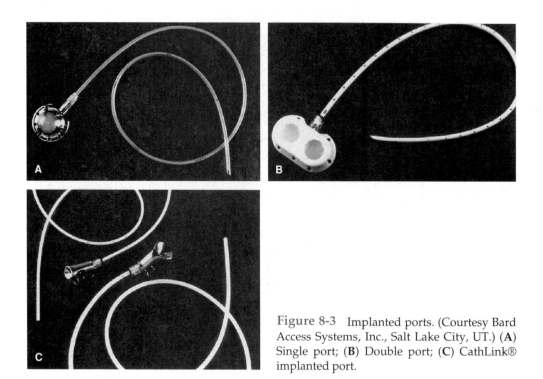

Figure 8-3   Implanted ports. (Courtesy Bard Access Systems, Inc., Salt Lake City, UT.) (**A**) Single port; (**B**) Double port; (**C**) CathLink® implanted port.

above the wrist and is used to administer medication and draw blood. Because it is flushed with heparin or saline periodically or after use to keep it from clotting, a 5 mL discard tube should be drawn prior to collection of blood specimens. Drawing coagulation test specimens from heparin locks is not recommended. Only specially trained personnel should draw blood from a heparin lock.

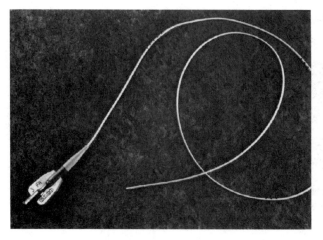

Figure 8-4   Groshong® peripherally inserted central catheter. (Courtesy Bard Access System, Inc., Salt Lake City, UT.)

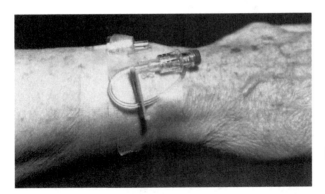

Figure 8-5   Peripheral heparin lock with extension tubing added for accessibility.

Arteriovenous (AV) Shunt

An AV shunt is an artificially created connection between an artery and a vein. It is most commonly created to provide access for dialysis. Never apply a blood pressure cuff or tourniquet to or perform venipuncture on an arm with a shunt.

External AV Shunt or Cannula

An **external AV shunt** or **cannula** (Fig. 8-6) is a temporary surgical connection between an artery and a vein used for dialysis and blood drawing. Tubing of the cannula extends to the outside surface of the arm and has a rubber diaphragm cap through which a needle may be inserted to draw blood. A discard tube must be drawn prior to drawing specimen tubes. Drawing blood from a cannula should be performed only by specially trained personnel with the permission of the patient's physician.

Internal AV Shunt or Fistula

An **internal AV shunt** or **fistula** (Fig. 8-7) is created by a surgical procedure which fuses a vein and artery together permanently. The connection is close to the surface of the skin and the loop created can usually be easily seen and felt. It is used for dialysis and should not be used for phlebotomy procedures. Specimens should be drawn from the other arm.

COMPLICATIONS ASSOCIATED WITH BLOOD COLLECTION

The phlebotomist must be aware of complications associated with blood collection procedures. Complications may affect the patient, the integrity of the specimen, or both. Some complications are unavoidable; others can be avoided by employing proper collection technique or can be minimized by the alert response of a knowledgeable phlebotomist.

Complications Affecting the Patient
ALLERGIES TO ANTISEPTICS, ADHESIVES, OR LATEX

Occasionally, a patient is allergic to the antiseptic used in skin preparation prior to venipuncture or skin puncture. In this case, an alternate antiseptic should be used.

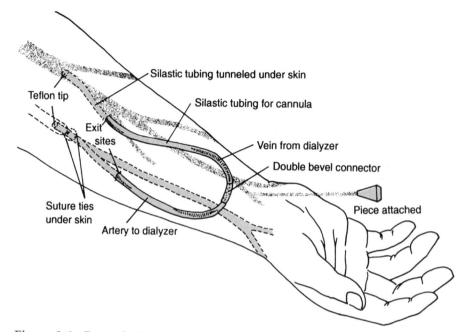

Silastic tubing tunneled under skin

Teflon tip

Silastic tubing for cannula

Exit
sites

Vein from dialyzer

Double bevel connector

Suture ties
under skin

Artery to dialyzer

Piece attached

Figure 8-6   External AV shunt (cannula) (Slockbower JM, Blumenfeld TA).

Some patients are allergic to the glue used in adhesive bandages. Usually paper tape placed over a folded gauze square can be used instead. If the patient is also allergic to paper tape, the area can be wrapped with gauze and fastened with paper tape over the gauze.

Increasing numbers of individuals are developing allergies to latex. Most are seemingly minor and involve irritation or rashes from physical contact with latex products such as gloves. Others are so severe that being in the same room where latex materials are used can set off a life-threatening reaction. If a patient is known to have a severe allergy to latex, there may be a warning sign on the patient's door. It is important that no items made of latex be brought into the room. This means the phlebotomist must wear nonlatex gloves and use a nonlatex tourniquet when in the room, whether collecting blood from the patient or the patient's roommate.

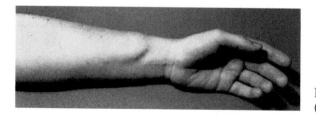

Figure 8-7   Internal AV shunt (fistula).

EXCESSIVE BLEEDING

Normally, a patient will stop bleeding from the venipuncture site within a few minutes. Some patients, particularly those on anticoagulant therapy, may take longer to stop bleeding. Pressure must be maintained over the site until the bleeding stops. If the bleeding continues after 5 minutes, notify the nurse. Do not leave until bleeding has stopped or the nurse takes charge of the situation.

FAINTING (SYNCOPE)

Some patients become faint at the thought of or sight of their blood being drawn, especially if they are ill. A patient who feels faint or has a history of fainting (syncope) should be asked to lie down for the procedure. Inpatients who are already lying down rarely faint during blood draws. Outpatients are more likely to faint, because they are usually sitting up during venipuncture. If a patient starts to faint during venipuncture, the following steps should be taken:

1. Remove the tourniquet.
2. Withdraw the needle as quickly as possible.
3. Talk to the patient to divert attention away from the procedure as well as to help keep him or her alert.
4. Have the patient lower his or her head and breathe deeply, while physically supporting the patient to prevent injury in case of collapse.
5. Loosen a tight collar or tie if possible.
6. Apply a cold compress or washcloth to the forehead and back of the neck.
7. Use an ammonia inhalant to bring an outpatient around if necessary.
8. Alert the laboratory pathologist if the patient does not respond.

Once the patient has recovered, he or she must remain in the area for at least 15 minutes. The patient should be instructed *not* to operate a vehicle for at least 30 minutes. It is important for the phlebotomist to document the incident (following hospital policy) in case of future litigation.

HEMATOMA

A hematoma or bruise is caused by blood leaking into the tissues around the venipuncture site. It is identified by swelling at or near the venipuncture site. A hematoma is painful, unsightly, and can damage underlying nerves. If a hematoma should start to form while the phlebotomist is attempting to draw a specimen, the phlebotomist should immediately release the tourniquet, withdraw the needle, and hold pressure over the site. Reasons a hematoma may form include the following:

1. The vein is fragile or too small for the needle size.
2. The needle penetrates all the way through the vein.
3. The needle is only partly inserted into the vein.
4. Excessive or blind probing is used to locate the vein.
5. The needle is removed while the tourniquet is still on.
6. Pressure is not adequately applied following venipuncture.

INADVERTENT ARTERIAL PUNCTURE

If accidental puncture of an artery is suspected during a venipuncture procedure, it is important to hold pressure over the site for a full 5 minutes. A phlebotomist can usually recognize arterial blood by its bright red color or the fact that it spurts or pulses into the tube. The arterial blood can usually be submitted for testing, rather than redrawing the patient. However, if an arterial specimen is submitted to the lab for testing, it should be labeled as arterial since some lab values are different for arterial specimens.

INFECTION

Infection at the site following venipuncture is not unheard of, but is rare. Using proper aseptic technique and reminding the patient to keep the bandage on for at least 15 minutes should minimize the risk of infection.

NAUSEA/VOMITING

A patient who becomes nauseous should be reassured and made comfortable. A feeling of nausea often precedes vomiting, so it is a good idea to give the patient an emesis basin to hold as a precaution. Ask the patient to breathe slowly and deeply. Apply a cold, wet washcloth to the patient's forehead. If the patient is an inpatient, ask for assistance from the nurse before proceeding to collect the specimen.

NERVE DAMAGE

Excessive or blind probing while performing a venipuncture can lead to injury of a main nerve (such as the median cutaneous nerve), causing permanent damage. Injuries such as this may result in a lawsuit.

PAIN

A small amount of pain is associated with routine venipuncture and skin puncture. Putting the patient at ease prior to blood collection helps relax the patient and seems to make the procedure less painful. Warning the patient prior to needle insertion will avoid a startle reflex by the patient. If extreme pain occurs, *remove the needle immediately* and choose another site.

A stinging sensation upon venipuncture can be avoided by allowing the alcohol to dry completely prior to needle penetration.

Excessive, deep, or blind probing with the needle can be very painful to the patient and should be avoided.

PETECHIAE

Petechiae are small, nonraised red spots which appear on the patient's skin when a tourniquet is applied. These spots may be due to a defect of the capillary walls or platelet defects. They are *not* an indication that the phlebotomist has used incorrect procedure. However, they are an indication that the venipuncture site may bleed excessively.

REFLUX OF ANTICOAGULANT

In rare instances, it is possible for blood to backflow (**reflux**) into the patient's veins from the collection tube during the venipuncture procedure. Some patients have had adverse reactions to tube additives, particularly EDTA, owing to reflux. Reflux can occur when the contents of the collection tube are in contact with the tube stopper while the specimen is being drawn. To prevent reflux reactions, keep the patient's arm in a downward position so that the collection tube remains below the venipuncture site and fills from the bottom up. Back-and-forth movement of the contents of the tube should also be avoided until the tube is removed from the evacuated tube holder. An outpatient can be properly positioned by having him or her lean forward and extending the arm downward over the arm of the drawing chair. Proper positioning of an inpatient can be achieved by raising the head of the bed and extending the patient's arm over the side of the bed or supporting the arm with a rolled towel.

SEIZURES

In the rare event that a patient should have a seizure while the phlebotomist is drawing a blood specimen, it is important to remove the needle as quickly as possible. Try to hold pressure over the site without completely restricting the patient's movement. Do not try to put anything into the patient's mouth.

VEIN COLLAPSE

Too much vacuum for the size of the vein can cause the vein to collapse. This can result from using too large of an evacuated tube or from pulling too forcefully on the plunger of a syringe when drawing blood from a small or fragile vein. Another reason for vein collapse may be a tourniquet that is tied too tightly or too close to the venipuncture site. Sometimes veins of elderly patients are fragile and will collapse when the tourniquet is removed during a blood draw.

VEIN DAMAGE

Properly performed, an occasional venipuncture will not impair the **patency** (state of being freely open) of a patient's veins. Numerous venipunctures in the same area over an extended period of time, however, will eventually cause a buildup of scar tissue and increase the difficulty of performing subsequent venipuncture. Blind probing and improper technique when redirecting the needle can also damage veins and impair patency.

Collection Technique Factors Affecting Specimen Integrity

Sometimes the character or integrity of a specimen can be compromised by the methods (techniques) used in collection. The fact that the integrity of a specimen has been compromised is not always discernible by the phlebotomist or other laboratory personnel. However, a poor-quality specimen will generally yield poor-quality results and affect the care of the patient. Obviously, this is to be avoided. Consequently, it is very important for the phlebotomist to be aware of the following pitfalls of collection.

HEMOCONCENTRATION OR VENOUS STASIS

Prolonged application of the tourniquet causes stagnation of the normal blood flow (**venous stasis**). When venous stasis occurs, the plasma portion of the blood filters into the tissues, causing hemoconcentration, or an increase in nonfilterable blood components such as RBCs, enzymes, iron, and calcium.

Hemoconcentration can also be caused by vigorous hand pumping, probing, long-term IV therapy, and sclerosed or occluded veins.

HEMOLYSIS

Hemolysis results from the destruction of RBCs and the liberation of hemoglobin into the fluid portion of the specimen. When this happens, the specimen is said to be **hemolyzed**. Hemolysis of a specimen causes the serum or plasma to be pink (slight hemolysis) to red (gross hemolysis) in color. Because hemolysis will affect certain tests, such as enzymes and potassium (K^+), a hemolyzed specimen may have to be redrawn.

Hemolysis can be caused by the following:

1. Mixing additive tubes too vigorously or using rough handling during transport.
2. Drawing blood from a vein that has a hematoma.
3. Pulling back the plunger on a syringe too quickly.
4. Using a needle with too small of a bore for venipuncture.
5. Using too large a tube when using a small-diameter butterfly needle.
6. Frothing of the blood caused by improper fit of the needle on a syringe.
7. Forcing the blood from a syringe into an evacuated tube.
8. Not wiping away the first drop of blood (which may contain alcohol residue) from a skin puncture.
9. Excessive squeezing of the site when obtaining a skin puncture specimen.

PARTIALLY FILLED TUBES

It is important to fill anticoagulant and other additive tubes until the vacuum is exhausted to obtain the proper ratio of blood to additive for which the tube was designed. Although in some cases a partially filled tube may be accepted for testing by the laboratory, it will not have the proper ratio, which may lead to erroneous test results.

The blood-to-anticoagulant ratio is especially critical for light blue sodium citrate tubes used for coagulation studies. Partially filled tubes for coagulation tests will not be accepted by most laboratories. If the tube is not filled properly, the specimen will have to be recollected.

Inadvertent partial filling of tubes may result from loss of vacuum and may indicate that a tube is cracked or has been dropped. Cracked tubes present a safety hazard because they may leak or break with further handling. Never use a tube that is cracked or has been dropped: discard it instead. In addition, *never* pour two partially filled anticoagulant tubes together in order to fill one tube, as this will also affect the blood-to-anticoagulant ratio.

SPECIMEN CONTAMINATION

There are a number of ways a phlebotomist may inadvertently contaminate a specimen. One way is to use the wrong antiseptic to clean the site prior to specimen collection. For example, using alcohol to clean the site can contaminate an ethanol (blood alcohol) specimen. Using povidone–iodine (*eg*, Betadine) to clean a skin puncture site can contaminate the specimen with povidone–iodine and cause erroneously high levels of uric acid, phosphate, and potassium.

Using the correct antiseptic, but not allowing it to dry, can also cause contamination. Antiseptic contamination of blood cultures can occur if the antiseptic is not dry when the needle is inserted into the vein or into the culture bottles. Traces of the antiseptic in the culture media may inhibit growth of bacteria and cause false-negative blood culture results. Alcohol that is not dry when a skin puncture is performed can cause hemolysis of the specimen and affect test results.

Microbial contamination of blood cultures can result from improperly cleaning the site or culture bottles or from touching the site after it has been prepped (cleaned).

Powder from gloves can contaminate blood films on slides and skin puncture specimens, especially neonatal screening specimens.

Study & Review Questions

1. Values for this test are normally highest in the morning.
   a. Cortisol
   b. White blood count
   c. Iron (Fe)
   d. Eosinophil count

2. What tests may be affected most if the patient is not fasting?
   a. CBC and protime
   b. Glucose and triglycerides
   c. RA and cardiac enzymes
   d. Blood culture and thyroid profile

3. Drugs known to interfere with urine tests should be stopped
   a. 4 to 24 hours prior to the test.
   b. 24 to 36 hours prior to the test.
   c. 48 to 72 hours prior to the test.
   d. not at all; drugs do not interfere with urine tests.

4. Veins that feel hard and cordlike when palpated are called
   a. collapsed veins.
   b. fistulas.
   c. sclerosed veins.
   d. young venules.

5. A hematoma may result from all of the following *except*
   a. the needle bevel is only partly inserted into the vein.
   b. not enough pressure is applied to the site following venipuncture.
   c. the tourniquet is released before needle withdrawal.
   d. the needle has penetrated all the way through the vein.

6. Small, red spots that appear on a patient's arm when the tourniquet is applied are called
   a. edema.
   b. hematoma.
   c. hemolysis.
   d. petechiae.

7. When fingers and hands of the patient are swollen with excess fluids, the condition is called
   a. atherosclerosis.
   b. edema.
   c. hemoconcentrated.
   d. hypertensive.

8. A fistula is
   a. always a congenital problem.
   b. part of the dialysis machine.
   c. a good source of arterial blood.
   d. the fusion of a vein and artery.

Suggested Laboratory Activities

1. Prioritize a list of tests with special timing or circumstances involved.

2. Change specimen integrity by improper handling and evaluate results.

3. Collect a specimen from a student who has just eaten and check for lipemia.

4. Ask a lab to evaluate specimens taken before and after a change in basal state, for example, draw a CK before and after jogging.

BIBLIOGRAPHY AND SUGGESTED READINGS

Bishop, M. L., Duben-Engelkirk, J. L., & Fody, E. P. (1996). *Clinical chemistry: Principles, procedures, correlations* (3rd ed.). Philadelphia: Lippincott-Raven.

Byrne, C. J., & Saxton, D. (1986). *Laboratory tests: Implications for nursing care.* San Francisco: Addison-Wesley.

National Committee for Clinical Laboratory Standards, H3-A3. (July 1991). *Procedures for the collection of diagnostic blood specimens by venipuncture* (3rd ed.). Villanova, PA: NCCLS.

National Committee for Clinical Laboratory Standards, H4-A3. (July 1991). *Procedures for the collection of diagnostic blood specimens by skin puncture* (3rd ed.). Villanova, PA: NCCLS.

National Committee for Clinical Laboratory Standards, H21-A2. (1991). *Collections, transport and preparation of blood for coagulation testing and performance of coagulation assays.* Villanova, PA: NCCLS.

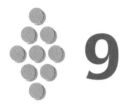

9

Venipuncture Collection Procedures

KEY TERMS

bedside manner	ID band	needle sheath	pediatric tubes
collapsed vein	ID card	palpate	resheathing
concentric circles	Luer adapter	patient	sclerosed
dorsal hand vein	MR number	identifcation	test requisition

OBJECTIVES

Upon successful completion of this chapter, the reader will be able to:

1. Describe the process involved in requesting a test, identify the types of requisitions used, and list required requisition information.

2. Describe proper bedside manner and how to handle special situations associated with patient contact.

3. Explain the importance of proper patient identification and describe what information is verified, how to handle discrepancies, and what to do if a patient's ID band is missing.

4. Describe how to prepare patients for testing, how to answer inquiries concerning tests, and what to do if a patient objects to the test.

5. Describe how to verify diet information and what to do when diet requirements have not been followed.

6. Describe each step in the venipuncture procedure.

7. List necessary information found on specimen tube labels.

8. Describe the situations that may lead to failure to obtain blood and list the acceptable reasons for inability to collect a specimen.

9. Describe collection procedure when using a butterfly and syringe and how to dispense blood into tubes following syringe collection.

(continued)

10. Identify the challenges of pediatric venipuncture and describe how to deal with the patient and parents or guardians, select a method of restraint, and determine which equipment to use for blood collection.

11. Describe how to perform pediatric antecubital and dorsal hand vein venipuncture.

INTRODUCTION

1) Doctors' request/order.

In addition to tests on inpatients, many hospital laboratories perform tests on outpatients from doctor's offices, clinics, and so forth. The following procedures refer to inpatient test collection. Outpatient procedures are the same, if applicable, unless otherwise indicated.

Preparation procedures covered in this chapter are necessary for all blood collection procedures, including venipuncture, skin puncture, and arterial puncture.

health unit coordinator AKA health unit clerk/secretary fills out paper work/enters order in computer

INITIATION OF THE TEST REQUEST

The test collection process begins when the physician orders or "requests" a test to be performed on a patient. All laboratory testing must be requested by a physician, and results must be reported to a physician.

In a hospital setting, a **health unit coordinator** (Fig. 9-1), also known as a **health unit clerk** or **secretary,** fills out the paper work or enters the order in the computer under the direction of the patient's nurse.

In an outpatient setting, the physician's office may call and inform the lab of the order, or the patient may arrive at the lab with order in hand from the physician's office.

Test requistion: 1) computer generated form 2) manuel form

Test Requisitions

The form on which the test is ordered and sent to the lab is called the **test requisition**. The requisition may be a computer generated form or a manual form.

Computer requisitions (Fig. 9-2) usually contain the actual labels that are to be placed on the specimens once they have been collected. There are a number of different

Computer requisitions: 1) contain actual labels to be placed on collected specimen. — contains pt ID info — indicates type of tube — important pt info (potential bleeder)

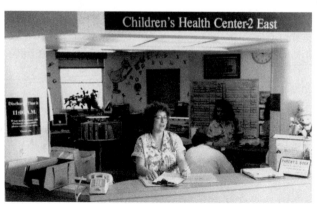

Children's Health Center-2 East

Figure 9-1   Health unit clerk at nurses station.

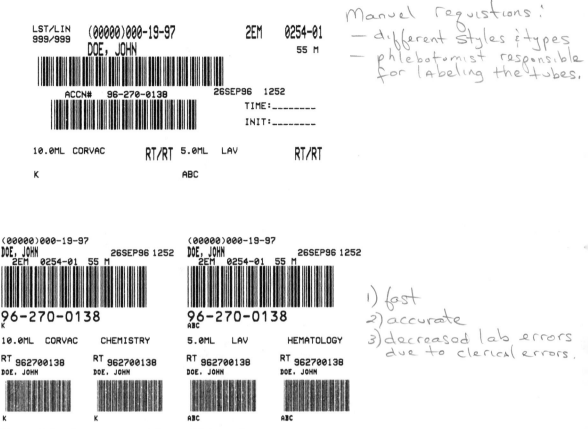

Figure 9-2 Computer requisition with barcode.

types of computer requisitions. Besides the pertinent patient identification information, many also indicate the type of tube needed for the specimen as well as other patient information such as "potential bleeder" or "no venipuncture right arm."

Manual requisitions (Fig. 9-3) come in many different styles and types. Some laboratories require separate requisitions for each department. There are often different colors for each department so that they can be easily distinguished. Many institutions have gone to using one large form with separate sections for the different departments. Some requisitions are a three-part form that serves as a request, a report, and a billing form. When a manual requisition is used, the phlebotomist is responsible for labeling the specimen tube with the required patient information.

Either type of requisition may contain a barcode. A barcode is a series of black and white stripes of varying widths corresponding to letters and numbers; the stripes can be grouped together to represent patient names, identification numbers, or laboratory tests. Barcode information can be scanned into a computer using a special light or laser. Barcode systems allow for fast, accurate processing and their use has been shown to decrease laboratory errors due to clerical mistakes.

Whatever the system used, it is essential for the phlebotomist to become familiar with the various forms in order to be able to interpret them quickly and accurately.

SONORA Laboratory Sciences
3401 E. HARBOUR DRIVE PHOENIX, AZ 85034
602/470-0000 800/766-6721 (800-SONORA-1)

2549672 2549672
2549672 2549672
2549672 2549672

2549672 ACCOUNT INFORMATION

PATIENT I.D. / ROOM NO.
REFERRING PHYSICIAN
COLLECTION DATE / / COLLECTION TIME ☐ A.M. ☐ P.M.
PATIENT LAST NAME (PLEASE PRINT) FIRST NAME MI
BIRTH DATE / / AGE SEX PATIENT SOCIAL SECURITY NO.
ADDRESS (REQUIRED)
CITY STATE ZIP CODE PHONE
TOTAL DUE $ PAID AMOUNT DUE INITIAL
CC TO: DR: ADDRESS CITY, STATE, ZIP
CALL RESULTS TO ☐ FAX RESULTS TO ☐ ☐ STAT INDICATE TEST(S) NEEDED: DRAWING FEE ☐
☐ FASTING ☐ NON-FASTING CLINICAL DATA/COMMENTS

INSURANCE INFO
☐ PHYSICIAN CLIENT ☐ PATIENT ☐ INSURANCE ☐ MEDICARE ☐ AHCCCS
RESPONSIBLE PARTY RELATIONSHIP ☐ SELF ☐ SPOUSE ☐ DEPENDENT
POLICY, I.D. OR MEDICARE # GROUP #
INSURANCE COMPANY
ADDRESS
CITY STATE ZIP
EMPLOYER NAME:
PHOTOCOPY BOTH SIDES OF INSURANCE CARD AND STAPLE TO REQUISITION DIAGNOSIS CODE ICD-9# REFERRAL/AUTHORIZATION #

WRITTEN TESTS CUSTOM PROFILES - CONTACT LABORATORY FOR ADDITION OF CUSTOM PROFILES

PROFILES AND TEST COMBINATIONS ** SEE LAB USERS GUIDE OR FEE LIST FOR SEPARATELY BILLED CPT-4 CODES

☐ 2950	CHEM30 (80019, 82977, 83540)	S	☐ 2958	CHEM BASIC (80019)	S	☐ 2002	CARDIAC RISK (CHOL, TRIG, HDL, DIRECT LDL, VLDL, CHOL/HDL RATIO)	2S
☐ 2067	CHEM30, CBC	S,W	☐ 4794	CHEM BASIC, CBC	S,W	☐ 6165	COCCI PANEL (COCCI IgM, IgG COMP FIX IF IND)	S
☐ 4849	CHEM30, CBC, UA	S,W,U	☐ 4855	CHEM BASIC, CBC, UA	S,W,U	☐ 2455	ELECTROLYTES (NA, K, CL, CO2, GAP)	S
☐ 4736	CHEM30, CBC, SED RATE	S,W	☐ 4856	CHEM BASIC, CBC, SED RATE	S,W	☐ 6006	EPSTEIN BARR-WITH INTERP (IgG, IgM, EBNA)	2S
☐ 2072	CHEM30, CBC, T7	S,W	☐ 4857	CHEM BASIC, CBC, T7	S,W	☐ 4750	HEPATITIS ABC (HAAB IgM, HBSAG, HBCAB IgM, HCAB)	3S
☐ 4850	CHEM30, CBC, T7, UA	S,W,U	☐ 4858	CHEM BASIC, CBC, T7, UA	S,W,U	☐ 2164	HEPATITIS PANEL (HBSAG, HBSAB, HBCAB IgM, HAAB IgM)	3S
☐ 4851	CHEM30, CBC, T7, TSH	2S,W	☐ 4859	CHEM BASIC, CBC, T7, TSH	S,W	☐ 2165	HEPATITIS ACUTE (HBSAG, HBCAB IgM, HAAB IgM)	3S
☐ 2022	CHEM30, DIRECT CARDIAC RISK (DCR)	2S	☐ 4681	CHEM BASIC, CALC CARDIAC RISK (CCR)	S	☐ 2254	HYPOTHYROID PROFILE (T7, TSH)	S
☐ 2069	CHEM30, DCR, CBC	2S,W	☐ 4682	CHEM BASIC, CCR, CBC	2S,W	☐ 2700	LH/FSH	S
☐ 2214	CHEM30, DCR, CBC, UA	2S,W,U	☐ 4683	CHEM BASIC, CCR, CBC, UA	2S,W,U	☐ 1017	PRENATAL 1 (ABO/RH, AB SCR, CBC, RPR, RUBELLA)	S,CT,W
☐ 4852	CHEM30, DCR, CBC, SED RATE	2S,W	☐ 4688	CHEM BASIC, CCR, CBC, SED RATE	2S,W	☐ 1018	PRENATAL 2 (ABO/RH, AB SCR, CBC, RPR, RUBELLA, UA)	S,CT,W,U
☐ 2071	CHEM30, DCR, CBC, T7	2S,W	☐ 4684	CHEM BASIC, CCR, CBC, T7	2S,W	☐ 1019	PRENATAL 3 (ABO/RH, AB SCR, CBC, RPR, RUBELLA, HBSAG)	S,CT,W
☐ 4853	CHEM30, DCR, CBC, T7, UA	2S,W,U	☐ 4686	CHEM BASIC, CCR, CBC, T7, UA	2S,W,U	☐ 2855	PSA/PAP	S
☐ 4954	CHEM30, DCR, CBC, T7, TSH	2S,W	☐ 4860	CHEM BASIC, CCR, CBC, T7, TSH	2S,W	☐ 2023	THYROID GROUP (T7)	S

MICROBIOLOGY/VIROLOGY (* = COMPLETE VIROLOGY INFO SHEET)

☐ 6130 CHLAMYDIA CULTURE*	☐ 6016 CHLAMYDIA EIA*
☐ 6265 HERPES CULTURE*	☐ VIRUS CULTURE*
☐ 6240 GC GENPROBE	☐ 6375 OVA & PARASITES

******CULTURES-ALWAYS INDICATE SOURCE WHEN ORDERING CULTURE******

☐ 6010 AFB CULTURE	☐ 6080 BETA STREP CULTURE
☐ 6225 FUNGUS CULTURE	☐ 6230 GC CULTURE
☐ 6570 ANAEROBIC CULTURE	☐ ROUTINE CULTURE

SOURCE: ______

MANY TESTS AND PROFILES CONTAIN SEPARATELY BILLABLE CPT-4 CODES. ALL TESTS BILLED TO PATIENTS AND THIRD PARTY PAYORS INCLUDING MEDICARE AND AHCCCS WILL BE BILLED ACCORDING TO THEIR RESPECTIVE CODES. SEE YOUR FEE LIST, LAB USER'S GUIDE OR THE REVERSE SIDE OF THIS PAGE FOR SEPARATE CODES.

INDIVIDUAL TESTS

☐ 1050	ABO/RH TYPE	CT	☐ 2465	GLUCOSE (FASTING)	S	☐ 6315	MONOTEST	S	☐ 4290	SED RATE (WEST)	W
☐ 2220	AMYLASE	S	☐ 2510	GLUCOSE (RANDOM)	S	☐ 2790	POTASSIUM	S	☐ 2013	THEOPHYLLINE	S
☐ 6040	ANA	S	☐ 2030	GLUCOSE-2HR PP	S	☐ 2915	PREGNANCY, SERUM	S	☐ 2985	T3 (TOTAL)	S
☐ 2250	BUN	S	☐	GLUCOSE TOL HRS ______	S	☐ 2102	PSA	S	☐ 2995	T3 UPTAKE	S
☐ 4075	CBC (AUTO DIFF)	W	☐	GESTATIONAL TOL HRS ______	S	☐ 4255	PROTIME (INR)	P(F)	☐ 2043	T4	S
☐ 2305	CEA	S	☐ 2520	GLYCOHEMOGLOBIN	W	☐ 4020	PTT	P(F)	☐ 2118	TSH	S
☐ 2395	CREATININE	S	☐ 2530	HDL CHOL	S	☐ 6415	RPR	S	☐ 4370	URINALYSIS	U
☐ 2430	DIGOXIN	S	☐ 6260	HIV (SEE BACKER PAGE 3)	S	☐ 6440	RUBELLA IgG	S			

SPECIMEN REQUIREMENT CODES

SST		
S - SERUM OR SST	W - WHOLE BLOOD	U - RANDOM URINE
CT - CLOTTED TUBE	- (LAVENDER TOP TUBE)	(F) - SPIN, FREEZE IN PLASTIC VIAL
P - PLASMA (BLUE TOP)	U24 - 24 HOUR URINE	(R) - SUBMIT AT ROOM TEMPERATURE

I AUTHORIZE SONORA LABORATORY SCIENCES TO BILL ME FOR CHARGES NOT COVERED BY MEDICARE OR MY INSURANCE COMPANY.

DRAWN ____ OPEN ____ TR ____ LABEL ____ VERIFY ____ CHANGE ____ PATIENT SIGNATURE ____

SEND FIRST 2 COPIES TO LABORATORY

Figure 9-3 Manual requisition (Courtesy Sonora Laboratory Sciences, Phoenix, AZ).

Information Needed on the Requisition
- Ordering physician's name
- Patient's name
- Patient's medical record number
- Patient's date of birth
- Room number and bed (if inpatient)
- Type of test to be performed
- Date test is to be performed
- Test status (*eg*, timed, fasting, priority)
- Billing information (if outpatient)

Receipt of Test Requisition by the Lab

Computer requisitions are usually printed out at a computer terminal at the phlebotomist station in the laboratory. Manual requisitions are sent by courier or pneumatic tube system or are collected during "sweeps" by members of the phlebotomy team. A phlebotomist is then in charge of sorting the requisitions according to date, time, and priority of collection, as well as location of the patient.

Preparing to Collect Requested Specimens

When it is time to collect the specimens, the phlebotomist checks the requisitions to see that all of the needed equipment is on the blood-collecting tray or cart. The phlebotomist then proceeds to the first patient.

PATIENT CONTACT

Entering the Patient's Room

Doors to patient's rooms are usually open. If the door to the room is closed, the phlebotomist should knock lightly, open the door slowly, and say something like "good morning," before proceeding into the room. Even if the door is open, it is a good idea to knock lightly to make occupants aware that you are about to enter. Curtains are often pulled when nurses are working with patients or when patients are using bedpans or urinals. Making your presence known to patients before proceeding or opening the curtain may avoid embarrassing them.

Watching for Signs

It is important to watch for signs containing information concerning your patient. Signs are typically posted on the door to the patient's room or on the wall behind the patient's bed. Signs commonly encountered include those that signify infection control precautions to follow when entering the room, limit the number of visitors allowed in the room at one time, indicate that fall precautions are to be observed for patients, and warn that a patient has a severe allergy (*eg*, to latex or flowers).

A sign with a picture of a fallen leaf with a teardrop is sometimes used on obstetric wards to indicate that a patient has lost a baby. A sign with only the letters DNR means that the patient has a **"Do Not Resuscitate"** order. A Do Not Resuscitate order, also called a "no-code," usually means that no code is to be called and no heroic measures are to be taken if the patient stops breathing. A sign of particular importance to a phlebotomist is one that prohibits blood pressures or blood draws from a particular arm (Fig. 9-4).

Identifying Yourself

Identify yourself to the patient by stating your name, that you are from the lab, and why you are there (eg, "Good morning. My name is Joe Smith. I'm from the lab and I'm here to collect a blood specimen ordered by your doctor."). If you are a student, communicate this information to the patient as well. This is a part of informed consent and patient rights. The patient has a right to refuse to have blood drawn by a student.

Handling Special Situations

IF THE PATIENT IS ASLEEP

If the patient is asleep, as is often the case on early morning rounds, wake him or her gently. Try not to startle the patient. (Startling can cause a change in test results.) Nudge the bed rather than the patient. Speak softly but distinctly, and avoid turning on bright overhead lighting, at least until the patient's eyes have adjusted to being open. *Never* attempt to collect a blood specimen from a sleeping patient. Such an attempt may startle the patient and cause injury to the patient or the phlebotomist. In addition, drawing blood from a sleeping patient violates the patient's right to informed consent.

IF THE PATIENT IS UNCONSCIOUS

Unconscious patients are often encountered in emergency rooms and intensive care units. When patients are unconscious, permission for procedures has usually been given by next of kin. If the patient is unconscious, continue to speak to the patient. Identify yourself and inform the patient of your intent just as you would an alert patient. Unconscious patients can often hear what is going on around them even though they are unresponsive. They may also be able to feel pain and may move when you insert the needle to draw the specimen. It may therefore be necessary to have someone assist you in holding an unconscious patient's arm during the blood draw.

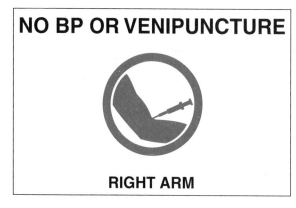

Figure 9-4   Warning sign indicating "No blood pressures or venipuncture in right arm."

IF A PHYSICIAN OR MEMBER OF THE CLERGY
IS WITH THE PATIENT

If the patient's physician or a member of the clergy is with the patient, don't interrupt. The patient's time with the physician or clergy is private and limited. Proceed to the next patient and come back to that patient later. If the request is for a stat or timed specimen, excuse yourself, explain why you are there, and ask permission to proceed.

IF THE PATIENT IS NOT IN THE ROOM

If the patient is not in the room, check at the nurses' station to find out where the patient is. If the patient has been taken to another department such as x-ray, you may still be able to collect the specimen from the patient in the waiting area of that department, before procedures have begun.

Every attempt should be made to find the patient, especially if the test is timed. If the patient cannot be located or is unavailable, or if you are unable to obtain the specimen for any other reason, it is the policy of most laboratories to have you fill out a form stating that you were unable to obtain the specimen at the requested time, as well as the reason why. The original copy of this form is left at the nurses' station and a copy goes back to the lab.

Handling Family and Visitors

Often there are family members or visitors in the room when you arrive to collect a specimen. It is best to ask them to step outside the room until you are finished. Most will prefer to do so. Occasionally a family member, especially a spouse, is willing to assist you if needed. It is generally acceptable to let a willing family member help steady the arm or hold pressure over the site while you label tubes.

PATIENT IDENTIFICATION

Importance of Proper Identification

The most important step in specimen collection is **patient identification**. Obtaining a specimen from the wrong patient can have serious, even fatal, consequences, as in the case of specimens for type and crossmatch prior to blood transfusion. Misidentification of a patient can be grounds for dismissal of the person responsible and could even lead to a malpractice lawsuit against that person.

Determining the Patient's Name and Date of Birth

When identifying a patient, ask the patient to state his or her name and date of birth. For example, *never* say "Are you Mrs. Smith?" A person who is very ill, hard of hearing, or on heavy medication may say "yes" to anything. Using a "memory jogger" such as having a patient spell an unusual name, or commenting in some positive way about a name, will help you remember that you verified it.

Checking the Patient's Identification Bracelet

If the patient's response matches the information on the requisition, proceed to check the patient's **identification (ID)** bracelet (Fig. 9-5) (also called **ID band**, **arm band**, or **wrist band**).

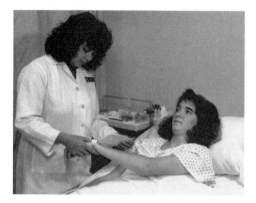

Figure 9-5   Phlebotomist at bedside checking patient identification band.

All hospital patients are required to wear an ID band, usually on the wrist. The ID band lists the patient's name and hospital identification number or **medical record (MR) number** (Fig. 9-6). Additional information includes the patient's birth date or age, room number and bed designation, and physician's name.

It is important that the patient's name, MR number, and birth date information on the ID band match the information on the requisition *exactly*. It is not unusual to have patients with the same or similar names in the hospital at the same time. (Examples are patients with common last names, fathers and sons, multiple birth babies, and relatives involved in tissue transplant procedures.) There have even been instances where two patients shared the same full name and birth date. Two patients will *not*, however, have the same hospital or medical record number, although it may be similar.

Identification protocol may vary slightly from one health care institution to another. Generally, additional ID information such as room number, bed number, and physician's name are important but are allowed to differ. For instance, occasionally a room number will differ because the patient has been moved. In addition, the name of the ordering physician may be different since it is not unusual for a patient to be under the care of several different physicians at the same time.

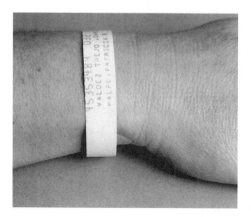

Figure 9-6   Typical identification bracelet.

How to Handle ID Discrepancies

If there is a discrepancy between the name, MR number, or date of birth information on the ID band and the information on the requisition, the patient's nurse should be notified. The specimen should not be obtained until the discrepancy is addressed and the patient's identity is verified.

If the ID Band Is Missing

If there is no ID band on the patient's wrist, check to see if it is on an ankle. Intravenous lines in patient's arms often infiltrate the surrounding tissues and cause swelling that necessitates removal of the ID band. When this occurs, especially on a patient with IV lines in both arms, nursing personnel will often place the ID band around the ankle.

In some instances, harried personnel remove ID bands from IV-infiltrated arms, or while other procedures are being performed on patients, and place them on the night table by the patient's bed. An ID band on a night table could belong to a patient who previously occupied that bed. It is also not unusual for a new patient to occupy a bed before the nursing staff has a chance to attach his or her ID band. For this reason, identification should *never* be verified from an ID band that is *not* attached to the patient. In such instances, as well as when no ID band can be found, it is necessary to ask the patient's nurse to attach an ID band before the specimen is drawn. In an emergency situation where there is no time to wait for attachment of the ID band, the name or initials of the nurse making the ID verification should be written on the requisition.

Emergency Room Identification Procedures

It is not uncommon for an emergency room (ER) to receive an unconscious patient with no identification. Specimens should not be collected without some way to connect the specimen positively with the patient. In many institutions, the phlebotomist will attach a special three-part identification band, such as a Typenex Blood Recipient ID band (Fenwal Laboratories, a division of Travenol Laboratories, Deerfield, IL), to an unidentified ER patient's wrist. The same number is on all three parts. The first part becomes the patient's ID band. The second part is attached to the specimen. The third part is used if the patient needs a transfusion, and is attached to the unit of blood.

Identification of Infants and Young Children

Infants can be identified by the ID band, which is usually located on the ankle. The phlebotomist should be very careful when identifying as-yet-unnamed newborn infants. They are commonly identified, for example, as "Baby Boy Jones." Be especially careful when identifying twins or other multiple-birth babies. They are commonly identified, for example, as Jones, twin A or B. *Never* rely on the name card on the infant's bed for identification purposes. Always check the ID band.

The identification of young children can be confirmed by a parent or relative. Identity of young children who are missing ID bands should be confirmed by the patient's nurse, and an ID bracelet should be attached in the same way as for adults.

Identification of Outpatients

Outpatients do not normally have ID bands. However, they may have an **ID card**. Some clinics give their patients ID cards from which specimen labels can be imprinted using an address-o-graph machine.

Outpatients often arrive with the order from their doctor in hand. The outpatient area receptionist will verify the identity of the patient and fill out the proper lab requisition or generate one via computer. Some labs supply the doctors that use their services with the proper lab forms so that the patient arrives with the lab requisition already filled out.

Even if the patient has been properly identified by the receptionist, the phlebotomist must verify the patient's ID once the patient is actually called into the blood-drawing area from the waiting room. Simply calling a person's name and having someone respond is not verification enough. Anxious or hard-of-hearing patients may think that they heard their name called, when in fact the phlebotomist called a similar name. There could also be two patients in the waiting area with the same name. The phlebotomist should ask an outpatient his or her name and date of birth, in the same manner described for inpatients, before obtaining the specimen.

PREPARING THE PATIENT FOR TESTING

Bedside Manner

Gaining the patient's trust and confidence and putting the patient at ease are important aspects of **bedside manner**. The phlebotomist who has a professional appearance and who behaves in a professional manner will more easily gain a patient's trust. A confident phlebotomist will convey that confidence to the patient.

A cheerful and pleasant manner and an exchange of small talk with the patient will help to put a patient at ease, as well as divert attention from any discomfort associated with the procedure.

Handling Difficult Patients

A phlebotomist's cheerful and pleasant manner may not be echoed by the patient. Hospitalization is usually a stressful situation for a patient. A patient may be lonely, scared, fearful, or just plain disagreeable and may react in a negative manner toward the phlebotomist. The phlebotomist should remain calm and professional and treat the patient in a caring manner under all circumstances.

Explaining the Procedure

Most patients have had a blood test before. To them the phlebotomist's statement of intent to perform a blood test is usually sufficient for them to understand what is about to occur. To a patient who has never had a blood test, a more detailed explanation may be necessary. Special procedures may require additional information.

If a patient does not speak or understand English, the phlebotomist may have to use sign language or other nonverbal means to demonstrate what is to occur. If this fails, an interpreter must be located. Speaking slowly and distinctly, using sign language, or writing down information may be necessary for patients with hearing problems.

In any event, as part of informed consent the phlebotomist must always inform the patient of the procedure and determine that the patient understands what is about to take place before proceeding.

Handling Patient Inquiry About Tests

Some hospitals will allow the phlebotomist to tell the patient the name of the test or tests to be performed. Others prefer that all inquiries be directed to the patient's physician. Because a particular test may be ordered to rule out a number of different problems, an attempt by the phlebotomist to explain the purpose of a test could be very misleading and unduly alarming to the patient. The phlebotomist usually handles such inquiries by stating that the doctor has ordered the tests as part of the patient's care and that the doctor will be happy to explain the tests to him or her if asked.

In cases where bedside testing is being performed (such as glucose monitoring), if the patient is already aware of the type of test being performed and asks about results, the phlebotomist should check with the patient's nurse to see if it is acceptable to tell the patient the results.

If the Patient Objects to the Procedure

Most patients understand that blood tests are needed in the course of their treatment. Occasionally a patient will object to the procedure. Reminding the patient that the test was ordered by the doctor as part of his or her care will sometimes convince the patient to cooperate. If not, often the patient's nurse may be able to convince the patient to cooperate. It is not up to the phlebotomist to attempt to badger the patient into cooperating, nor should a conscious, mentally alert adult patient be restrained in order to obtain a specimen. Remember, the patient has the right to refuse to have the test done.

When it has been determined that a patient truly refuses to cooperate, the phlebotomist should write on the requisition that the patient has refused to have blood drawn. The phlebotomist should also notify the patient's nurse and the phlebotomy supervisor that the specimen was not obtained owing to patient refusal.

Verifying Diet Restrictions

Once the patient has been properly identified and has consented to the procedure, the phlebotomist should verify that the patient has followed any special diet instructions or restrictions. The most common diet requirement is for the patient to fast (refrain from eating) for a certain period of time, commonly overnight or "nothing past midnight."

If the phlebotomist determines that the patient did not fast or otherwise follow diet instructions, the nursing staff (or patient's physician, in the case of an outpatient) should be informed so that a determination can be made as to whether or not to proceed with the test. In the event that the phlebotomist is told to proceed with collecting the specimen, the phlebotomist should write "non-fasting" on the specimen requisition and the specimen label.

Proceeding With Specimen Collection

Once the patient has been properly identified and informed, compliance with diet restrictions has been determined, and the patient has consented to the procedure, the phlebotomist can proceed to collect the test specimen.

ROUTINE VENIPUNCTURE PROCEDURE

Most laboratory tests require collection of a blood specimen by means of a routine venipuncture. Performance of a venipuncture is often referred to as "drawing blood." A routine venipuncture involves the following steps. (*Note:* The following steps were written using guidelines established by the National Committee for Clinical Laboratory Standards [see National Standards, Chapter 1]. In a clinical setting, there may be some variation in methods because of individual technique and special circumstances.)

Review the Test Requisition

Check to see that all information on the requisition is complete. Verify the time and date of collection, and any special circumstances such as diet restrictions or priority of test collection. Identify the tests to be collected and make certain the blood collection tray or cart is stocked with the necessary equipment.

Identify Patient

The most important step in the venipuncture procedure is proper patient identification. Identify the patient in the manner previously described in this chapter.

Verify Diet Restrictions

Verify that the patient has followed diet restrictions, if applicable, following procedures described earlier in the chapter.

Assemble Equipment and Supplies

A routine venipuncture requires the following equipment and supplies (Fig. 9-7):

1. Gloves
2. Tourniquet

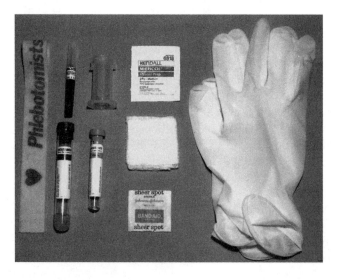

Figure 9-7 Routine venipuncture equipment.

3. 70% isopropanol (alcohol) prep pads or preferred antiseptic for the test (*eg*, povidone–iodine for blood cultures, non–alcohol-containing antiseptic for blood alcohol); alternate antiseptic such as green soap or soap and water for a patient allergic to the preferred antiseptic
4. Gauze pads or cotton or Dacron balls
5. Needle and evacuated tube holder (assembled) (Fig. 9-8)
6. Appropriate tubes for the tests, arranged in proper order of draw with the first tube inserted into the evacuated tube holder (Expiration dates on the tubes must be checked to make certain that they have not expired.)
7. Needle disposal (sharps) container
8. Adhesive bandages or other bandaging materials
9. Permanent marker or pen

Wash Hands and Put on Gloves
Proper hand washing followed by glove application is a very important part of the venipuncture procedure. Hands may be washed in a downward motion, scrubbing from wrists to fingertips, which prevents backflow of contaminated water and soap. A circular scrubbing motion using plenty of friction will help dislodge surface debris and bacteria. It is important to pay particular attention to areas between the fingers and around the nails. Hands should be rinsed from wrists to fingertips also and dried with a clean paper towel. Once the hands have been dried, the water can be shut off using a clean, dry paper towel. The phlebotomist then puts on a clean pair of gloves.

Reassure Patient
Reassuring the patient is a part of bedside manner. If the patient is worried about the amount of pain associated with the procedure, be honest and tell him or her that there will be a small amount of discomfort, but it will be of short duration. *Never* tell a patient that it won't hurt. Even children expect to be told the truth.

Explain to the patient the importance of holding the arm very still. A child's cooperation can be gained by having him or her take an active part in the process, such as holding the gauze pad. Rewards such as stickers, character badges, or smiley face bandages will help leave the child with a positive memory of the procedure.

Position Patient
A patient should be either seated or lying down while having blood drawn. A patient should *never* be standing or seated on a high stool.

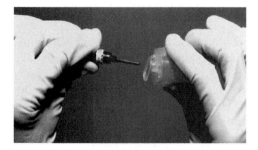

Figure 9-8   Needle and holder assembly.

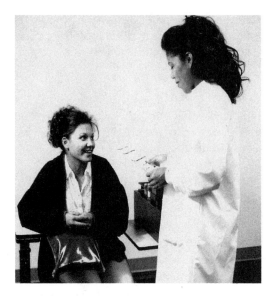

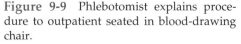

Figure 9-9 Phlebotomist explains procedure to outpatient seated in blood-drawing chair.

SEATED PATIENT

Outpatients are most commonly seated in a special blood-drawing chair (Fig. 9-9). When seated, a patient's arm should be supported firmly on a slanted armrest and extended downward in a straight line from the shoulder to the wrist. The arm should *not* be bent at the elbow. Straightening the arm at the elbow helps fix the vein and make it easier to locate. A downward position allows gravity to help the veins enlarge and become more prominent. In addition, a downward position helps assure that blood collection tubes fill from the bottom up, which is necessary to prevent reflux of tube contents and additive carryover between tubes.

SUPINE PATIENT

Inpatients normally have blood drawn in a supine position. An outpatient in a weakened condition or one who has fainted previously when having a blood test should also have blood drawn lying down. As with the seated patient, the arm should be extended in a straight line from shoulder to wrist and not bent at the elbow. In proper position, the hand should be lower than the elbow. A pillow or a rolled towel may be used to support and position the arm if necessary.

OTHER CONSIDERATIONS

Bed rails may be let down, being careful not to catch IV lines, catheter bags and tubing, or other patient apparatus.

Bed rails *must* be raised again when the phlebotomist is finished. If the phlebotomist lowers a bed rail and forgets to replace it when finished, and a patient subsequently falls out of bed and is injured, the phlebotomist can be held liable. Many phlebotomists have learned to collect specimens with bed rails in place so as not to forget to put them back up.

A patient should not be eating, drinking, or chewing gum or have a thermometer, toothpick, or any other foreign object in the mouth when having blood drawn. Objects

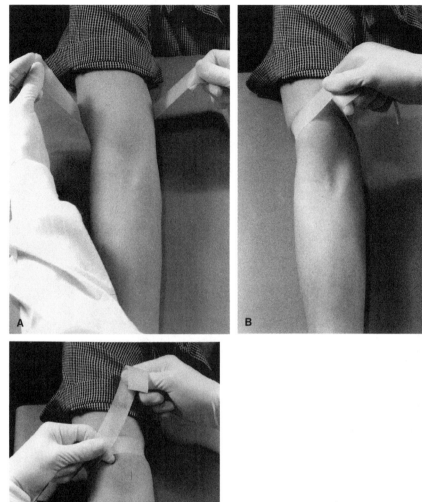

Figure 9-10 Tourniquet application. (**A**) Proper tourniquet placement with tension applied. (**B**) Both tourniquet sides grasped between thumb and forefinger of the right hand. (**C**) Left side of tourniquet crossed over the right side with both sides held between the thumb and index finger of the left hand. (*continued*)

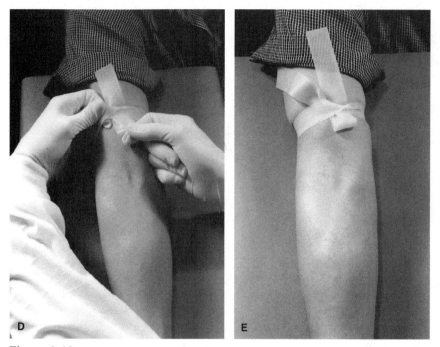

Figure 9-10 (*Continued*)   (**D**) Left end of tourniquet tucked under right side, forming loop. (**E**) Properly tied tourniquet.

in the mouth can cause choking. A bite reflex could break a thermometer and injure a patient.

Apply Tourniquet

A tourniquet is applied to increase pressure in the veins and aid in vein selection (Fig. 9-10). It should be applied tightly enough to slow the venous flow without affecting the arterial flow. This allows more blood to flow into the area than out, which causes the veins to enlarge, making them easier to find and penetrate with a needle. If a patient has prominent veins, tourniquet application can wait until after cleansing, just prior to needle insertion.

The tourniquet is applied 3 to 4 inches above the intended venipuncture site. If it is tied too close to the site, the vein may collapse as blood is withdrawn. If it is tied too far above the site, it may be ineffective. If a patient has sensitive skin or dermatitis, the tourniquet may be applied over a sleeve or dry washcloth or gauze wrapped around the arm.

- *Do not* apply a tourniquet over an open sore. Choose another site.
- *Do not* apply a tourniquet to an arm on the side of a recent mastectomy without the permission of the patient's physician.

Apply a latex strip tourniquet by positioning it around the arm with each hand grasping one side of the tourniquet a few inches from the end and applying a small amount of tension (see Fig. 9-10*A*). While continuing to maintain tension, bring the two sides of the tourniquet together, and grasp both between the thumb and forefinger of the right hand (see Fig. 9-10*B*). Reach over the right hand with the left hand and grasp the right side of the tourniquet between the thumb and forefinger of the left hand, releasing it from the grip of the right hand. The tourniquet ends will now be held in opposite hands. Cross the left end over the right end where it crosses the left index finger, grasping both sides together between the thumb and forefinger of the left hand, close to the patient's arm (see Fig. 9-10*C*). While the two sides are still grasped securely, tuck a portion of the left side of the tourniquet under the right side, using either the left middle finger or right index finger, and pull the tucked portion into a loop (see Fig. 9-10*D*). The ends of a properly tied tourniquet will point toward the shoulder (see Fig. 9-10*E*). A slight tug on the tourniquet end on the right (the side forming the loop) should easily release it from the patient's arm (Fig. 9-11*D*).

The tourniquet should feel slightly tight to the patient. It should not be rolled or twisted and it should not be so tight that it pinches or hurts. It should not be so tight that the arm turns red or purple.

A tourniquet that is tied too tightly may prevent arterial blood flow into the area and result in failure to obtain blood. A tourniquet that is too loose will be ineffective. To minimize the effects of stasis and hemoconcentration, the tourniquet should *never* be left in place longer than 1 minute (see NCCLS document H3-A3, National Committee for Clinical Standards, 771 E. Lancaster Ave., Villanova, PA 19085).

Select Venipuncture Site

Venipuncture is most commonly performed in the antecubital area of the arm where the median cubital, cephalic, and basilic veins lie fairly close to the surface. This area should be examined first. Some veins are easily visible, others will have to be located by feel. A patient will generally have the most prominent veins in the dominant arm.

Having the patient make a fist will help make the veins more prominent. Vigorous **pumping** (opening and closing) of the fist should be avoided as it may cause erroneous results in a number of tests due to hemoconcentration.

Use the tip of the index finger to **palpate** (feel) the vein (Fig. 9-11*A*). Palpating will help to determine the size, depth, and direction of the vein. Select a vein that is large and well anchored or fixed (does not move to the side easily or "roll").

If you have trouble feeling a vein, close your eyes while feeling. (Closing your eyes enhances your sense of touch.) A vein has a bounce or resilience to it. An artery will pulsate. To avoid inadvertently puncturing an artery, *do not* select a vein that overlies or is close to an artery. In addition, *do not* select a vein that feels hard and cord-like or lacks resilience. Such veins are said to be **sclerosed**. Sclerosed veins are hard to penetrate, roll easily, and may not have adequate blood flow to yield a representative blood sample. A **thrombosed** vein (a vein containing a thrombus or clot) will also feel hard and should not be used for venipuncture.

Once you have selected a vein, try to visualize mentally the location of the vein. It often helps to note the position of the vein in reference to a freckle, mole, hair, skin crease, or other skin structure to make relocation easier after cleansing the site.

One way to remember the location of a hard-to-find vein is to mark the vein's position in the following manner. First, locate the vein with the index finger. Keeping your

(text continues on page 212)

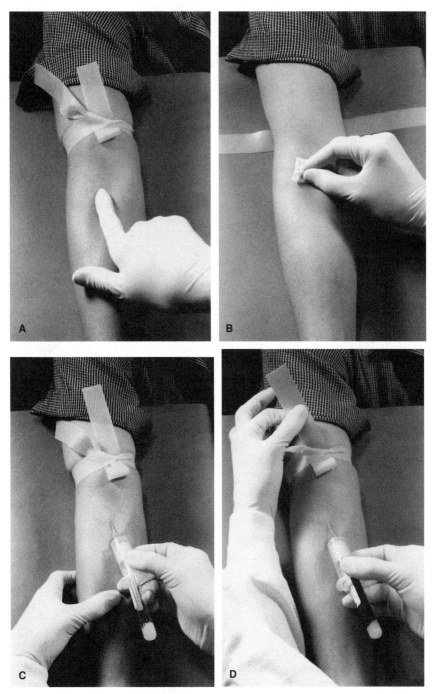

Figure 9-11 Venipuncture procedure. (**A**) Palpating (feeling) for a vein. (**B**) Cleaning the site (note: the tourniquet has been removed for this procedure). (**C**) Entering the vein with the needle while the thumb pulls the skin taut (note: the tourniquet has been retied). (**D**) Removing the tourniquet: one hand steadies the tube holder as the tube fills with blood; the other pulls the end of the tucked side of the tourniquet to release it from the patient's arm. (*continued*)

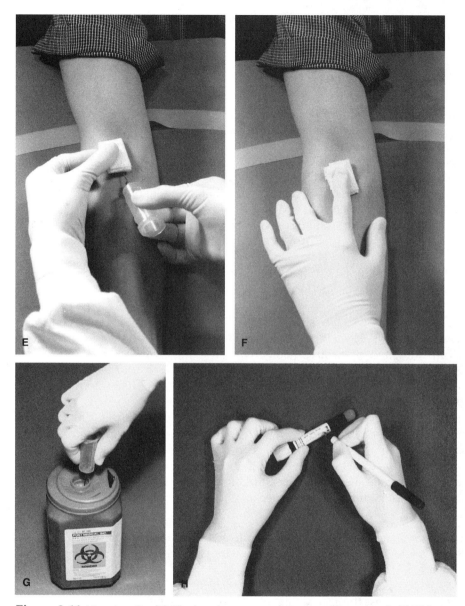

Figure 9-11 (*Continued*)   (**E**) Placing the gauze prior to needle removal. (**F**) Phlebotomist holding pressure over the venipuncture site. (**G**) Disposing of the needle. (**H**) Labeling the specimen tube.

finger over the site, use the other hand to align the corner of a clean alcohol pad over the vein, near your finger (Fig. 9-12*A*). Slide the pad away from the site, paralleling the direction of the vein and keeping the corner of the pad pointing in the direction of the vein (see Fig. 9-12*B*). Keep the pad far enough away from the site so as not to be in the way or disturbed when cleaning the site (see Fig. 9-12*C*).

If no suitable antecubital vein can be found, check the other arm. When no suitable antecubital vein can be found in either arm, check for wrist or hand veins. If a suitable vein still cannot be found, wrap a warm, wet towel around the arm or hand for a few minutes. Warming the site will increase blood flow and help to make veins more prominent.

Ankle veins should only be used as a last resort and after checking with the patient's physician. Blood flow to the extremities, especially in bedridden patients and patients with coagulation problems, is not representative of the general circulation and may yield erroneous results. Ankle vein puncture of a patient with coagulation problems may have dangerous consequences such as thrombus (blood clot) formation and impaired circulation.

Release Tourniquet

If the tourniquet was applied during vein selection it should be released during the cleansing process (see NCCLS document H3-A3).

Cleanse the Site

Cleansing the venipuncture site (see Fig. 9-11*B*) with an antiseptic helps prevent microbial contamination of the specimen and the patient. However, it will *not* sterilize the site. The recommended antiseptic is 70% isopropyl alcohol. Most health care institutions use a commercially prepared, sterile, prepackaged alcohol pad referred to as an **alcohol prep pad**.

Clean the site using a circular motion, starting at the center of the site and moving outward in ever widening **concentric circles**. Use sufficient pressure to remove surface dirt and debris. If the site is especially dirty, clean it again with another alcohol prep pad.

Allow the area to dry for 30 seconds to 1 minute. The evaporation and drying process helps to destroy microbes. In addition, penetrating the site with a needle while the alcohol is wet may cause hemolysis of the specimen as well as a burning sensation in the patient.

- *Do not* recontaminate the site by drying the alcohol with unsterile gauze.
- *Do not* blow on the site. Blowing or fanning it with your hand may introduce airborne contaminants.
- *Do not* touch the site after cleaning. If it is necessary to repalpate the vein, the site must be cleaned again unless the gloved finger has first been cleaned in the same manner as the arm.

Verify Equipment and Tube Selection

Check to see that the correct tubes and other equipment have been selected for the tests ordered. Make certain that the needle is securely fastened to the evacuated tube holder and the first tube is properly seated in the holder.

- *Do not* push the tube past the guideline on the holder or loss of vacuum may result.
- *Do not* remove the **needle sheath** (cover) until just prior to needle insertion.

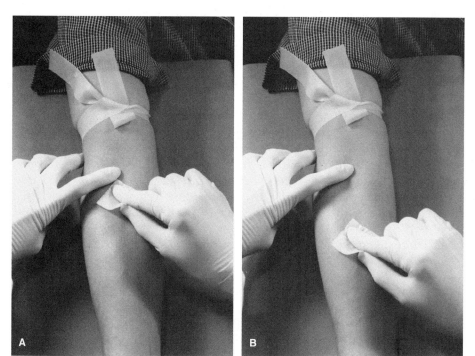

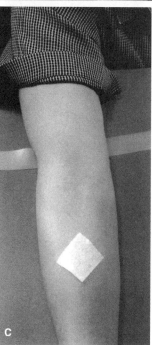

Figure 9-12 Marking the site with an alcohol pad. (**A**) Aligning the corner of a clean alcohol pad over the vein located by the index finger. (**B**) Sliding the pad away from the site, paralleling the direction of the vein and keeping the corner of the pad pointing in the direction of the vein. (**C**) Alcohol pad pointing in the direction of the vein.

- Place blood-drawing equipment within easy reach. Make certain that extra equipment or the blood collecting tray, as well as the sharps container, are within easy reach.
- *Do not* place the blood collection tray on the patient's bed.

Reapply Tourniquet

Reapply the tourniquet, being careful not to touch the cleansed area. Have the patient make a fist if necessary.

Pick Up Blood-Drawing Equipment and Remove Needle Sheath

Hold the blood-drawing apparatus in your dominant hand with the thumb on top of the evacuated tube holder and the fingers underneath. (Some phlebotomists like to position the index finger near the hub of the needle during vein entry; however, the finger *must not* touch the needle.) Verify that the tube is positioned in the evacuated tube holder. A properly positioned tube is pushed onto the needle just far enough to hold the tube and keep it from falling out of the holder, but not far enough to release the vacuum of the tube. (Most tube holders contain a guideline beyond which the tube should not be pushed.) If the tube tries to prematurely push off of the needle in the tube holder, it is acceptable to wait until the needle is inserted in the patient's vein to put the tube into the holder.

Remove the needle cover. Visually inspect the needle tip for obstructions, imperfections, or barbs. Do not let the needle touch anything prior to venipuncture. If it does, it must be removed and replaced with a new needle.

Anchor the Vein

Grasp the patient's arm with your nondominant hand, using your thumb to pull the skin taut 1 to 2 inches below the intended venipuncture site. This **anchors** the vein and helps keep it from moving or rolling to the side upon needle entry. (If the vein rolls, the needle may slip beside the vein, not into it.) The fingers of the same hand can be used to support the back of the arm in the area of the elbow. This helps keep the patient from pulling away as the needle enters the vein.

For safety reasons, using both the index finger and the thumb for anchoring the vein (two-finger technique) is not recommended, because it is not uncommon for an apprehensive patient to suddenly pull back the arm as the needle is inserted. If two-finger technique is used, there is the possibility that the needle may come out of the patient's arm and into the phlebotomist's finger. If the phlebotomist is anchoring with the thumb and the fingers are wrapped around the arm, the patient is less likely to pull completely away from the phlebotomist's grasp and the needle is more likely to stay in the vein.

Insert the Needle Into the Vein

Have the patient make a fist. This step can be eliminated on patients with prominent veins that are easily anchored. Line the needle up with the vein with the bevel of the needle facing up and pointing in the same direction as the venous flow. The direction of needle insertion should follow the path of the vein. Warn the patient by saying something like "There is going to be a little poke now." Insert the needle into the skin at a 15- to 30-degree angle, using one smooth motion to penetrate first the skin and then the vein (see Fig. 9-11C). Do not push down on the needle or use a scooping motion as the needle is inserted. When the needle enters the vein, you will feel a slight "give" or decrease in resistance. As soon as you sense that the needle is in the vein, stop advancing the needle and securely anchor the tube holder.

At this point, some phlebotomists switch to holding the blood-drawing apparatus in their nondominant hand so that tube changes can be made with their dominant hand. This is accomplished by gently slipping the fingers of the opposite hand under the holder and placing the thumb atop the holder as the other hand lets go. Another method is to grasp the holder between the thumb and index finger, with the hand resting on the patient's arm over (but not touching) the needle. Other phlebotomists, particularly those who are left handed, do not change hands but continue to steady the holder in the same hand and change tubes with the opposite.

Whatever the method, it is important to hold the blood-drawing apparatus steady so there is minimal needle movement. If the holder is not securely anchored, the needle can push through the back of the vein or pull out of the vein when tubes are changed during the draw. When the tube holder is securely anchored, the knuckles of the anchoring fingers are pressed against the patient's arm.

Fill the Tubes

With the tube holder securely anchored, advance the evacuated tube to the end of the holder, using your thumb to push the tube while your index and middle fingers grasp the flange of the tube holder. Blood should begin to flow freely into the evacuated tube. If not, exert constant forward pressure on the end of the tube in case the rubber needle sleeve is trying to push the tube off of the needle.

As soon as blood flows into the tube, *release the tourniquet* (see Fig. 9-11D) and have the patient release his or her fist, if applicable. *Do not* leave the tourniquet on for more than 1 minute. When the tourniquet is released, blood should continue to flow and multiple tubes can still be collected. *Exception:* On elderly patients and others with fragile veins that might collapse, or in other difficult draw situations where release of the tourniquet might cause stoppage of blood flow, the tourniquet is sometimes left on until the last tube is filled and released just prior to needle withdrawal. Three or four tubes can usually be filled in under 1 minute if the tourniquet was properly applied just prior to needle insertion.

Steady the needle in the vein. Try not to pull up or press down on the needle while it is in the vein. Both actions can be painful to the patient and may enlarge the hole in the vein, resulting in leakage of blood and hematoma formation.

Try to maintain the arm and the tube in a downward position so that blood fills the tube from the bottom up and does not contact the needle in the tube holder. This will help to prevent reflux (flow of blood from the tube back into the vein) as well as carryover of additives to other tubes by means of blood left on the needle as tubes are changed.

To ensure a proper ratio of additive to blood, let the tube fill until the vacuum is exhausted and blood ceases to flow. Tubes will not fill completely to the top. Remove the tube, using a twisting and pulling motion while bracing the thumb against the flange of the holder.

If the tube contains an additive, mix it immediately by *gently* inverting it 5 to 8 times (depending upon the type of additive and manufacturer's recommendations) before putting it down. Vigorous mixing of anticoagulant tubes or shaking of tubes can cause hemolysis. Lack of or inadequate mixing can lead to clot formation. Nonadditive tubes do not require mixing.

If other tubes are to be drawn, place them into the holder and push them all the way onto the needle. Steady the tube holder so that the needle does not pull out or penetrate through the vein as tubes are placed and removed. Be certain to follow the proper order of draw (see Chapter 7).

When the last tube has been filled, it must be removed from the holder and mixed (if applicable) before the needle is removed from the arm. If the tube is still attached to the needle when it is removed from the arm, the needle will drip blood and cause needless contamination.

Withdraw the Needle

After the last tube has been removed from the holder, fold a clean gauze square in fourths and place it directly over the site where the needle enters the vein (see Fig. 9-11E). A clean cotton ball may be used over the site instead of gauze, however, cotton balls tend to stick to the site and reinitiate bleeding when removed. *Do not* press down on the gauze while the needle is in the vein. (Applying pressure to the needle during removal is painful, and the needle may slit the vein and the skin as it is withdrawn.) Withdraw the needle in one smooth motion, and immediately apply pressure to the site with the gauze pad (see Fig. 9-11F) or cotton ball for 3 to 5 minutes or until the bleeding has stopped. Failure to apply pressure will result in leakage of blood and hematoma formation. It is acceptable to have the patient hold pressure while you proceed to label tubes, providing the patient agrees and is fully alert. *Do not bend the arm up.* Keep it extended or raised. If for some reason your sharps container has been moved out of reach (as sometimes happens in emergencies when others are working on the patient at the same time) and the patient is not able to hold pressure, it is generally acceptable to bend the patient's arm temporarily while locating the sharps container and disposing of the needle.

Dispose of the Needle

Dispose of the needle immediately (see Fig. 9-11G) by placing it in the proper slot of a biohazard sharps container and turning it clockwise until it unscrews from the evacuated tube holder. If the needle remains in the slot of the sharps container with the rubber guard sticking up out of the container, use the tube holder to push it to the side and into the container. *Do not* attempt to loosen it with your fingers. If the needle refuses to separate from the holder, throw the entire unit away. If using one of the new safety needle holders or sharps container systems, follow manufacturer's instructions.

Do not cut, bend, break, or recap needles. *Never* stick the needle into the patient's mattress. If you find yourself in a situation where a sharps container is not readily accessible, a **one-handed** resheathing technique or a **resheathing** device may be used according to the national standards outlined in NCCLS document M29-T2.

Label the Tubes

Label the tubes with an indelible pen. Specimen tube labels (see Fig. 9-11H) should contain the following information as a minimum:

- Patient's name
- Hospital number (if applicable) or date of birth

- Time of collection
- Date
- Phlebotomist's initials

Additional pertinent information such as "fasting" or "nonfasting" should also be included on the label. If using a preprinted computer label, the date, time, and phlebotomist's initials and other pertinent information must be hand written on the label. Compare the information on the label with the patient's ID band and the requisition before leaving the patient.

- *Do not* label tubes prior to venipuncture.
- *Do not* leave the room before labeling the tubes.
- *Do not* dismiss an outpatient before labeling is completed.
- *Do not* label tubes with a pencil.

Observe Any Special Handling Instructions

Follow recommended special handling procedures for each specimen, such as putting it in crushed ice to cool (*eg*, ammonia), keeping it warm (*eg*, cold agglutinin), and protecting from it from light (*eg*, bilirubin).

Check the Patient's Arm and Apply Bandage

Examine the patient's arm to see if bleeding has stopped. If the bleeding has stopped, apply an adhesive bandage (or tape over several folded gauze squares) over the site. Instruct the patient to remove the bandage after a minimum of 15 minutes to avoid irritation by the bandage. If the patient is allergic to adhesive bandages, apply paper tape over a clean folded gauze square or cotton ball.

If the patient has sensitive skin or is allergic to the paper tape, wrap gauze around the arm and place the tape over the gauze.

Some hospitals prefer *not* to bandage the site because bandages tend to irritate the skin and leave a sticky residue, which interferes with subsequent venipuncture. Follow hospital protocol.

Instruct an outpatient not to carry a purse or other heavy object or lift heavy objects with that arm for approximately 1 hour.

Dispose of Contaminated Materials

Dispose of contaminated materials in proper biohazard containers. Do not leave other materials such as needle caps and wrappers in the patient's room. Check to see that you have your tourniquet and other equipment before exiting the patient's room.

Thank the Patient

Thanking patients for their cooperation is courteous and helps to leave the patient with a positive feeling about the laboratory.

Remove Gloves and Wash Hands

Remove gloves aseptically by grasping one glove at the wrist and pulling it inside out and off of the hand, ending up with it in the palm of the still-gloved hand. Slip your ngloved fingers under the second glove at the wrist and pull it off of the hand, ending with one glove inside the other with the contaminated surfaces inside. Dispose of the gloves in a biohazard waste container. *Wash your hands before proceeding to the next patient.*

Check Specimen Collection Logs

Check the patient's name off of the specimen collection and diet restriction logs at the nursing station if applicable. In an outpatient setting, inform the patient that it is all right to go ahead and eat if no other tests are scheduled that require fasting.

Transport the Specimen to the Lab

Transport specimens to the laboratory in a timely fashion. Enter specimens into the computer system or log book. Collection of laboratory specimens must be documented or verified. The specimen collection process is not complete until the appropriate patient and specimen collection information is entered into a computer or manually recorded in a log book.

FAILURE TO OBTAIN BLOOD

Failure to obtain blood can be caused by any one of a number of factors. Being aware of these factors and how to correct for them may determine whether you obtain blood on the first try or have to repeat the procedure. If you fail to obtain blood, it is important to remain calm so that you can clearly analyze the situation. The following sections outline items that you should check.

Tube Position and Vacuum

Check the tube to see that it is properly seated and the needle has penetrated the stopper. Reseat the tube to make certain the needle sleeve is not pushing the tube off of the needle. If you suspect that the tube may have lost its vacuum, try another tube.

Needle Position

A seasoned phlebotomist uses visual cues to help determine proper needle position (Fig. 9-13A). Try to determine visually if any of the following have occurred.

NEEDLE BEVEL AGAINST THE VEIN WALL

Blood flow can be impaired if the needle bevel is up against either the upper or lower wall of the vein (see Fig. 9-13B and C). This is very hard to tell. Try rotating the bevel slightly. If blood flow is established, this was probably the case.

NEEDLE TOO DEEP

The needle may have gone too deeply and penetrated all the way through the vein (see Fig. 9-13D). This can happen on needle insertion or as the tube is pushed onto the needle if the tube holder is not held steady. If this is the case, withdrawing the needle slightly should establish blood flow. If the needle position is not corrected quickly, blood will leak into the tissues and form a hematoma.

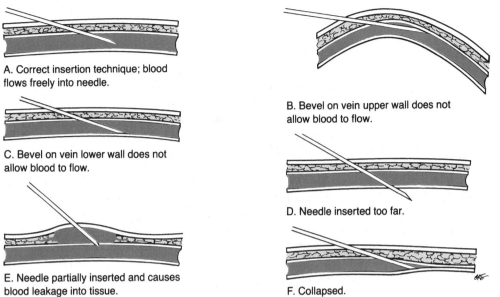

A. Correct insertion technique; blood flows freely into needle.

B. Bevel on vein upper wall does not allow blood to flow.

C. Bevel on vein lower wall does not allow blood to flow.

D. Needle inserted too far.

E. Needle partially inserted and causes blood leakage into tissue.

F. Collapsed.

Figure 9-13   Proper and improper needle positioning.

NEEDLE NOT DEEP ENOUGH

If the needle is not completely inserted into the vein (see Fig. 9-13E), blood may fill the tube very slowly. By pushing the needle gently into the vein, correct blood flow should be established. Partial needle insertion can also cause blood to leak into the tissue and start to form a hematoma. If this occurs, immediately remove the tourniquet and withdraw the needle.

NEEDLE HAS SLIPPED BESIDE THE VEIN

Veins are fairly tough, and if a vein is not anchored well, it may move slightly and the needle may slip to the side of the vein instead of penetrating it. Sometimes the needle ends up to the side and slightly under the vein. In this situation, slip the tube off of the needle so that you do not risk losing the vacuum, and withdraw the needle until just the bevel is under the skin. Anchor the vein securely and redirect the needle into the vein.

NEEDLE POSITION CANNOT BE DETERMINED

If you cannot determine the position of the needle and the above solutions do not help, you may have to use your fingers to relocate the vein. Remove the tube from the needle and withdraw the needle until the bevel is just under the skin.

If your gloved finger has been cleaned with alcohol you may feel the arm above the point of needle insertion and try to determine needle position. *Do not* feel too close to the needle as this is painful to the patient.

Once you have relocated the vein, redirect the needle into the vein and proceed with the venipuncture. If you cannot relocate the vein, withdraw the needle in the proper manner and hold pressure over the site.

Do not blindly probe the arm in an attempt to locate a vein. Probing is painful to the patient and may cause damage to nerves and other tissues. It can also lead to inadvertent puncture of an artery.

Collapsed Vein

Sometimes the vacuum draw of a tube or the pressure created by pulling on a plunger of a syringe can be too much for a vein and cause it to collapse (see Fig. 9-13*F*). You can often tell that a vein has collapsed because it will disappear as soon as the needle penetrates it. Tighten the tourniquet if possible by grasping the ends with one hand and twisting them together. That may be enough to reestablish blood flow. If the tourniquet cannot be retightened, use your finger to apply pressure to the vein several inches above the needle. Remove the tube from the needle and wait a few seconds for the blood flow to reestablish. Try using a smaller-volume tube or if using a syringe, pull more slowly on the plunger. If the blood flow does not reestablish, you will have to withdraw the needle and attempt a second venipuncture at another site.

PROCEDURE FOR INABILITY TO OBTAIN A SPECIMEN

A phlebotomist who is unable to obtain a specimen on the first try should try again. If the second attempt is unsuccessful, the phlebotomist should *not* try a third time. Another phlebotomist should take over. Unsuccessful venipuncture attempts are frustrating to the patient as well as the phlebotomist. Unless it is a stat specimen, if the second phlebotomist is also unsuccessful, it is a good idea to give the patient a rest and come back at a later time.

There are times when a phlebotomist is not be able to obtain a specimen from a patient without even attempting venipuncture. Occasionally, a patient will refuse to allow the phlebotomist to draw the specimen. Other times, the patient is unavailable because he or she has gone to surgery, or to another department, such as radiology, for testing. Sometimes the patient has already been discharged from the hospital. The following are acceptable reasons for inability to obtain a specimen:

1. Patient refusal
2. Patient unavailable
3. Phlebotomist attempted but was unable to draw blood

If the specimen cannot be obtained, the patient's nurse or physician should be notified. In addition, most hospitals require the phlebotomist to fill out a form stating that the specimen was not obtained and the reason why. The original form is delivered to the nurses' station to be placed in the patient's chart. A copy of the form is retained by the laboratory.

PROCEDURE FOR USING A BUTTERFLY

The phlebotomist may elect to use a **winged infusion** set or **butterfly** when attempting to draw blood from antecubital veins of infants and small children or when drawing blood from difficult adult veins, such as small antecubital veins or wrist or hand veins (Fig. 9-14*A*).

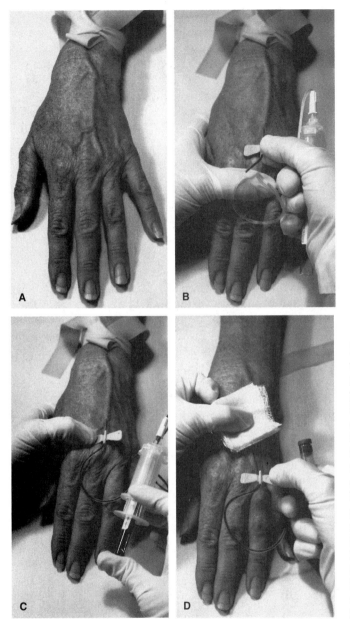

Figure 9-14 Procedure for using butterfly in a hand vein. (**A**) Hand with tourniquet in place reveals prominent vein. (**B**) With the skin pulled taut over the knuckles, the needle is inserted into the vein until there is a "flash" of blood in the tubing. (**C**) Using the non-dominant hand, a wing of the butterfly is held against the patient's hand to steady the needle while the blood collecting tube is pushed onto the blood collecting needle. (**D**) Once the proper tubes have been drawn, gauze is placed over the vein and the needle is removed.

Equipment Selection

There are butterfly needles that can be attached directly to a syringe; however, a butterfly needle with a threaded multiple sample **Luer adapter** that can be attached directly to an evacuated tube holder is preferred. A 23-gauge needle will easily penetrate small veins and not rupture or "blow" them. Choose small-volume **pediatric tubes** to collect the specimen. Large-volume tubes may create too much vacuum draw on the vein and cause it to collapse. In addition, large-volume tubes used with a 23-gauge needle may cause hemolysis of the specimen.

Procedure

Assemble the equipment while the site is drying and the tourniquet is off. Remove the butterfly device from the package. (Retain the package to place the needle in when resecuring the tourniquet.) The tubing will be coiled somewhat because it was coiled in the package. Extend the tubing its full length and stretch slightly to help keep it from coiling back up. Attach the butterfly collection device to the evacuated tube holder. Seat the first tube in the holder.

When drawing the specimen from an antecubital vein, proceed as you would a routine venipuncture, being certain to anchor the vein securely. If drawing from a hand or wrist vein, apply the tourniquet to the wrist proximal to the wrist bone. Have the patient either make a fist or bend the fingers slightly. Make certain the hand is well supported on the bed, a rolled towel, or an armrest. Choose a vein and cleanse the site. Anchor the vein by pulling the skin taut over the knuckles with the thumb.

Cradle the tube holder and tubing in the palm of your dominant hand or lay it next to the patient's hand. Hold the needle between your thumb and index finger or fold the wings together upright and grasp it by the folded wings.

With the needle bevel facing up and lined up with the vein, enter the vein at shallow angle between 10 and 15 degrees. Be careful not to penetrate all the way through the vein. A "flash" of blood will appear in the tubing (see Fig. 9-14B) when the needle is in the vein. "Seat" the needle by threading it up the lumen (central area) of the vein slightly so that the needle will not twist out of the vein if you let go of the needle. If the needle tries to twist out of the vein, hold it with the thumb of the opposite hand (see Fig. 9-14C).

Push the blood-collecting tube to the end of the holder. Release the tourniquet when blood begins to flow into the tube. (Because butterfly draws are usually performed on difficult veins, the tourniquet is sometimes left in place until the last tube is filled, as long as the draw takes less than 1 minute.)

Keep the tube and holder in a downward position so that the tube fills from the bottom up (see Fig. 9-14C), as in a regular venipuncture procedure. Follow the proper order of draw.

When the last tube has been filled, remove it from the holder. Place gauze and apply pressure after needle removal (see Fig. 9-14D) in the same manner as a routine venipuncture. Remove the needle by grasping one of the butterfly wings near where it is attached to the needle and carefully withdraw it from the vein. If the needle has a safety cover, hold the needle by the cover. Once the needle is out of the vein, slide the cover over the needle. If the draw was difficult and the tube was not completely filled, it may be replaced in the needle holder and advanced onto the needle to draw the remaining blood out of the tubing, if it is done immediately.

Dispose of the needle and tubing by dropping the needle into the sharps container while holding onto the still-attached tube holder. *Do not* allow the tubing to dangle its full length above the sharps container, or the needle may spring back and poke your hand or arm. Release the tubing from the Luer adapter with a twisting motion and let it fall into the sharps container. The multiple sample Luer adapter may then be released from the tube holder in the same manner as when removing a regular needle. If the tube holder contains a needle release system, the entire unit will release from the holder directly into the sharps container.

SYRINGE VENIPUNCTURE PROCEDURE

Although the preferred method of obtaining venipuncture specimens is the evacuated tube method, use of a needle and syringe or butterfly and syringe may be necessary if the patient has fragile or weak veins that collapse easily. The vacuum pressure of the evacuated tube may be too great for such veins. This is often the case with elderly patients and newborn infants. When using a syringe, the phlebotomist can control the pressure by pulling slowly on the syringe plunger.

When drawing blood by syringe, follow the same identification, patient preparation, and site selection and preparation procedures as for a routine venipuncture. To comply with OSHA regulations, use a needle-locking syringe (*eg*, Luer lock). Prepare the needle or butterfly needle and syringe by removing them from their sterile wrappers. Pull on the syringe plunger to see that it moves freely, and reseat it (push it all the way back into the barrel of the syringe) before removing the syringe cap. Securely attach the needle to the syringe. *Do not* remove the needle cover.

Apply the tourniquet. Remove the needle cap and visually inspect the needle for defects.

Enter the vein (Fig. 9-15*A*) bevel up in the same manner as routine venipuncture. When the vein has been entered, you will see blood appear in the hub of the needle. Release the tourniquet.

Steady the syringe as you would the evacuated tube holder (see Fig. 9-15*B*). (Some phlebotomists switch hands at this point.) Slowly pull back on the plunger of the syringe and allow the barrel of the syringe to fill with blood (see Fig. 9-15*C*). When an adequate amount of blood has been collected, withdraw the needle in the same manner described for routine venipuncture (see Fig. 9-15*D*).

Filling More Than One Syringe

Filling more than one syringe is not recommended but can be done if absolutely necessary.

To fill a second syringe, place several thicknesses of gauze under the syringe at the point of the needle or butterfly attachment to the syringe. While holding the needle very steady, twist the syringe off of the needle and quickly attach the second syringe. When a butterfly needle is used, pinch the tubing to stop the blood flow, remove the first syringe, and attach the second. It is best to have someone assist with the procedure by filling the tubes from the first syringe while you are collecting blood in the second. Otherwise, the blood in the first syringe may clot before you have a chance to transfer it to the evacuated tubes. When an adequate amount of blood has been collected in the second syringe, withdraw the needle in the same manner described for routine venipuncture.

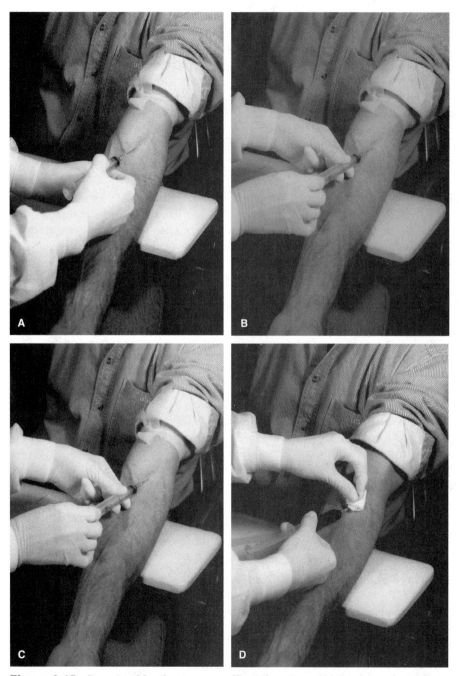

Figure 9-15 Drawing blood using a needle and syringe. (**A**) Inserting the syringe needle into the vein. (**B**) Switching hands and steadying the syringe. (**C**) Filling the syringe with blood by slowly pulling on the syringe plunger. (**D**) Withdrawing the needle from the vein.

Transferring Blood From a Syringe to Evacuated Tubes

Place the tubes needed for the required tests in a rack or slot in the blood collecting tray.

Penetrate the stopper of the tube to be filled with the syringe needle (Fig. 9-16). Let the tube fill using the vacuum draw of the tube.

- To minimize the chance of hemolysis, slant the needle to the side of the tube so that the blood runs down the side of the tube.
- To avoid needlesticks, *never* hold the tubes in hand while filling from a syringe.
- *Do not* force the blood into the tube by pushing on the syringe plunger. Forcing the blood into the tube by pushing the syringe plunger can cause hemolysis of the specimen. It may also cause the creation of an aerosol of blood as the needle is removed from the tube. In addition, pushing the plunger may force the stopper to pop off of the tube, splashing the contents.

If the tube is not to be filled completely, pull back on the plunger to stop the flow. Fill the tubes following the proper order of draw for the syringe method as outlined in Chapter 7.

Dispose of the syringe and needle as one unit by dropping it into a sharps container.

PEDIATRIC VENIPUNCTURE

Collecting blood by venipuncture from infants and children may be necessary for tests that require large amounts of blood (*eg*, cross-matching and blood cultures) and

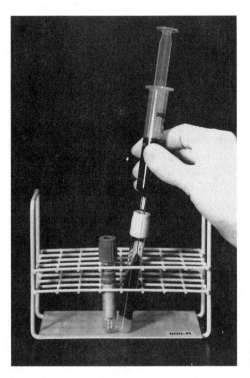

Figure 9-16 Filling an evacuated tube from a syringe.

tests that cannot be performed by skin puncture (*eg*, ammonia levels and most coagulation studies).

Venipuncture in children under the age of 2 years should be limited to superficial veins and not deep, hard-to-find veins. Normally, the most accessible veins of infants and toddlers are the veins of the antecubital fossa and forearm. Other venipuncture sites are the medial wrist, the dorsum of the foot, the scalp, and the medial ankle. The use of **dorsal hand vein** technique for neonate blood collection is increasing in popularity.

Challenges

Performing venipuncture on pediatric patients presents special challenges and requires the expertise and skill of an experienced phlebotomist. In addition, every attempt should be made to collect the minimum amount of blood required for testing because of the small blood volume of infants and children. Removal of more than 10% of an infant's blood volume at one time can lead to cardiac arrest. Removal of large amounts of blood over an extended period can lead to anemia and may require the infant to undergo a blood transfusion.

Dealing With the Parents or Guardians

If parents or guardians are present, it is important for the phlebotomist to earn their trust before attempting the procedure. A phlebotomist who behaves in a warm and friendly manner and displays a calm, confident, and caring attitude will more easily earn that trust and limit parental anxiety as well. Give parents the option of staying in the room during the procedure or waiting outside until you are finished.

Dealing With the Patient

With older children, it is important to gain their trust as with adults. Remember that children have wider zones of comfort. Approach them slowly and gain their trust before handling equipment or touching their arms to look for a vein.

It is best to answer a child's questions honestly. Remember, *never* tell a child that it will not hurt. Tell her or him that it will hurt just a little bit, but will be over quickly. Help the child to understand the importance of holding still. Give the child a job to do such as holding the gauze or bandage. Offer the child a reward for being brave. However, *do not* put conditions on whether or not he or she receives the reward, such as "You can only have the reward if you don't cry." Some crying is to be anticipated, however, it is important to calm the child as soon as possible, because the stress of crying and struggling can alter blood components and lead to erroneous test results.

Selecting a Method of Restraint

Immobilization of the patient is a critical aspect in obtaining an adequate specimen from infants and children. Physical restraint is usually required.

Toddlers are most easily restrained by having them sit upright on a parent's lap (Fig. 9-17). The arm to be used for venipuncture is extended to the front and downward. The parent places an arm around the toddler over the arm that is not being used. The other arm supports the venipuncture arm from behind, at the bend of the elbow. This helps steady the child's arm and prevents the child from twisting the arm during the draw.

Older children may sit by themselves in the blood-drawing chair, but a parent or another phlebotomist should help steady the arm.

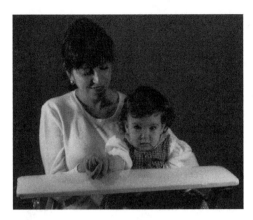

Figure 9-17   Seated adult restraining a toddler for venipuncture.

If the child is drawn in a supine position, the parent or another phlebotomist leans over the child from the opposite side of the bed. One arm reaches around and holds the venipuncture arm from behind, and the other reaches across the child's body, holding the child's other arm secure against his or her torso.

Equipment Selection

Because infants and children have small blood volumes and small veins, it is important to select the smallest tubes and needles allowed to collect the required specimen. In addition, you may need to use a pediatric-sized tourniquet.

Procedures

Follow proper identification requirements and cleansing procedures outlined earlier in the chapter. You may be required to wear a mask, gown, and gloves in the newborn nursery.

ANTECUBITAL VEIN

Venipuncture of an antecubital vein is most easily accomplished using a 23-gauge butterfly attached to an evacuated tube holder or syringe. The tubing of the butterfly allows for flexibility if the child struggles or twists during the draw. Using the evacuated tube method of collection is preferred because it minimizes chances of clotted specimens and inadequately filled tubes. However, the smallest tubes available should be used to reduce the risk of creating too much vacuum draw on the vein, leading to vein collapse.

DORSAL HAND VEIN

Dorsal hand veins are favored sites for venipuncture in neonates (newborns) and infants under 2 years of age. Collecting blood specimens by dorsal hand vein venipuncture is more efficient and less time consuming than skin puncture collection because specimens can be collected quickly from a single venipuncture, as opposed to the multiple sticks often required to collect skin puncture specimens. In addition, specimens are less likely to be diluted with tissue fluids or hemolyzed. Infant dorsal hand vein venipuncture (Fig. 9-18) is performed as follows:

INFANT DORSAL HAND VEIN VENIPUNCTURE

- Put on mask and gown, if applicable, and gloves.
- Identify the infant.
- Immobilize the infant by wrapping snuggly in a blanket.
- Check for the most visible vein in either hand.
- Encircle the wrist with your thumb underneath and index finger on top. Apply pressure with your index finger to enlarge the vein. (Use of a tourniquet is not necessary.)
- Flex the wrist downward, being careful not to bend it too much or the vein may flatten out and be harder to see. It may also collapse when punctured.
- Once the vein is selected, release your grasp and clean the site with alcohol.
- Allow the alcohol to air dry. Select an appropriate needle for the size of the vein. 23-to-25–gauge transparent hub syringe needles are commonly used.
- Encircle the wrist as before and bend the hand slightly downward. Create pressure on the vein with your index finger.
- Line the needle up parallel to the vein. Slip the needle into the vein at an approximate 15° angle with the skin. Advance the needle slowly until blood appears in the hub.
- Fill microcollection tubes directly from the hub. Avoid bumping the hub or putting pressure on the needle. Release finger pressure intermittently to encourage blood flow.
- After collecting the specimen, place gauze, withdraw the needle, and apply pressure until bleeding stops. Immediately dispose of the needle in a sharps container.
- Do not apply a bandage because it may tear the skin when removed later.
- Label the specimen in the proper manner and follow any special handling instructions for specimens.
- Discard all used supplies in the proper containers. Remove mask, gown, and gloves, and wash hands. Enter collection information in the nursery log book.
- Deliver the specimen to the lab.

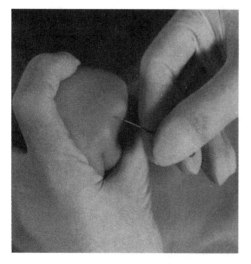

Figure 9-18   Positioning the needle for dorsal hand vein punctures on an infant.

Study & Review Questions

1. The most important step in specimen collection is
   a. entering the patient's room correctly.
   b. handling visitors.
   c. identifying the patient.
   d. identifying yourself to the patient.

2. An ID band should include all of the following patient information except
   a. diagnosis.
   b. medical record number.
   c. name.
   d. physician's name.

3. If a patient adamantly refuses to have blood drawn, the phlebotomist should
   a. convince the patient to cooperate.
   b. notify the patient's nurse and fill out a failure to obtain specimen form explaining what happened.
   c. restrain the patient and collect the specimen.
   d. write a note to the physician.

4. You are sent to collect a specimen on an inpatient. The patient is not wearing an ID band. What do you do?
   a. Ask the patient's name and collect the specimen if it matches the requisition.
   b. Have the patient's nurse put an ID band on the patient before drawing the specimen.
   c. Identify the patient by the name card on the door.
   d. Refuse to draw the specimen and return to the lab.

5. A tourniquet should be applied
   a. away from open sores.
   b. 8 to 10 inches above the intended venipuncture site.
   c. for at least 2 minutes before releasing.
   d. tight enough to stop all blood flow.

6. After cleaning the venipuncture site with alcohol, the phlebotomist should
   a. allow the alcohol to dry completely.
   b. blow on the site to help the alcohol dry.
   c. dry the site with a regular gauze pad or cotton ball.
   d. insert the needle quickly before the alcohol has a chance to dry.

7. Which of the following actions is *not* proper venipuncture technique?
   a. Allow the tube to fill until the vacuum is exhausted.
   b. Fill the tube from the stopper end first.
   c. Maintain the tube in a downward position throughout the draw.
   d. Remove the tourniquet as soon as blood flows freely into the tube.

8. Specimen collection tubes are labeled
   a. at the patient's bedside after collecting the specimen.
   b. at the patient's bedside before the specimen is collected.
   c. in the laboratory after collection.
   d. in the laboratory before the specimen is collected.

9. Failure to obtain a blood specimen may be caused by all of the following *except*
   a. the needle bevel has penetrated through the opposite wall of the vein.
   b. the needle bevel is against the vein wall.
   c. the needle bevel is centered in the lumen of the vein.
   d. the needle bevel is only partly inserted into the vein.

10. After penetrating a hand vein with a butterfly needle, the phlebotomist needs to "seat" the needle, meaning

   a. have the patient make a tight fist to keep the needle in place.

   b. keep the skin taut during the entire procedure.

   c. push the needle up against the back wall of the vein.

   d. slightly thread the needle up the central area of the vein.

11. Which of the following choices describes proper technique for filling tubes from a syringe?

   a. Fill serum tubes before anticoagulant tubes.

   b. Hold the collection tube tightly so that it does not slip out of your hand when inserting the syringe needle into the stopper.

   c. Insert the needle into the tube and slowly push the plunger of the syringe.

   d. Slant the needle so that blood runs down the inside wall of the tube.

12. What is the best approach to use with an 8-year-old child who needs to have blood drawn?

   a. Explain what you are going to do and ask the child to cooperate.

   b. Have someone restrain the child and collect the specimen before he or she has time to think about it.

   c. Offer the child a treat or toy, but only if he doesn't cry.

   d. Tell the child that it won't hurt and that only babies cry.

Suggested Laboratory Activities

1. Compare various types of manual and computer requisitions.

2. Fill in the required information on several types of requisitions.

3. Practice reading physician laboratory orders on patient charts.

4. Practice proper bedside manner by role-playing with another student.

5. Compare identification on sample requisitions with information on ID bands worn by students.

6. Practice assembling equipment for collecting various test specimens.

7. Demonstrate proper venipuncture site selection on a fellow student.

8. Practice routine venipuncture on an artificial arm.

9. Demonstrate proper venipuncture technique on a fellow student.

10. Practice the use of a butterfly needle to obtain a blood specimen from a hand vein on an artificial arm.

11. Practice proper syringe usage on an artificial arm.

12. Practice proper restraint methods on a child-size dummy or doll.

BIBLIOGRAPHY AND SUGGESTED READINGS

Bishop, M. L., Duben-Engelkirk, J. L., & Fody, E. P. (1996). *Clinical chemistry: Principles, procedures, correlations* (3rd ed.). Philadelphia: Lippincott-Raven Publishers.

College of American Pathologists (CAP). (1994). *So you're going to collect a blood specimen: An introduction to phlebotomy* (6th ed.). Northfield, IL: Author.

Lotspeich-Steininger, C. A., Stiene-Martin, E. A., & Koepke, J. A. (1992). *Clinical hematology: Principles, procedures, correlations.* Philadelphia: Lippincott-Raven Publishers.

National Committee for Clinical Laboratory Standards, H3-A3. (July 1991). *Procedures for the collection of diagnostic blood specimens by venipuncture* (3rd ed.). Villanova, PA: NCCLS.

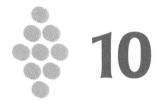

10

Skin Puncture Equipment and Procedures

KEY TERMS

arterialized
blood smears
calcaneus
capillary blood gases
Caraway tubes
clay sealant
cyanotic
differential

feather
interstitial fluid
intracellular fluid
lancet
microcollection
    containers
microhematocrit tubes
Natelson tubes

newborn screening
osteochondritis
osteomyelitis
phenylketonuria (PKU)
plantar surface
reference (normal)
    values
whorls

OBJECTIVES

Upon successful completion of this chapter, the reader will be able to:

1. List and describe the various types of equipment needed to perform skin puncture.

2. State the composition of skin puncture blood, identify which tests have different reference values when collected by skin puncture methods, and name tests that cannot be performed by skin puncture.

3. State indications for performing skin puncture on adults, infants, and children.

4. Describe the proper procedure for selecting a skin puncture site and indicate precautions associated with site selection.

5. Describe the proper procedure for collecting skin puncture specimens from adults, infants, and children.

6. List the order of draw for collecting skin puncture specimens.

7. Describe the procedure for making both routine and thick blood smears and reasons for making them at the collection site.

SKIN PUNCTURE EQUIPMENT

In addition to general blood collection equipment described in Chapter 7, the following special equipment may be required for skin puncture procedures.

Lancets

A **lancet** (Fig. 10-1) is a sterile, disposable, sharp-pointed instrument used to pierce the skin to obtain droplets of blood used for testing. The type of lancet selected for skin puncture should not be capable of puncturing to a depth that penetrates bone. A revolutionary new device, the Laser Lancet (Venisect, Inc., Little Rock, AR), perforates skin without the use of conventional instruments. This lancet vaporizes a minute hole to the capillary bed by means of a laser pulse delivered through a disposable tip.

A number of companies manufacture conventional skin puncture devices which control the puncture depth. Examples are the Microtainer Brand Safety Flow Lancet (Becton Dickinson, Franklin Lakes, NJ) in sizes for heelstick and finger stick and the Tenderfoot

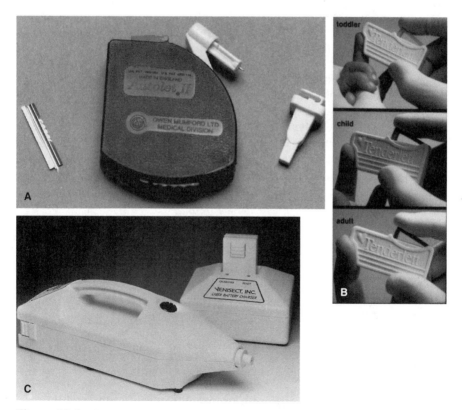

Figure 10-1 Several types of skin puncture lancets. (**A**) Metal lancet; Autolet (Ulster Scientific Inc., New Paltz, NY); Safety Flow Lancet (Becton Dickinson, Franklin Lakes, NJ). (**B**) Tenderlett Toddler, Junior, and Adult lancet devices (International Technidyne Corp., Edison, NJ). (**C**) Laser Lancet System (Venisect, Inc., Little Rock, AR).

for neonates (newborns), Tenderlett Toddler, and Tenderlett Junior for children (International Technidyne Corp., Edison, NJ). Also available are the Autolet II and Autolet Lite Clinisafe (Ulster Scientific, Inc., New Paltz, NY) spring-activated, reusable puncture devices that both feature a removable, single-use lancet and platform. The platform, which is positioned over the site prior to puncture, controls depth of puncture and is available in three color-coded depths: white (1.8 mm), yellow (2.4 mm), and orange (3.0 mm). The Autolet Lite Clinisafe has a safety mechanism that prevents reuse of the device unless the lancet and platform are replaced.

Collection Devices

MICROCOLLECTION CONTAINERS

A number of companies manufacture special **microcollection containers** (Fig. 10-2) to be used for obtaining blood from skin punctures. These small containers are often referred to as "bullets" because of their size and shape. They are made of plastic and have color-coded stoppers, which indicate the presence or absence of an additive, as well as the type of additive if present. Color coding corresponds to that of blood collection tubes used in venipuncture. Examples of microcollection tubes include Microtainers and Microcuvettes (Becton Dickinson, Franklin Lakes, NJ), Capiject tubes (Terumo, Somerset, NJ), and Samplette capillary blood collectors (Sherwood Medical, St. Louis, MO).

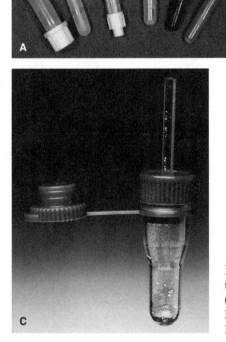

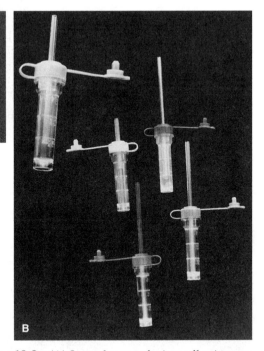

Figure 10-2   (**A**) Several types of microcollection containers. (**B**) SAFE-DRAW™ microcollection device. (Courtesy Hematronix, Inc., Plano, TX.) (**C**) SAFE-T-FILL™ capillary blood collection device. (Courtesy RAM Scientific, Needham, MA.)

Special microcollection containers designed with safety in mind combine capillary tubes with collection containers to facilitate collection of specimens. Examples are the SAFE-DRAW microcollection device (see Fig. 10-2*B*) (Hematronix, Inc., Plano, TX) and the SAFE-T-FILL capillary blood collection device (see Fig. 10-2C) (RAM Scientific, Needham, MA).

MICROHEMATOCRIT TUBES

Microhematocrit tubes (Fig. 10-3) are disposable, narrow-bore glass or plastic capillary tubes designed to hold 50 to 75 microliters of blood. These tubes are primarily used for hematocrit (packed cell volume) determinations on micro samples. They fill with blood by capillary action. They are designed to be used with special centrifuges. Microhematocrit tubes are also used to collect other micro specimens. Microhematocrit tubes come coated with ammonium heparin for hematocrit determinations and tests requiring plasma, or plain for collection of serum specimens. Ammonium-heparin–coated tubes have a red band at one end of the tube; plain tubes have a blue band. Special plain capillary tubes are available for capillary coagulation tests.

Special microhematocrit tubes designed to be used exclusively with special centrifuges from Statspin Technologies require as little as 9 microliters of blood and are gaining popularity for use in screening programs and pediatric clinics.

CARAWAY TUBES AND NATELSON TUBES

Caraway and **Natelson tubes** (see Fig. 10-3) are disposable, glass microcollection tubes. They can be used for most tests performed on skin puncture blood. They are tapered at one end and come with or without an anticoagulant. Anticoagulated tubes for plasma determinations come with a yellow circular band at the nontapered end and usually contain lithium heparin. Nonanticoagulated tubes have a blue band. Caraway tubes are 75 mm in length and have a capacity of approximately 350 microliters. Natelson tubes are around 147 mm in length and have a capacity of approximately 250 microliters.

Capillary Blood Gas Collection Equipment

Capillary blood gas collection equipment (Fig. 10-4) is used to collect blood gas specimens by skin puncture. The following special equipment, often assembled together in kit form, is commonly used:

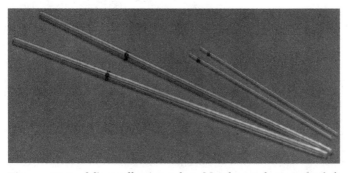

Figure 10-3   Microcollection tubes: Natelson tubes on the left and microhematocrit tubes on the right.

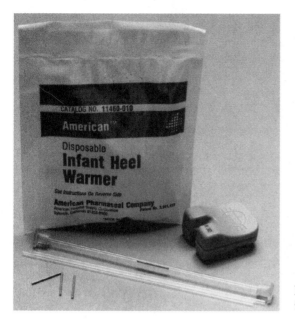

Figure 10-4   Capillary blood gas collection equipment.

- *Collection tubes:* **Capillary blood gas collection tubes** vary according to volume requirements for different testing methods and instrumentation. Tubes of 100 mm in length with a capacity of 100 microliters are most common. A color-coded band identifies the type of anticoagulant that coats the inside of the tube; it is usually green, indicating sodium heparin.
- *Stirrers:* **Metal stirrers** (often referred to as **"fleas"**) are inserted into the tube after collection of a capillary blood gas specimen to aid in mixing the anticoagulant.
- *Magnet:* A **magnet** is required to aid in mixing capillary blood gas specimens after collection. The magnet often has a hole in the center so that it can be slipped over the capillary tube. It then is moved back and forth along the tube length, pulling the metal stirrer with it and mixing the anticoagulant into the blood specimen.
- *Plastic/clay sealant:* **Plastic** or **clay sealants** are commonly used to seal one end of microhematocrit tubes as well as tubes for chemistry determinations. Both ends of capillary blood gas tubes need to be sealed in order to maintain specimens under anaerobic (without air) conditions.
- *Plastic caps:* **Plastic end caps** or **closures** are available in place of clay to seal microcollection tubes. Capillary blood gas collection tubes often come with their own caps.

Micropipet Dilution Systems

A **micropipet dilution system** (Fig. 10-5) serves as both a collection device and a dilution unit for the blood sample. Components of this disposable system are a sealed plastic reservoir that contains a premeasured amount of reagent; a detachable glass, self-filling capillary pipet; and a pipet shield, which also serves as a device to puncture the reservoir covering or diaphragm prior to adding the sample.

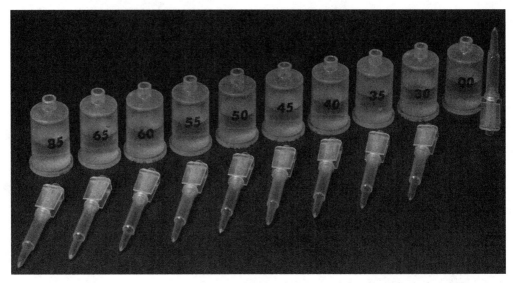

Figure 10-5   Unopette system (Courtesy Becton Dickinson and Co., Franklin Lakes, NJ).

Warming Devices

Warming the area prior to skin puncture can increase the blood flow as much as seven times. This is especially important when performing heelsticks on newborns. Several **heel warming devices** (see Fig. 10-4) are commercially available. In order to avoid burning the patient, these devices provide a uniform temperature that does not exceed 42° C. A towel or diaper wet with warm tap water can also be used to wrap the hand or foot prior to skin puncture. However, care must be taken not to get the water so hot that it scalds the patient.

SKIN PUNCTURE PRINCIPLES

Composition of Skin Puncture Blood

Blood obtained through skin puncture is a mixture of arterial blood (from arterioles), venous blood (from venules), and capillary blood, along with **interstitial** and **intracellular fluids** from the surrounding tissues. It contains a higher proportion of arterial blood than venous blood because of the pressure with which the arterial blood enters the capillaries. Composition of skin puncture blood, therefore, more closely resembles arterial blood than venous blood. This is especially true if the area has been warmed, since warming increases arterial flow into the area.

Reference Values for Skin Puncture Blood

Because skin puncture blood differs in composition from regular venous blood, **reference (normal) values** for certain tests will be different for skin puncture blood. The most notable differences are for glucose, which is higher in skin puncture blood; and total protein (TP), calcium (Ca^{++}), and potassium (K^+), which are lower in skin puncture blood. Some studies, however, have shown that potassium values are more likely to be falsely elevated in skin puncture specimens owing to tissue fluid contamination and hemolysis of the specimen.

Tests That Cannot Be Performed by Skin Puncture

Although today's technology allows many tests to be performed on very small quantities of blood, and a wide selection of devices are available to make collection of skin puncture specimens relatively safe and easy, some tests cannot be performed on skin puncture specimens. These include most erythrocyte sedimentation rate (ESR) methods and coagulation studies, blood cultures, and tests that require large volumes of serum or plasma.

Indications for Performing Skin Puncture

ADULTS

Skin puncture is performed on adults when there are no accessible veins, to save veins for other procedures such as chemotherapy, when the patient has thrombotic or clot-forming tendencies, and for certain bedside and home-testing procedures such as glucose monitoring.

INFANTS AND CHILDREN

Skin puncture is the preferred method of obtaining blood from infants and children. Obtaining blood from infants and children by venipuncture is difficult and may damage veins and surrounding tissues. Because infants and young children have such a small blood volume, removing large quantities of blood can also lead to anemia. Large quantities removed rapidly can cause cardiac arrest. In addition, some tests, such as screening tests for **phenylketonuria (PKU)** and several other inherited diseases, are designed to be performed on skin puncture blood only.

Site Selection for Skin Puncture

GENERAL CRITERIA

Skin puncture sites should be warm, pink, and free of scars, cuts, bruises, or rashes.

Do not choose a site that is cold, **cyanotic** (bluish in color), or **edematous** (swollen).

INFANTS

The heel is the recommended site for collection of skin puncture specimens on infants less than 1 year old. However, it is important that the puncture be performed in an area of the heel where there is little risk of puncturing the bone.

Puncture of the bone can cause painful **osteomyelitis** (os"te-o-mi"el-i'tis) or bone infection, as well as **osteochondritis** (os"te-o-kon-dri'tis), inflammation of the bone and cartilage. Additional punctures through previous puncture sites may spread the infection.

Studies have shown that the **calcaneus** (kal-ka'ne-us) or heel bone of premature infants may be as little as *2.4 mm* below the skin surface (Fig. 10-6) on the **plantar surface** (bottom) of the heel and half that distance at the **posterior curvature** (back) of the heel. For this reason, guidelines were developed to determine the safest areas as well as the optimal depth for performing heel puncture. According to the guidelines recommended

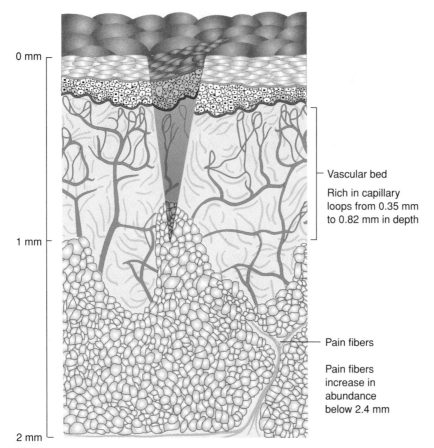

Figure 10-6 Cross section of full-term infant's heel, showing lancet penetration depth needed to access capillary bed.

by NCCLS, document H4-A3 (National Committee for Clinical Laboratory Standards, 771 E. Lancaster Ave., Villanova, PA 19805), to avoid puncturing bone, heel puncture should only be performed on the plantar surface of the heel, medial to an imaginary line extending from the middle of the great (big) toe to the heel or lateral to an imaginary line drawn from between the fourth and fifth toes to the heel (Fig. 10-7). In addition, the puncture should not exceed 2.4 mm in depth.

- *Do not* puncture deeper than 2.4 mm.
- *Do not* puncture through previous puncture sites.
- *Do not* puncture the area between the imaginary boundaries.
- *Do not* puncture the posterior curvature of the heel.
- *Do not* puncture in the area of the arch.
- *Do not* puncture areas of the foot other than the heel.

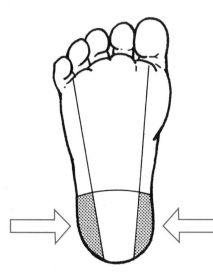

Figure 10-7 Infant heel. Shaded areas indicated by arrows represent recommended areas for infant heel puncture.

OLDER CHILDREN AND ADULTS

The recommended site for skin puncture on adults and older children is the palmar surface of the **distal segment** (end segment) of the middle or ring finger of the nondominant hand. The puncture should be made in the central, fleshy portion of the finger, slightly to the side of center and perpendicular to the **whorls** (grooves) of the fingerprint (Fig. 10-8).

- *Do not* puncture the side or very tip of the finger. The distance between the skin surface and the bone is half as much at the side and tip as it is in the central portion of the end of the finger.
- *Do not* puncture parallel to the grooves of the fingerprint. A puncture parallel to or along the lines of the fingerprint will cause blood to run down the finger rather than form a rounded drop, which makes collection difficult.
- *Do not* puncture the index finger. The index finger is more calloused and, therefore, harder to poke than the other fingers. Also, the patient will use that finger more and will notice the pain longer.
- *Do not* puncture the fifth or little finger. The amount of tissue between skin surface and bone is the thinnest in this finger.
- *Do not* puncture fingers of infants and very young children. The amount of tissue between skin surface and bone is so small that bone injury is very likely.

SKIN PUNCTURE PROCEDURE

Identify the Patient

Follow identification and preparation procedures outlined in Chapter 9.

Assemble Skin Puncture Equipment

1. 70% Isopropyl alcohol prep pads
2. Sterile gauze pads

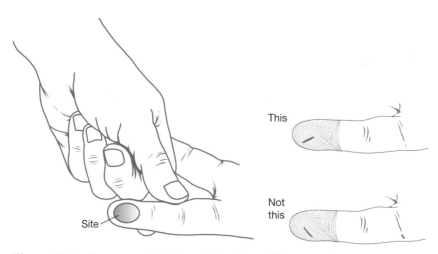

Figure 10-8   Recommended site and direction of finger puncture.

3. Sterile lancet or automated skin puncture device
4. Warming device (if applicable)
5. Collection devices (capillary tubes, microtainers, slides, etc.)

Warm the Site

Blood flow can be increased up to seven times by warming the site prior to skin puncture. Because warming primarily increases arterial flow into the area, the specimen obtained will be referred to as an **arterialized** specimen. When collecting pH or blood gas specimens by skin puncture, warming is an essential part of the procedure.

Warming can be accomplished by wrapping the site for a minimum of 3 minutes with a towel or diaper that has been moistened with comfortably warm water (no warmer than 42° C or 108° F). Commercial heel warmers are also available.

Clean the Site

Skin puncture sites should be cleaned with 70% isopropanol. *Do not* use povidone iodine to clean skin puncture sites. Povidone–iodine should not be used because it greatly interferes with a number of tests, most notably bilirubin, uric acid, phosphorous, and potassium. These tests can be more easily remembered by associating them with the word "**BURPP**," where B stands for bilirubin, UR stands for uric acid, and the two Ps stand for phosphorous and potassium.

Once cleaned, the site must be allowed to air dry to minimize the chance of alcohol contamination of the specimen. Alcohol residue, in addition to causing a stinging sensation, causes rapid hemolysis of red blood cells. Alcohol residue has also been shown to interfere with glucose testing.

Perform Skin Puncture

FINGER PUNCTURE (FINGER STICK)

To perform a finger puncture, support the arm on a firm surface and have the patient extend the hand with the palmer surface facing up. Select and clean the site (Fig. 10-9*A*) and allow it to air dry.

Grasp the finger firmly between your thumb and index finger and perform the puncture (see Fig. 10-9*B*) perpendicular to the whorls (lines) of the fingerprint. This will allow the blood to form a bead or drop that is easily collected. A puncture along the lines (parallel) to the fingerprint will allow the blood to run down the finger and make collection difficult.

HEEL PUNCTURE (HEELSTICK)

Grasp the heel firmly, but gently, with the index finger wrapped around the foot supporting the arch and the thumb wrapped around the ankle and below the puncture site (Fig. 10-10). Perform the puncture perpendicular to the lines of the footprint, using a recommended heel puncture device.

FINGER PUNCTURE AND HEEL PUNCTURE

Continue both heelsticks and finger sticks in the following manner:

- Dispose of the puncture device promptly in a sharps container.
- Apply firm pressure toward the site.
- Wipe away the first drop of blood with a dry gauze (see Fig. 10-9*C*). (The first drop is usually contaminated with tissue fluid.) This also gets rid of any remaining alcohol residue which could hemolyze the specimen, as well as keep the blood from forming a well-rounded drop.
- Position the site downward and continue to apply moderate pressure proximal to the puncture site. *Do not* squeeze or massage the site vigorously. Such activities introduce excess tissue fluid into the specimen and may also cause hemolysis of the specimen.
- Proceed to collect the blood using devices appropriate for the type of test to be performed. Collect slides (see Fig. 10-9*D*), platelet counts, and other hematology specimens first to avoid the effects of platelet aggregation (clumping). Collect other anticoagulant containers next. Collect serum specimens last.
- Touch the collection device to the drop of blood formed on the surface of the skin. Capillary pipets (see Fig. 10-9*E*) will fill by capillary action. When filled, seal the ends of capillary pipets with clay.
- Touch the "scoop" of microcollection tubes (see Fig. 10-9*F*) to the drop of blood and let the drop of blood run down the walls of the tube. Tap the tube gently now and then to encourage the blood to settle to the bottom of the tube. *Do not* use a scooping motion against the surface of the skin. Scraping the scoop against the skin activates platelets and may also cause hemolysis. Cap microcollection containers with the cap provided and mix additive tubes 8 to 10 times.
- When collection is finished, apply pressure to the site with a clean gauze until bleeding stops. Keep the site elevated while pressure is applied.

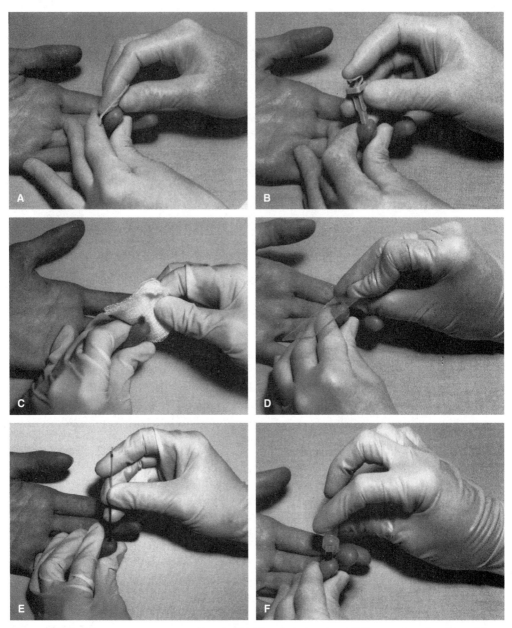

Figure 10-9   Finger puncture procedures. (**A**) Cleaning the site. (**B**) Puncturing the skin with an automatic safety lancet. (**C**) Wiping the first drop. (**D**) Making a slide from skin puncture by touching the slide to the drop of blood. (**E**) Collecting skin puncture blood in a capillary tube. (**F**) Collecting skin puncture blood in a microtainer.

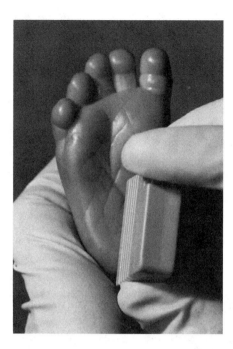

Figure 10-10 Infant heel puncture using Tenderfoot® automatic incision device. (International Technidyne Corp., Edison, NJ.)

- *Do not* apply bandages to infants and children under 2 years old. They may become a choking hazard to the infant or child. In addition, bandages may stick to the paper-thin skin of newborns and tear the skin when removed later.
- Label the specimens with the appropriate information (see Chap. 9). Labels can be directly affixed to microcollection containers. Hematocrit containers can be "flagged" (Fig. 10-11) or placed in a plain red top tube and the tube labeled.
- Follow any special specimen handling requirements.
- Thank the patient.
- Dispose of contaminated gauze in a biohazard container and remove all equipment from the area.
- Remove gloves and wash hands.
- Transport the specimen to the lab.

SPECIAL SKIN PUNCTURE PROCEDURES

Routine Blood Film (Smear) Preparation

Some tests require evaluation of a blood film or smear made from a fresh drop of blood from a fingertip. An example is a leukocyte alkaline phosphatase (LAP) stain or score, which usually requires four fresh **peripheral** (skin puncture or venous) **blood smears**. Skin puncture collection of peripheral smears is preferred. In addition, some hematologists prefer blood smears from blood that has not been in contact with anti-coagulant. When collected with other skin puncture specimens, blood smears should be collected first to avoid effects of platelet clumping.

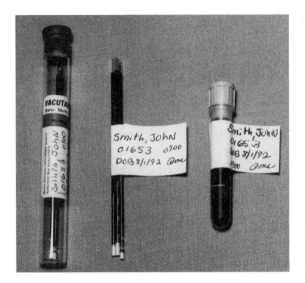

Figure 10-11 Labeled microcollection devices (left to right): capillary tubes inserted into labeled red top evacuated tube, flagged capillary tubes, and flagged microcollection container.

A blood smear is also needed when a manual **differential** is part of a complete blood count or when an abnormal platelet count must be confirmed by looking at or manually counting platelets in the blood film. Two blood smears are normally prepared and submitted for testing. These blood smears are rarely made at bedside. They are generally made in the hematology department from the EDTA specimen tube. They are often made using an automated machine that makes a uniform smear from a single drop of blood. Blood smears from EDTA-anticoagulated blood should be made within 1 hour of collection to eliminate cell distortion caused by the anticoagulant.

A routine blood smear is made in the following manner:

- Select two clean glass **slides**, free of cracks or chipped edges.
- Wipe away the first drop of blood in the normal manner. Touch the slide to the second drop in such a manner that the drop ends up ½ to 1 inch from the end of the slide or on the clear area of the slide just next to the frosted area, if applicable. The drop should be about 1 to 2 mm in diameter and centered on the slide.
- To make a smear manually from an anticoagulated blood specimen, the tube of blood must first be mixed for a minimum of 2 minutes to insure a uniform specimen. A capillary tube or pipet is then used to dispense a drop of blood from the specimen tube onto the slide. A device called DIFF-SAFE (Fig. 10-12) (Alpha Scientific, Malvern, PA) allows a slide to be made from an EDTA tube without removing the tube stopper. The device is inserted through the rubber stopper of the specimen tube and is then pressed against the slide to deliver a uniform drop of blood.
- Hold the blood drop slide in the nondominant hand between the thumb and forefinger with the blood drop at the thumb end, grasp the blood drop end between the thumb and forefinger, or place the slide on a flat surface and hold it steady with the index finger of the nondominant hand. Use the dominant hand to rest a second (or spreader) slide in front of the drop at approximately a 30-degree angle (Fig. 10-13A)

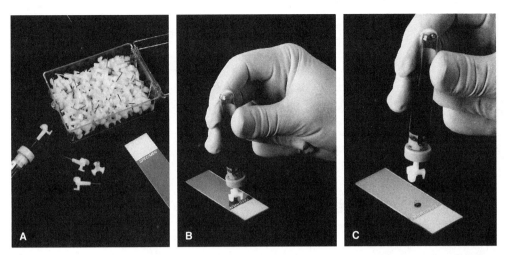

Figure 10-12   (**A**) DIFF-SAFE blood delivery device. (**B**) Applying blood drop to slide using DIFF-SAFE device. (**C**) Blood drop on slide. (Courtesy Alpha Scientific, Malvern, PA.)

with the first slide. The spreader slide is held at one end, between the thumb and index finger in either a vertical or horizontal position.

- Pull the spreader slide back to the edge of the blood drop. Stop the spreader slide as soon as it touches the drop and allow the blood to spread along its entire width (see Fig. 10-13*B*).
- As soon as the blood has spread its entire width, push the spreader slide forward (away from the thumb) in one smooth motion, carrying the entire length, all the way off the end of the blood drop slide. *Do not* push down on the spreader slide. Let the weight of the spreader slide carry the blood and make the smear.
- Place the drop of blood for the second smear on the spreader slide from the first smear. Use the slide containing the first smear as the spreader slide for the second smear. This way, two smears can be made using only two slides.
- Allow the blood films to dry naturally. *Never* blow on a slide to dry it because this results in red blood cell distortion.
- Label frosted blood slides by writing the patient information in pencil on the frosted area. *Do not* use ink as it may be dissolved during the staining process. Attach paper labels containing patient information in the space left at the blood drop end of slides that are not frosted.
- *Remember*, all blood smears are considered infectious until fixed or stained.

Making a good blood smear is a skill that takes practice to perfect. Improperly made blood smears will not contain a normal, even distribution of blood cells and may produce erroneous results. An acceptable smear (see Fig. 10-13C) will cover about one half to three fourths of the surface of the slide and have no holes, lines, or jagged edges. It will have the appearance of a **feather** in that there will be a smooth gradient from thick to thin when held up to the light. The thinnest area of a properly made smear, often referred to as the "feather," is one cell thick and is the most important area because that is where a differential is performed.

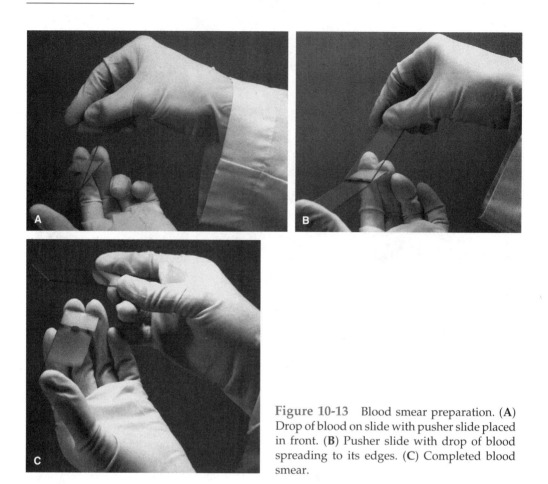

Figure 10-13 Blood smear preparation. (**A**) Drop of blood on slide with pusher slide placed in front. (**B**) Pusher slide with drop of blood spreading to its edges. (**C**) Completed blood smear.

Smears that are uneven, too long (cover the entire length of the slide), too short, too thick, or too thin are not acceptable. The length and thickness of the smear can usually be controlled by the size of the drop and the angle of the spreader slide.

Holes in the smear can be caused by fingerprints or dirt on the slide, fat globules, or lipids. Ragged edges can be caused by a chipped pusher slide, a blood drop that has started to dry, or uneven pressure as the smear is made. (See Table 10-1 for common problems associated with routine blood smear preparation.)

Thick Blood Smear Preparation

Thick blood smears are most often requested to detect the presence of malaria, which is caused by four species of parasitic sporozoan (types of protozoa) organisms called plasmodia. These organisms are transmitted to humans by the bite of infected female anopheles mosquitoes. Symptoms of malaria include serial bouts of fever and chills at regular intervals, related to the multiplication of certain forms of the organism within the red blood cells and the consequent rupture of those cells. The

Table 10-1
Common Problems Associated With Routine Blood Smear Preparation

Problem	Probable Cause
Absence of feather	Spreader slide lifted before the smear was completed
Holes in the smear	Dirty slide, fat globules in the blood, blood contaminated with glove powder
Ridges or uneven thickness	Too much pressure applied to spreader slide
Smear is too thick	Blood drop too big, spreader slide angle too steep, patient has high red blood cell count
Smear is too short	Blood drop too small, spreader slide angle too steep, spreader slide pushed too quickly, patient has high red blood cell count
Smear is too long	Blood drop too large, spreader slide angle too shallow, spreader slide pushed too slowly, patient has low hemoglobin
Smear too thin	Blood drop too small, spreader slide angle too shallow, patient has low hemoglobin value
Streaks or tails in feathered edge	Blood drop started to dry out, edge of spreader slide dirty or chipped, spreader slide pushed through blood drop, uneven pressure applied to spreader slide

progressive destruction of red blood cells in certain types of malaria causes severe anemia.

Malaria is diagnosed by the presence of the organism in a peripheral blood smear. Diagnosis often requires the evaluation of both regular and thick blood smears. Presence of the organism is observed most frequently in a thick smear, however, identification of the species requires evaluation of a regular blood smear. The smears may be ordered stat or at timed intervals and are most commonly collected just prior to the onset of fever and chills.

To prepare a thick smear, a very large drop of blood is placed in the center of a glass slide and spread with the corner of another slide or coverslip until it is the size of a dime. It is then allowed to dry for a minimum of 2 hours before staining with fresh diluted Giemsa stain. The water-based Giemsa stain lyses the red blood cells and makes the organism easier to see.

Capillary Blood Gases (Arterialized Skin Puncture Blood Gases)

Arterial punctures can be hazardous to infants and young children. For this reason, blood gas determinations on infants and young children are usually performed on arterialized skin puncture (capillary) specimens.

Skin puncture blood is less desirable for blood gases not only because of its partial arterial composition, but also because it is temporarily exposed to air during collection, possibly altering blood gas results. Proper collection techniques are essential to minimize this exposure.

Skin puncture specimens for blood gas determinations are collected from the same sites as routine skin puncture specimens. Warming the site for 5 to 10 minutes prior to skin puncture helps increase blood flow and arterialize the specimen.

CAPILLARY BLOOD GAS SPECIMEN COLLECTION PROCEDURE

1. Assemble equipment and supplies.
2. Select and warm the site.
3. Perform the skin puncture following routine skin puncture procedures.
4. Wipe away the first drop and collect the blood in a special heparinized glass capillary tube. Collect the blood carefully to prevent introduction of air bubbles into the capillary tube while obtaining the specimen. (Exposure of the blood to air for as little as 10 seconds can cause erroneous results.) Fill the capillary tube completely.
5. After collecting the specimen, immediately seal one end of the tube with clay or a special cap.
6. Depending on the type of equipment used, place a small magnetic mixing bar or several magnetic "fleas" into the capillary tube.
7. Quickly seal the opposite end and mix the specimen by running a magnet from one end of the tube to the other several times. (This procedure mixes the heparin with the specimen to prevent clotting.)
8. Label the specimen and immediately place it horizontally in a mixture of ice and water to prevent changes in pH and blood gas values.
9. Transport the specimen to the lab immediately.

Neonatal Bilirubin Collection

Neonates (newborns) are commonly tested to detect and monitor increased bilirubin levels caused by overproduction or impaired excretion of bilirubin. Overproduction of bilirubin occurs from accelerated red blood cell hemolysis associated with hemolytic disease of the newborn (HDN). Impaired excretion is often the result of temporary abnormal liver function commonly associated with premature infants. Bilirubin can cross the blood–brain barrier in infants, accumulating to toxic levels that may cause permanent brain damage or even death. A transfusion may be needed if levels increase at a rate equal to or greater than 5.0 mg/dL per hour or when levels exceed 18.0 mg/dL.

High levels of bilirubin result in jaundice (yellow skin color). Because bilirubin breaks down in the presence of light, jaundiced infants are often placed under special ultraviolet lights to lower bilirubin levels. The light should be turned off when a bilirubin specimen is being collected.

Proper collection of bilirubin specimens is crucial to the accuracy of results. Specimens are normally collected by heel puncture. They must be collected quickly to minimize exposure to light and must be protected from light during transportation and handling. Specimens are often collected in amber-colored microcollection containers which reduce light exposure. Specimens must be collected carefully to avoid hemolysis, which could falsely decrease bilirubin results. Because determination of the rate of increase in bilirubin levels depends on accurate timing, specimens should be collected as close as possible to the time ordered.

Newborn Screening

Newborn screening is performed to test for the presence of genetic, or inherited, diseases such as phenylketonuria (fen'il-kee'to-nu'ree-ah) or PKU, hypothyroidism, galactosemia, homocystinuria, maple syrup urine disease, and sickle cell. In the United States, newborn screening to detect PKU and hypothyroidism are required by law.

PHENYLKETONURIA (PKU)

The incidence of PKU in the United States is approximately 1 in 14,000 births. PKU results from a defect in the enzyme responsible for the conversion of the amino acid phenylalanine to tyrosine. Phenylalanine accumulates in the blood and is slowly metabolized by an alternate pathway resulting in increased phenylketones in the urine. Because phenylalanine is not being metabolized properly, phenylalanine levels can rise to toxic levels. PKU cannot be cured but it can usually be treated with a diet low in phenylalanine. If left untreated or not treated early, PKU can lead to brain damage and mental retardation. PKU testing requires the collection of two specimens, one shortly after an infant is born and the other after the infant is 10 to 15 days old.

HYPOTHYROIDISM

Congenital hypothyroidism occurs at the rate of approximately 1 in 4,000 births and is the result of insufficient levels of thyroid hormones. Some forms of neonatal hypothyroidism are not inherited. Newborn screening tests detect both inherited and noninherited forms. In the United States and Canada, the newborn screening test for hypothyroidism measures total thyroxine (TT_4). Positive results are confirmed by measuring thyroid stimulating hormone (TSH) levels.

COLLECTION PROCEDURE

Blood samples for PKU, hypothyroidism, and other newborn screening tests are commonly collected by absorption onto a special filter paper which is part of the test requisition. The filter paper contains printed circles which must be filled with blood (Fig. 10-14). The circles are filled by touching the paper to drops of blood obtained by heel puncture. A large drop of blood must be applied from only one side of the paper and blood must soak completely through to the other side. Blood should *not* be applied more than once or layered with successive drops in the same collection circle. The drops should not be smeared or touched. The phlebotomist must also be careful not to touch the filter paper with gloves or any other object or substance. The specimen should be allowed to air dry in an elevated horizontal position away from heat or sunlight. Specimens should not be stacked together before or after the drying process, as cross-contamination between specimens may result.

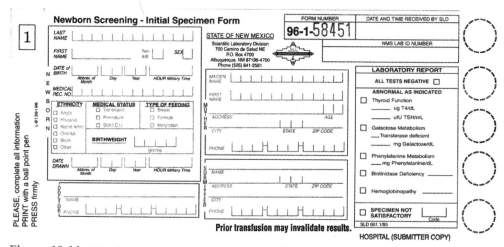

Figure 10-14   Newborn screening specimen form. (Courtesy Daniel Gray, State of New Mexico Scientific Laboratory, Albuquerque, NM.)

Study & Review Questions

1. Skin puncture blood
    a. is venous.
    b. is arterial.
    c. contains interstitial fluid.
    d. all of the above.

2. Which of the following has a higher concentration in capillary blood than in venous?
    a. Blood urea nitrogen
    b. Carotene
    c. Glucose
    d. Total protein

3. A blood test that cannot normally be performed by skin puncture is
    a. CBC.
    b. erythrocyte sedimentation rate.
    c. potassium.
    d. thyroid panel.

4. The least hazardous area of an infant's foot on which to perform skin puncture is the
    a. arch.
    b. central area of the heel.
    c. posterior curvature of the heel.
    d. medial or lateral area of the plantar surface of the heel.

5. It is necessary to control the depth of lancet insertion during heel puncture to avoid
    a. puncturing a vein.
    b. excessive bleeding.
    c. bone injury.
    d. bacterial contamination.

6. Povidone–iodine used to clean a skin puncture site is known to cause erroneous results for with of the following tests?
    a. Albumin
    b. Bilirubin
    c. CBC
    d. Triglycerides

7. When collecting skin puncture tests, which of the following should be collected first?
    a. CBC
    b. Electrolytes
    c. Glucose
    d. Phosphorus

8. A blood smear "pusher slide" should be at a
   a. 15-degree angle.
   b. 30-degree angle.
   c. 45-degree angle.
   d. 60-degree angle.

Suggested Laboratory Activities

1. Identify the proper sites for adult skin puncture on a fellow student.

2. Identify the proper sites for skin puncture on an infant, using an infant anatomic model.

3. Perform a finger puncture on another student and collect the blood using the various types of microcollection equipment.

4. Practice proper collection of blood for newborn screening, substituting blood obtained by finger puncture to fill the circles.

5. Practice making and labeling blood smears.

BIBLIOGRAPHY AND SUGGESTED READINGS

Bishop, M. L., Duben-Engelkirk, J. L., & Fody, E. P. (1996). *Clinical chemistry: Principles, procedures, correlations* (3rd ed.). Philadelphia: Lippincott-Raven.

Lotspeich-Steininger, C. A., Stiene-Martin, E. A., & Koepke, J. A. (1992). *Clinical hematology: Principles, procedure, correlations*. Philadelphia: J. B. Lippincott.

National Committee for Clinical Laboratory Standards, H4-A3. (July 1991). *Procedures for the collection of diagnostic blood specimens by skin puncture* (3rd ed.). Villanova, PA: NCCLS.

National Committee for Clinical Laboratory Standards, H14-A2. (July 1990). *Devices for collection of skin puncture blood specimens* (2nd ed.). Villanova, PA: NCCLS.

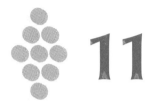

11

Special Procedures and Point-of-Care Testing

KEY TERMS

activated coagulation
   time (ACT)
aerobic
anaerobic
ancillary blood glucose
   testing (ABGT)
antimicrobial therapy
bacteremia
bleeding time (BT)

chain of custody
compatibility
fever of unknown
   origin (FUO)
forensic
   specimen
glucose tolerance
   test (GTT)
peak level

point-of-care testing
   (POCT)
postprandial (PP)
septicemia
skin antisepsis
therapeutic drug
   monitoring (TDM)
tolerance test
trough level

OBJECTIVES

Upon successful completion of this chapter, the reader will be able to:

1. Explain the principle behind and list any special equipment required and the steps involved for each of the special collection procedures.

2. Describe patient identification and specimen labeling procedures, and identify the type of specimen required for bloodbank tests.

3. Explain and state the importance of sterile technique in the collection of blood cultures, and identify the reasons why a physician might order them.

4. Identify and describe how to properly collect coagulation specimens and specimens that require cooling, light protection or transportation at body temperature.

5. Name and compare and contrast the various types of tolerance tests.

6. Describe chain of custody procedures and identify the tests that may require them.

7. State the importance of peak and trough levels in therapeutic drug monitoring.

8. Define point-of-care testing (POCT), identify and explain the principle behind the tests commonly performed as POCT, and list special equipment required and the steps involved for each of the POCT tests.

SPECIAL PROCEDURES

Blood specimens for most laboratory tests can be collected using routine venipuncture or skin puncture procedures. Some tests, however, require special or additional collection procedures. Collecting specimens for these tests may require special preparation, equipment, handling, or timing. The following sections describe some of the most commonly encountered special blood test procedures.

Blood Bank Specimens

SPECIMEN REQUIREMENTS

Most blood bank tests require a large plain (no serum separator gel) red stopper tube or a large lavender stopper EDTA tube. Strict procedures must be followed when identifying the patient and labeling the specimen. Specimens with incomplete or inaccurate information are not accepted by blood bank.

LABELING REQUIREMENTS

Blood bank specimens require the following identification information:

1. Patient's full name (including middle initial)
2. Patient's hospital identification number (or social security number for outpatients)
3. Patient's date of birth
4. Date and time of collection
5. Phlebotomist's initials
6. Room number and bed number (optional)

BLOOD TYPE AND CROSSMATCH SPECIMENS

One of the most common tests performed by the blood bank is a blood type and crossmatch. A blood type and crossmatch is performed to determine the **compatibility** of blood to be used in a transfusion. A transfusion of incompatible blood can be fatal because of **agglutination** (clumping) and **lysis** (rupturing) of the red blood cells within the patient's circulatory system (see Chapter 5). For this reason, hospitals require *strict* identification and labeling procedures when obtaining specimens for crossmatch.

SPECIAL IDENTIFICATION SYSTEMS

There are a number of different blood bank identification systems available. One procedure requires the attachment to the patient's wrist of a special identification (ID) bracelet such as the Typenex Blood Recipient Identification Band (Fenwal Biotech Division, a division of Travenol Laboratories, Chicago, IL) (Fig. 11-1).

In this procedure, the patient's identity is confirmed and the information written on a self-carbon adhesive label on the special bracelet, which contains an ID number. The adhesive label containing the ID number is peeled from the bracelet, leaving the carbon copy of the information, including the ID number, on the bracelet. The adhesive label is placed on the specimen drawn from the patient. Additional ID number labels from the bracelet are sent to the lab with the specimen to be used in the crossmatch process and eventually attached to the unit of blood used for transfusion. Before the transfusion is

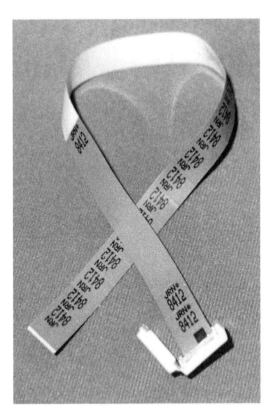

Figure 11-1　Typenex blood recipient identification band. (Fenwal Laboratories, a division of Travenol Laboratories, Chicago, IL.)

given, the nurse *must* match the number on the patient's identification bracelet with the number on the unit of blood.

Another identification system for blood bank patients, the Blood-Loc Safety System (Fig. 11-2) from Novatek Medical Inc. (Greenwich, CT), consists of four elements: a unique three-letter code printed on a colored adhesive sticker; a single-use plastic combination lock designed to seal the opening of a plastic bag; a back-plate that works in conjunction with the lock; and a 5 × 13-inch clear plastic bag. On admission to the hospital, a coded sticker is applied to the patient's ID band. When a specimen is drawn for a crossmatch, the phlebotomist must copy this unique code onto the specimen label. The code is circled so it is not confused with the phlebotomist's initials on the label. The specimen is then sent to the lab and the crossmatch is performed. When the unit of blood is needed for transfusion, it is put into a bag and sealed with the disposable lock, which is then permanently set with the patient's unique code. Before the unit is given to the patient, the nurse must use the code from the patient's wristband to be able to remove the unit from the plastic bag.

BLOOD DONOR COLLECTION

Blood donor collection involves collecting blood in amounts referred to as units to be used for transfusion purposes rather than for diagnostic testing. Donor collection requires special training and exceptional venipuncture skills. Facilities that provide

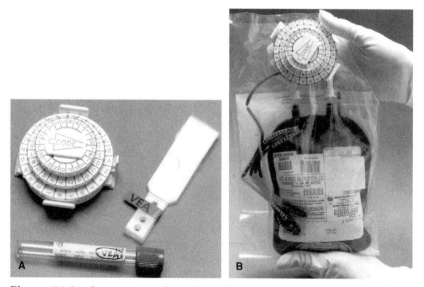

Figure 11-2   Components of the Blood-Loc® safety system showing: (**A**) the blood bag combination lock, a wrist band with unique code, and a tube with the code circled; (**B**) a Blood-Loc® safety bag with lock in place containing a unit of blood.

blood donor services are called blood banks. Blood banks follow guidelines of the American Association of Blood Banks (AABB).

Donor Eligibility

Anyone wishing to donate blood must be interviewed to determine eligibility to donate blood, as well as to obtain information for the records that must be kept for all blood donors. To donate blood, a person must be within the ages of 17 and 66 years and weigh at least 110 lb. Minors must have written permission from their parents. Adults over the age of 66 years may be allowed to donate at the discretion of the blood bank physician. A brief physical examination, as well as a complete medical history, is needed to determine the patient's state of health. This information is needed each time a person donates, no matter how many times a person has donated before. All donor information is strictly confidential. In addition, the donor must give written permission for the blood bank to use his or her blood.

Procedure

Donor units are normally collected from a large antecubital vein. The vein is selected in a similar manner as for routine venipuncture. Skin preparation involves a two-step cleaning process with a povidone–iodine preparation in a similar manner to blood culture collection. The collection unit is a sterile, closed system consisting of a bag to contain the blood connected by a length of tubing to a sterile needle. A 16-gauge, thin-wall needle is most commonly used. The bag fills by gravity and must be placed lower than the patient's arm. The collection bag contains an anticoagulant, generally a citrate phosphate dextrose solution, and is commonly placed on a mixing unit as the blood is being drawn. The unit is normally filled by weight but generally contains around 450 mL when full. Only one needle puncture can be used to fill a unit. If the unit only partially fills and the procedure must be repeated, and an entire new unit must be used. Average time to collect a unit is around 7 minutes. *450 -500 mL total*

A unit of blood can be separated into several components: red blood cells, plasma, and platelets. All components of the unit must be easily traceable to the donor.

R B C
plasma
platelets

AUTOLOGOUS BLOOD DONATION

Autologous donation is the process by which a person donates blood for his or her own use. This is done for elective surgeries where it is anticipated that a transfusion will be needed. Using one's own blood eliminates many risks associated with transfusion, such as disease transmission and blood or plasma incompatibilities. Although blood is normally collected several weeks prior to the scheduled surgery, the minimum time between donation and surgery can be as little as 72 hours. To be eligible to make an autologous donation, a person must have a written order from a physician, be in reasonably good health, be able to regenerate red blood cells, and have a hemoglobin of at least 11 g. If the patient meets regular donor requirements and the blood is not used, the blood may be used for the general population with the donor's permission.

Blood Cultures *bottles/tubes contain nutrient media; one aerobic, one anaerobic*

Blood cultures are ordered by a physician when there is **fever of unknown origin (FUO)** or reason to suspect **bacteremia** or **septicemia** (pathogenic bacteria in the blood). Blood cultures help determine the presence and extent of infection, as well as indicate the type of organism responsible and the antibiotic to which it is most susceptible. Once septicemia is diagnosed and treatment is initiated, blood cultures are useful in assessing the effectiveness of antibiotic therapy.

Collecting blood cultures in a timely fashion is important, as cultures are commonly ordered immediately before anticipated fever spikes as well as immediately after. Bacteria are most likely to be present in the blood stream at these times.

Blood culture specimens are collected in special tubes or bottles (Fig. 11-3); containing nutrient media which encourage the growth of any organisms present in the blood. Blood cultures are commonly collected in sets of two: one **anaerobic** (without air), and one **aerobic**. Anaerobic culture bottles are filled first when a syringe is used to collect the blood. When a butterfly collection set is used to collect the specimen, some clinicians prefer to have the aerobic bottle filled first because the air in the tubing will be drawn into the first specimen collected. When more than one set is ordered for the same time, the second set should be obtained from a separately prepared site on the opposite arm. However, in some cases, "second-site" blood cultures are more useful when drawn 30 minutes apart. If timing is not specified on the laboratory slip, follow laboratory protocol.

Skin antisepsis is the most important part of the blood culture collection procedure. Failure to follow sterile technique can introduce skin surface bacteria into the blood culture bottle and interfere with interpretation of results. All microorganisms isolated from blood cultures must be reported by the laboratory. It is up to the patient's

Anaerobic 1st with syringe
Butterfly 1st with aerobic

Second set from
second site = other arm
30 mins apart

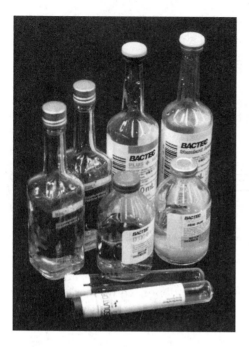

Figure 11-3   Blood culture bottles.

physician to determine whether the organism is clinically significant or merely a contaminant. If an organism is misinterpreted as pathogenic, it could result in inappropriate treatment.

Sterile technique methods for blood culture collection vary slightly from one laboratory to another. However, most methods require the use of povidone–iodine compounds in the form of swabsticks or special cleaning pad kits (Fig. 11-4) to clean

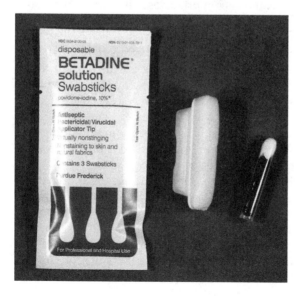

Figure 11-4   Two types of blood culture cleaning supplies; *left*, Povidone–iodine swabsticks (The Purdue Frederick Co., Norwalk, CT.); *right*, Frepp/Sepp povidone–iodine cleaning kit components.

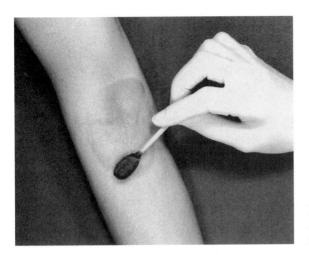

Figure 11-5 Scrubbing a blood culture collection site with a povidone–iodine swabstick.

the collection site. The procedure for one commonly accepted site cleaning method follows.

Blood culture

COLLECTION PROCEDURE

1. After selecting the venipuncture site, release the tourniquet (if applicable) and clean the site with an alcohol prep pad to initially rid the site of excess dirt and surface debris. Next, scrub the site for a minimum of 2 minutes, using a povidone–iodine swabstick (Fig. 11-5), covering an area 3 to 4 inches in diameter.
2. Clean the site again with a second povidone–iodine swabstick, beginning in the center and moving outward in concentric circles (Fig. 11-6) without going over any area more than once. Allow the area to air dry. Touching or palpating the site once it has been prepared is *not* recommended. However, if the patient has "difficult" veins and the necessity to repalpate is anticipated, the phlebotomist's gloved finger should be cleaned in the same manner as the venipuncture site. Note that antisepsis does not occur instantly. The scrubbing process in step 1, as well as the drying process in step 2, allows time for the antiseptic agent to be effective against skin surface bacteria.
3. While the area is drying, clean the tops of the blood culture containers with a third swabstick, using a different side of the swabstick for each bottle. Lay a clean alcohol

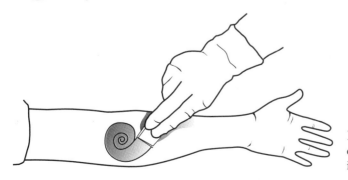

Figure 11-6 Pattern of concentric circles used when cleaning a blood culture site.

prep pad on top of each bottle. Blood culture containers equipped with plastic caps can be cleaned with 70% isopropyl alcohol after removing the cap and covered with an alcohol pad until ready to inoculate. Prepare venipuncture equipment, being careful to handle all equipment in an aseptic manner.

4. Reapply the tourniquet, taking care not to touch the prepped (prepared) area in the process. Perform the venipuncture.

5. Immediately prior to inoculation with blood, wipe the tops of the blood culture bottles with the alcohol pad to prevent introduction of iodine residue into the blood culture media. (Contamination of the media with iodine can inhibit growth of microorganisms and lead to false-negative culture results.)

6. Blood may be collected directly into blood culture media when using specially designed tubes or culture bottles that fit into the evacuated tube holder or a blood transfer system. Avoid backflow by keeping the culture bottle or tube lower than the collection site and preventing the culture media from contacting the stopper or needle during blood collection. Most blood culture bottles will draw 5 to 10 mL of blood. Pediatric bottles normally draw 1 to 3 mL. Mix each container after removing it from the needle holder. Keep track of which container was filled first. After filling both containers, remove the needle from the patient's arm and hold pressure over the site.

7. When the syringe method is used, the blood must be transferred to the bottles after the draw is completed. The practice of changing needles prior to this transfer is no longer recommended. Several recent studies have shown that changing needles has little effect on reducing contamination rates and may actually increase risk of needlestick injury to the phlebotomist. To help prevent accidental needlesticks when using a transfer set or needle and syringe, the culture bottle should *not* be held in the phlebotomist's hand during the inoculation process. In addition, when delivering blood to the bottles, direct the flow along the side of the container. Allow the blood to be drawn from the syringe by the vacuum of the container. Never push the plunger to expel the blood into the vial. This can hemolyze the specimen and cause aerosol formation when the needle is removed.

8. After collecting the specimen, clean the povidone–iodine from the patient's skin with an alcohol prep pad. Label the specimen containers with required identification information, including the site of collection (*eg*, right arm) and whether the specimen is aerobic or anaerobic.

ANTIMICROBIAL REMOVAL DEVICE (ARD)

It is not unusual for patients to be on **antimicrobial** (antibiotic) **therapy** at the time blood culture specimens are collected. Presence of the antimicrobial agent in the patient's blood can inhibit the growth of the microorganisms in the blood culture bottle. In such cases, the physician may order blood cultures to be collected in an **antimicrobial removal device** (ARD). The ARD contains a resin which removes antimicrobials from the blood. The blood can then be processed by conventional technique without the risk of inhibiting the growth of microorganisms. The ARD should be delivered to the lab for processing as soon as possible, as blood should not be exposed to the device for more than 2 hours. Some new blood culture media eliminate the need for special ARD media.

Coagulation Specimens

There are several important things to remember when collecting specimens for coagulation tests.

- If the coagulation specimen is the only specimen to be drawn, it is important to first draw a few milliliters of blood into a plain red stopper tube to eliminate tissue thromboplastin contamination picked up as the needle penetrates the skin. This tube can be thrown away if it is not needed for other tests and is referred to as a **"clear"** or **discard** tube.
- Sodium–citrate-containing tubes for coagulation studies must be filled until the vacuum is exhausted to obtain a *9 to 1 ratio of blood to anticoagulant.* Even when the tubes are properly filled, this ratio is altered if the patient has an abnormally high or low hemoglobin. In such cases, laboratory personnel may request collection of the test in a special tube which has had the volume of anticoagulant adjusted accordingly.
- *Never* pour two partially filled tubes together.
- Cooling may be required for some tests to protect the coagulation factors.

Cooled Specimens

Certain metabolic processes continue even after a specimen is drawn. Chilling the specimen slows down this metabolism. Specimens requiring chilling should be completely immersed in a slurry of crushed ice and water (Fig. 11-7). The use of large cubes of ice without water added prevents adequate cooling of the entire specimen and must therefore be avoided. In addition, placing a specimen in contact with a solid piece of ice can cause parts of the specimen to freeze, resulting in hemolysis and possible breakdown of the analyte. (Analyte is a general term for a substance undergoing analysis.) Specimens that require chilling are listed in Table 11-1.

Light-Sensitive Specimens

Some test components are broken down in the presence of light, causing falsely decreased values. The most common of these is **bilirubin.** Other tests in which the specimens are sensitive to light include **vitamin B$_{12}$, carotene, serum folate,** and **red cell folate**, as well as tests of urine specimens for **porphyrins** (see Table 11-1). Specimens can be easily protected from light by wrapping them in aluminum foil (Fig. 11-8). Light-inhibiting, amber-colored microcollection containers are available for collecting bilirubin specimens from infants.

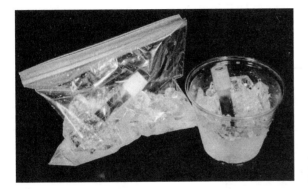

Figure 11-7   Blood samples in crushed ice for transport.

Table 11-1
Specimens That Require Special Handling

Crushed ice & water

temperature   3 C's

Specimens That Require Chilling	Specimens That Require Light Protection	Specimens Requiring 37°C Collection and Transportation
ammonia	bilirubin	cold agglutinin
arterial blood gases	carotene	cryofibrinogen
capillary blood gases	red cell folate	cryoglobulin (cryoprotein)
gastrin	serum folate	
glucagon	urine porphyrins	
lactic acid	vitamin B$_{12}$	
parathyroid hormone		
partial thromboplastin time	Aluminum fol	
protime		

Temperature-Sensitive (37° C) Specimens

Some specimens will precipitate or agglutinate if allowed to cool below body temperature (37° C) following collection. These specimens need to be transported at or near the normal body temperature of 37° C (see Table 11-1). In addition, most of these tests require the collection tube to be prewarmed to 37° C prior to collection of the specimen. Small, portable heat blocks that are kept in a 37° C incubator until needed and that hold this temperature for approximately 15 minutes after removal from the incubator are available for transporting such temperature-sensitive specimens. Temperature-sensitive specimens that can withstand temperatures higher than 37° C can be wrapped in an acti-

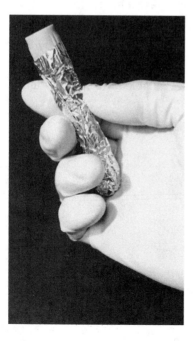

Figure 11-8　Light-sensitive specimen wrapped in aluminum foil.

vated heel warmer for transport (Fig. 11-9). Some of the most common body temperature specimens are as follows.

COLD AGGLUTININ

A **cold agglutinin** is an antibody that attaches to red blood cells and causes them to clump together or agglutinate at temperatures below body temperature. Cold agglutinin antibodies are present in the serum of persons with *Mycoplasma pneumonia* (atypical pneumonia) and certain blood diseases such as hemolytic anemia. To prevent the antibody from attaching to the red blood cells, a cold agglutinin specimen must be collected in a tube prewarmed to 37° C and kept at this temperature until the serum is separated from the cells.

CRYOFIBRINOGEN

Cryofibrinogen is an abnormal fibrinogen that precipitates when cooled and dissolves when brought back to body temperature.

CRYOGLOBULIN (CRYOPROTEIN)

A **cryoglobulin** is an abnormal protein, or globulin, that precipitates when cooled and dissolves when brought back to body temperature.

Paternity/Parentage Testing

Paternity testing is performed to determine the probability that a specific individual fathered a particular child. Generally, results of paternity testing can exclude the possibility of paternity, rather than prove paternity. Paternity testing may be requested by physicians, lawyers, child support enforcement bureaus, or, rarely, individuals. Tests performed usually include ABO and Rh typing, along with human leukocyte antigen (HLA) typing. Paternity testing generally requires special chain-of-custody protocol (see Forensic Specimens on p. 269) and specific identification procedures, which usually include fingerprinting. The mother, child, and alleged father are all tested.

Postprandial Glucose Testing

Postprandial (PP) means after a meal. Glucose levels in blood specimens obtained 2 hours after a meal are rarely elevated in normal persons, but may be significantly increased in diabetic patients. Therefore, a glucose test collected 2 hours after a meal, a

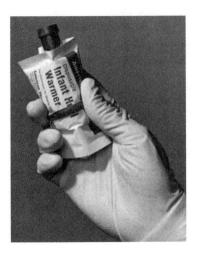

Figure 11-9   Temperature-sensitive specimen wrapped in heelwarmer for transport.

2-hour PP, is an excellent screening test for diabetes and other metabolism problems. The test is also used to monitor insulin therapy. Correct timing of specimen collection is very important. Glucose levels in specimens collected too early or late may be falsely elevated or decreased, respectively, leading to misinterpretation of results.

TEST PROCEDURE
1. Preparation for the test involves placing the patient on a high-carbohydrate diet for 2 to 3 days prior to the test.
2. It is important for the patient to be fasting prior to the test. This means no eating, smoking, or drinking other than water for at least 10 hours before the test.
3. The day of the test, the patient is instructed to eat a special breakfast containing the equivalent of 100 g of glucose.
4. A blood specimen for glucose determination is collected two hours after the patient finishes eating.

Therapeutic Phlebotomy

Therapeutic phlebotomy involves the withdrawal of a large volume of blood, usually measured by the unit (as in blood donation), or approximately 500 mL. It is performed by phlebotomists who have been specially trained in the procedure or in donor phlebotomy, in a manner similar to collecting blood from donors. It is used as a treatment for certain medical conditions such as polycythemia and hemochromatosis.

POLYCYTHEMIA
Polycythemia is a disease characterized by an overproduction of red blood cells that is detrimental to the patient's health. The patient's red blood cell levels are monitored regularly, usually by means of the hematocrit test. Periodic removal of a unit of blood when the hematocrit exceeds a certain level helps to keep the patient's red blood cell levels within the normal range.

HEMOCHROMATOSIS
Hemochromatosis is a disease characterized by excess iron deposits in the tissues. It can be caused by a defect in iron metabolism or as a result of multiple transfusions or excess iron intake. Periodic removal of single units of blood from the patient gradually causes depletion of excess iron stores as the body uses the iron to make new red blood cells to replace those removed.

Tolerance Tests
GLUCOSE TOLERANCE TEST
A **glucose tolerance test (GTT)** is performed to check for carbohydrate metabolism problems. The major carbohydrate in the blood is glucose. The two major types of disorders involving glucose metabolism are those in which the blood glucose level is increased (**hyperglycemia**), as in diabetes mellitus, and those in which the blood glucose levels are decreased (**hypoglycemia**). The enzyme insulin, produced by the pancreas, is primarily responsible for regulating blood glucose levels. The GTT evaluates insulin response to a measured dose of glucose by recording glucose levels collected at specific time intervals. Results are plotted on a graph creating what is referred to as a GTT curve (Fig. 11-10).

↑ blood glucose level = hyperglycemia
↓   "   "   "   "   = hypoglycemia

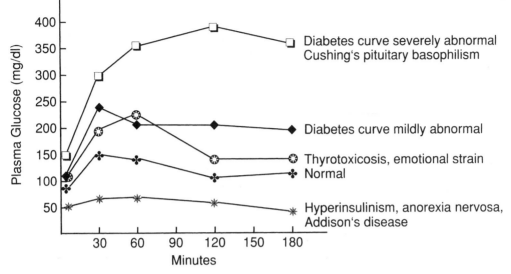

Figure 11-10 Glucose tolerance test (GTT) curves.

There are a number of variations of the GTT procedure, involving variations in doses of glucose and timing of collections. The standard procedure, on which most variations are based, follows.

Test procedure
Patient preparation for a GTT is very important. A patient should receive verbal as well as written instructions.

1. The patient is instructed to eat balanced meals containing approximately 150 g of carbohydrate for 3 days prior to the test.
2. The patient must then fast at least 12 hours preceding the test, but not for more than 16 hours. The patient is allowed and encouraged to drink water during the fast, since urine specimens are usually collected as part of the procedure. No other food or beverages are allowed. The patient is also not allowed to smoke or chew gum because these activities stimulate the digestive process and may cause erroneous test results.
3. A fasting blood specimen is drawn and checked for glucose. (If the fasting blood glucose is over 200 mg/dL, the test is usually not performed.) A fasting urine specimen may also be collected.
4. An adult patient is given a commercial glucose beverage, usually containing 75 or 100 g of glucose. Children and small adults are given approximately 1 g/kg of weight. The patient must consume the drink within 5 minutes.
5. Timing for the test is started as soon as the patient finishes the glucose beverage. Both blood and urine specimens are normally collected at 30 minutes, 1 hour, 2 hours, 3 hours, and so on, for the length of time specified by the physician; the test rarely exceeds 6 hours. Specimens should be labeled with both the exact time collected and the time interval of the test (*eg*, ½ hour, 1 hour).

6. No food, alcohol, smoking, or chewing gum is allowed throughout the test period. Water intake is allowed and encouraged.

In normal patients, blood glucose levels peak within 30 minutes to 1 hour following glucose ingestion. The peak in glucose levels triggers the release of insulin, which brings glucose levels back down to fasting levels within about 2 hours and no glucose spills over into the urine. Because diabetics have inadequate or absent insulin response, glucose levels peak at higher levels and are slower to return to fasting levels. If blood is not drawn on time, it is important for the phlebotomist to note the discrepancy so that the physician will take this into consideration.

The method used to collect GTT specimens should be consistent for all specimens. That is, if the first specimen is collected by venipuncture, all succeeding specimens should be venipuncture specimens. If skin puncture is used to collect the first specimen, all succeeding specimens should also be skin puncture specimens.

EPINEPHRINE TOLERANCE TEST

The **epinephrine tolerance test** is used to evaluate the amount and availability of **liver glycogen**. Glycogen is stored in the liver and converted to glucose when needed. Epinephrine accelerates the conversion of glycogen to glucose (glycogenolysis).

Test procedure
1. A fasting glucose specimen is collected.
2. A solution of epinephrine hydrochloride is injected intravenously by a physician or other qualified person.
3. A blood glucose specimen is collected 30 minutes later.

In a patient with normal glycogen stores, blood glucose levels at 30 minutes will increase at least 30 mg/dL above fasting levels. Little or no rise in blood sugar levels indicates depletion of glycogen stores or an interference in the conversion of available glycogen stores, such as caused by Von Gierke's disease.

GLUCAGON TOLERANCE TEST

A **glucagon tolerance test** also tests the presence and availability of liver glycogen stores. The test is conducted in the same manner as the epinephrine tolerance test, substituting glucagon for epinephrine. Results are also interpreted in the same manner.

LACTOSE TOLERANCE TEST

A **lactose tolerance test** is used to determine if a patient lacks the enzyme (mucosal lactase) that is necessary to convert the milk sugar lactose into glucose and galactose. A person lacking the enzyme suffers from gastrointestinal distress and diarrhea following ingestion of milk and other lactose-containing foods. Symptoms are relieved by eliminating milk from the diet.

Test procedure
1. A 3-hour GTT is performed the day before the lactose tolerance test.
2. A 3-hour lactose tolerance test is performed in the same manner as the GTT, however, an equal amount of lactose is substituted for the glucose.

3. Blood samples for glucose testing are drawn at the same times used in the GTT test the day before. If the patient has mucosal lactase, the resulting glucose curve will be similar to the GTT curve from the day before. If the patient lacks the enzyme (lactose intolerant), glucose levels will rise no more than 20 mg/dL from the fasting level, resulting in a "flat" curve. False-positive results have been demonstrated in patients with slow gastric emptying.

1st – best
grey top

Toxicology Specimens

BLOOD ALCOHOL (ETHANOL) SPECIMENS *2nd red, green*

Normally a **blood alcohol** (ethanol or ETOH) test is ordered by a patient's physician for medical reasons. Occasionally a blood alcohol test is requested by the police department for legal reasons. In such an event, special protocol, referred to as chain of custody, must be strictly followed (see the section on forensic specimens).

The 70% isopropyl alcohol used in skin preparation for routine venipuncture may interfere with test results of specimens drawn for blood alcohol determinations. Methanol can also affect results. In addition, tincture of iodine contains alcohol and likewise should not be used to clean the site. A non–alcohol-containing alternative antiseptic or regular soap and water should be used instead.

A **gray top, sodium fluoride tube**, with or without an anticoagulant depending upon the need for serum or plasma in the test procedure, is generally required for specimen collection, although red stopper serum tubes or green stopper heparin tubes are sometimes used. Because alcohol is volatile (easily vaporized or evaporated), the tube should be filled until the vacuum is exhausted and the stopper should *not* be removed until absolutely necessary.

FORENSIC SPECIMENS

Occasionally a blood, urine, or other body fluid specimen is requested by law enforcement officials for forensic or legal reasons. Tests most frequently requested are blood alcohol levels, drug levels, and specimens for DNA analysis. In such an event, special protocol, referred to as **chain of custody**, must be strictly followed. Chain of custody requires detailed documentation that tracks the specimen from the time it is collected until the results are reported. The specimen *must* be accounted for at all times. If documentation is incomplete, any legal action may be impaired.

A special form (Fig. 11-11) is used to identify the specimen and the person or persons who obtained and processed the specimen. Information on the form also includes the time, date, and place the specimen was obtained, along with the signature of the person from whom the specimen was obtained. Patient identification and specimen collection is performed in the presence of a witness, frequently a law enforcement officer. Special seals and containers may be required for the specimen. A phlebotomist involved in drawing a blood alcohol specimen for legal reasons can be summoned to appear in court.

DRUG SCREENING

Many health care organizations, sports associations, and major companies require **drug screening** of employees, prospective employees, or athletes. Table 11-2 lists drugs commonly detectable by drug screening, along with the length of time after

CHAIN OF CUSTODY REQUISITION FORM

SONORA Laboratory Sciences
3401 E. Harbour Dr., Phoenix, Arizona 85034
602 431-5000
800 SONORA-1
800 766-6721

ORDERING PHYSICIAN/COMPANY OR FACILITY

2013AC
SOEHS-T'BIRD SAMARITAN MEDICAL
CENTER   2013A
5555 W THUNDERBIRD RD
GLENDALE, AZ   85306
602 588-5555   *RT14

Failure to complete form properly could invalidate chain of custody.

DONOR INSTRUCTIONS   (To be completed by donor)

**************************** IDENTIFICATION IS REQUIRED AT TIME OF COLLECTION ****************************

DONOR AFFIDAVIT

I certify that the specimen identified by the ID number on this form was provided by me on this date and is not adulterated. In my presence, the specimen was sealed with an evidence seal taken from this form. The ID Number on the seal and on this form are identical. I have initialed the seal. By my signature I consent to the release of laboratory test results to the doctor, facility, individual or company shown on this form.

Donor Signature _____   Donor Name **(Print Clearly)** _____   Date _____

___/___/___
Birthdate _____   Social Security Number _____   Daytime Phone _____

You have the right to list any drugs, prescription or non prescription, that you may have taken in the last two weeks or other relevant medical information. Please do so, if desired, in the space provided: _____

COLLECTOR INSTRUCTIONS   (To be completed by collector)

1. Check donor identification **(preferably a picture I.D.)**
2. RECORD SPECIMEN TEMP: _____ (90° - 100°)
3. Specimen lid is tight, sealed properly with evidence seal, and initialed by donor.
4. I.D. number on specimen and form must match.
5. Place specimen in tamper-proof bag and seal in the presence of the donor.
6. Form is completed and signed by donor.
7. Collector signs this form, indicates date, time and collection site.

I certify that the specimen identified by this form was collected according to specified procedures, was properly identified and prepared for transport to the laboratory.

Collector Signature _____   Printed Name _____   Date _____   Collection Time _____

Collection Site _____   Address _____   Phone _____

COMMENTS: _____

LABORATORY USE ONLY

SPECIMEN RECEIVED BY: _____

SIGNATURE _____   PRINTED NAME _____   DATE _____

SPECIMEN SEAL CONDITION: ☐ INTACT   ☐ NOT INTACT

COMMENTS: _____

Check One Box
- ☐ Pre-Employment
- ☐ Post-accident
- ☐ Random
- ☐ Reasonable Cause
- ☐ Periodic
- ☐ Other _____

TESTS

[X] 2406 (FORENSIC COM-
PREHENSIVE)

SOCIAL SECURITY NUMBER

____ ____ ____

DEPT: _____

PHONE: _____

COLLECTION TIME/DATE

_____/_____

*********** SPECIMEN I.D. NUMBER 293012 ****************************

293012 293012   EVIDENCE SEAL   SPECIMEN I.D. NUMBER   EVIDENCE SEAL
293012 293012   293012
293012 293012   Donor Initials
                 EVIDENCE SEAL   ___/___/___   EVIDENCE SEAL
                                 Date

ORIGINAL TO LABORATORY

Figure 11-11   Chain of custody requisition form. (Courtesy Sonora Laboratory Sciences, Phoenix, AZ.)

Table 11-2
Drugs Commonly Detectable at Drug Screening

Drug or Drug Families	*Common Names*	*Detectable (time)*	*Comment*
Alcohol	—	2–12 hours	—
Amphetamines	methamphetamine, speed, crystal, crank, ice	1–3 days 2–7 days	Single/light use Frequent/chronic use
Barbiturates	downers, Seconal, Fiorinal, Tuinal, Phenobarbital	2 days to 4 weeks	Varies considerably with drugs in this class
Benzodiazepines	Valium, Librium, Xanax, Dalmane, Serax	1 week to >30 days	Varies considerably with drugs in this class
Cocaine (as metabolite)	crack	1–3 days 3–14 days	Single/light use Frequent use/freebase
Cannabinoids	marijuana, grass, hash	1–7 days >30 days	Single/light use Frequent/chronic use
Methadone	Dolophine	1–4 days	Single/light use
Opiates	heroin, morphine, codeine, Dilaudid hydrocodone	2–4 days >7 days	Single/light use Frequent/chronic use
Phencyclidine	PCP, angle dust	2–7 days >30 days	Single/light use Frequent/chronic use
Propoxyphene	Darvon, Darvocet	1–2 days >7 days	Single/light use Frequent/chronic use

Courtesy Tox Talk, Sonora Laboratory Sciences, Phoenix, AZ (1996).

use that the drug is detectable in the body. Whether it is performed for legal reasons or not, there are legal implications to drug screening that require use of the chain of custody protocol described in the earlier section on Forensic Specimens. Screening is often performed without prior notice. Drug screening requires the following special patient preparation and collection procedures defined by the **National Institute on Drug Abuse (NIDA):**

PATIENT PREPARATION REQUIREMENTS

- Explain the test purpose and procedure.
- Advise the patient of legal rights.
- Obtain a witnessed signed consent form.

SPECIMEN COLLECTION REQUIREMENTS

- A special area must be maintained for urine collection.
- A proctor is required to be present during urine collection to verify that the specimen came from the correct person.
- A split sample may be required for confirmation or parallel testing.
- The specimen must be labeled appropriately to establish a chain of custody.
- To avoid tampering, a specimen must be sealed and placed in a locked container during transport from the collection site to the testing site. Documentation must be carefully maintained from courier to receiver.

Therapeutic Drug Monitoring

Because the dosage of drug necessary to produce the desired effect varies widely among patients, **therapeutic drug monitoring (TDM)** is used by the physician to manage individual patient drug treatment. TDM helps the physician establish drug dosages, maintain dosages at beneficial levels, and avoid drug toxicity. Timing of specimen collection in regard to dosage administration is critical for safe and beneficial treatment and must therefore be consistent. A team effort is essential and requires coordination with pharmacy, nursing, and the lab. The phlebotomist is a key player in this team effort.

Some therapeutic drugs require the monitoring and evaluation of peak and trough drug levels in order for the physician to determine a safe and effective dosage for the patient (Fig. 11-12). Peak (or maximum) levels are collected when the highest serum concentration of the drug is anticipated, around 30 to 60 minutes after administration of the drug. Peak-level specimen collection requires careful coordination of sample collection with dosing. **Peak levels** screen for drug intoxication. Trough (or minimum) levels are easiest to collect, because they are collected when the lowest serum concentration of the drug is expected, usually immediately prior to administration of the next scheduled dose. **Trough levels** are monitored to ensure that levels of the drug stay within the therapeutic (or effective) range.

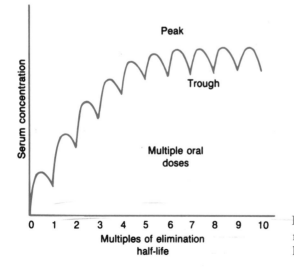

Figure 11-12   Dose–response curve after multiple oral doses of a drug given each half-life.

Collection timing is most critical for aminoglycoside drugs, such as amikacin, gentamicin, and tobramycin, which have short half-lives. (A half-life is the time required for the body to metabolize half the amount of the drug.) The timing is less critical for drugs that have longer half-lives, such as phenobarbital and digoxin.

Trace Elements *Royal blue — no additive*

Trace elements or metals include aluminum, arsenic, copper, lead, iron, and zinc. These elements are measured in such small amounts that traces of these substances commonly found in the glass and stopper material of evacuated tubes may leach into the specimen, causing falsely elevated test values. For this reason, these tests must be collected in special trace–element-free tubes made of materials that have been specially manufactured to be as free of trace elements as possible. An insert with each carton of tubes gives a detailed analysis of residual amounts of metals contained in the tubes. These tubes are usually royal blue in color and contain either no additive, EDTA, or heparin. The type of additive is indicated on the label; red for no additive, lavender for EDTA, and green for heparin.

POINT-OF-CARE TESTING

Point-of-care testing (POCT), also known as alternate site testing (AST) or ancillary, bedside, or near-patient testing, brings laboratory testing to the location of the patient. Its benefits include convenience to the patient and a short result turnaround time (TAT) to the health care facility. A short TAT allows health care providers to address crucial patient needs, deliver prompt medical attention, and help expedite patient recovery.

POCT is possible owing to advances in laboratory instrumentation that have led to the development of small, portable, and often hand-held testing devices. These devices allow testing to occur in a variety of hospital settings including the bedside, emergency room, operating suite, and intensive care unit, as well as other direct patient care settings such as physician's offices, nursing homes, clinics, patient service centers, and even the patient's own home. Health care personnel trained to perform POCT include phlebotomists, nurses (RNs and LPNs), nursing assistants (NAs), medical assistants (MAs), home health aids, patient-care technicians (PCTs), and respiratory therapy technicians (RTTs).

In addition to being able to operate the machine and perform the phlebotomy procedures required to collect the specimen, anyone performing POCT must understand quality assurance aspects of machine operation. Quality control and maintenance procedures are necessary to ensure that results obtained are accurate. At this time, no certification is required to perform POCT, however, anyone who performs POCT must meet the 1988 Clinical Laboratory Improvement Amendments qualifications.

Coagulation Monitoring
ACTIVATED COAGULATION TIME (ACT)

Activated coagulation time (ACT), also called activated clotting time, has always been a bedside test. It analyzes activity of the intrinsic coagulation factors and is used to monitor heparin therapy. Heparin is given intravenously to patients who have blood clots, to patients whose blood is apt to clot too easily, or as a precaution following certain surgeries. Effects on intravenous heparin administration are immediate, but difficult to control. Too much heparin can cause the patient to bleed, therefore, heparin therapy is closely monitored. Once a patient's condition is stabilized, the patient is placed on oral anticoagulant therapy such as coumarin, which can be monitored by the prothrombin test.

Prothrombin test

grey top

The test procedure involves expediting coagulation time by use of a clot-enhancing substance (activator) such as siliceous earth, silica, or celite contained in a special gray top tube. Other equipment needed to perform the test includes regular venipuncture equipment, a heat block or incubator, and stopwatch or timer. The procedure is as follows:

1. A routine venipuncture is performed and a 4-mL discard tube is drawn.
2. Blood is then drawn into a prewarmed tube containing the clot activator. A timer is started as soon as blood flows into the tube.
3. As soon as the tube vacuum is exhausted, the tube is mixed thoroughly and placed in the heat block for 60 seconds. *Note:* Although the tube may look like one that draws a larger volume, ACT tubes draw only a small volume of blood (approximately 2 cc).
4. At the end of 60 seconds, the tube is rocked gently back and forth and visually inspected for the first visible sign of a clot.
5. If no clot formation is seen, it is placed back in the heat block for 5 seconds after which it is removed and inspected again.
6. The procedure is repeated every 5 seconds until the first visible clot is observed, at which point the timer is stopped and the time recorded.
7. Results are recorded at the nurses' station and also reported to the coagulation department.

Sources of Error
1. Failure to start the timer as soon as the blood flow starts will decrease values.
2. Failure to mix the tube adequately will result in increased values.
3. A sample obtained by a traumatic draw, as well as an inadequate sample, will cause decreased values.
4. Anticoagulant drugs, antibiotics, steroids, and barbiturates can lead to erroneous results.

An automated variation of the ACT procedure, the Hemochron system (Fig. 11-13), is available from International Technidyne Corporation. With this system, a machine does the mixing and timing automatically. This system requires the use of a special tube with a black plastic cap. The tube is supplied by the manufacturer of the equipment.

BLEEDING TIME
The **bleeding time (BT)** test (Fig. 11-14) detects platelet function disorders by testing platelet plug formation in the capillaries. It is used in diagnosing problems with hemostasis and as a presurgical screening test.

Bleeding time is the time required for blood to stop flowing from a standardized puncture in either the earlobe, finger, or the inner surface of the forearm. Prolonged bleeding can be caused by abnormal platelet function or the ingestion of aspirin or other

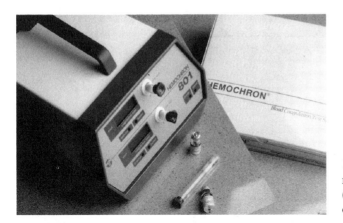

Figure 11-13 The Hemochron® machine for ACT determinations. (Courtesy International Technidyne Corp., Edison, NJ.)

salicylate-containing drugs within 2 weeks prior to the test. A number of other drugs such as ethanol, dextran, and streptokinase may also prolong bleeding time.

Bleeding time on the earlobe, originally described by Duke in 1910, is rarely ordered today. However, the test is still ordered by some facial surgeons who feel that the circulation of the ear more closely resembles that of the face.

The Duke bleeding time was modified by Ivy in 1941. The Ivy bleeding time is performed on the volar (inner) surface of the forearm utilizing a blood pressure cuff to maintain constant pressure. The incision is made with a sterile lancet.

Most laboratories today use a modification of the Ivy procedure, controlling the width and depth of the incision by use of an automated incision device such as the Sur-

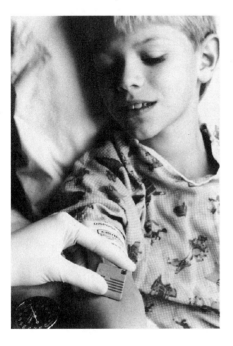

Figure 11-14 Bleeding time test being performed. (Courtesy International Technidyne, Edison, NJ.)

gicutt (Fig. 11-15) (International Technidyne Corp., Edison, NJ), Hemalet (Medprobe Laboratories, New York, NY), or Simplate II (Organon Teknika Corp., Durham, NC).

Materials needed for the modified Ivy are as follows:

1. Automated bleeding time device
2. Sphygmomanometer (blood pressure cuff)
3. Stopwatch, timer, or watch with sweep second hand
4. Filter paper (#1 Whatman or equivalent)
5. Alcohol prep pad
6. Butterfly bandage or steri-strip

Test procedure
1. Determine whether the patient has taken aspirin or any other salicylate-containing drug within the last 2 weeks. Advise the patient of the potential for scarring.
2. Support the patient's arm on a steady surface.
3. Select an area on the inner (volar) surface of the forearm, distal to the antecubital area and devoid of surface veins, scars, or bruises. The lateral aspect is preferred because using the medial aspect tends to cause more pain and has a higher incidence of scarring. It may be necessary to shave the test area lightly if it is covered with a large amount of hair.
4. Clean the selected area with alcohol and allow to dry.
5. Place the blood pressure cuff around the arm.
6. Remove the puncture device from its package, being careful not to touch or rest the blade slot on any unsterile surface.
7. Inflate the blood pressure cuff to 40 mm Hg. (Time between inflation of the blood pressure cuff and making the incision should be between 30 and 60 seconds.) This pressure *must* be maintained throughout the entire procedure.
8. Remove the safety clip and place the puncture device firmly on the forearm without pressing. A horizontal incision parallel to the antecubital crease is recommended.

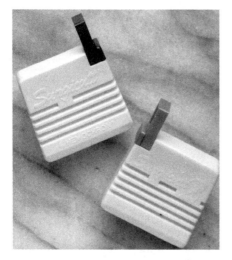

Figure 11-15 Surgicutt automated bleeding time device. (Courtesy International Technidyne Corp., Edison, NJ.)

9. Depress the trigger while simultaneously starting the timer. Remove the device from the arm as soon as the blade has retracted (approximately 1 second after the device has been triggered).
10. Blot the blood flow at 30 seconds by bringing the filter paper close to the incision and absorbing or "wicking" the blood onto the filter paper without touching the wound. (Touching the wound will disturb platelet plug formation!)
11. Continue to blot every 30 seconds until blood no longer stains the filter paper. Stop the timer and record the time to the nearest 30 seconds. If bleeding persists beyond 30 minutes, the test is usually stopped and the time is recorded as 30 minutes or greater.
12. Remove blood pressure cuff, clean the arm, and apply a butterfly bandage. Cover with an adhesive bandage. The patient is instructed not to remove either bandage for 24 hours.

Normal: Approximately 2 to 8 minutes depending on the method used.

Sources of error
1. Disturbing platelet plug formation will increase the bleeding time.
2. Failure to maintain 40 mm Hg will decrease the bleeding time.
3. Failure to start the timing as soon as the incision is made will decrease the bleeding time.

PROTHROMBIN TIME AND PARTIAL THROMBOPLASTIN TIME
Several instruments are available to perform both **prothrombin time (PT)** and **activated partial thromboplastin time (PTT or APTT)** at the bedside. The CIBA Corning Biotrack 512 coagulation monitor (CIBA Corning Diagnostics Corp., Medfield, MA) and the CoaguChek (Fig. 11-16) are hand-held instruments that perform the test on a single unmeasured drop of whole blood obtained by skin puncture. The TAS or Thrombolytic Assessment System (Cardiovascular Diagnostics Inc., Raleigh, NC) utilizes citrated blood added to a test well on a special test card previously inserted into the machine and warmed prior to testing. Each of these instruments provide results in under 5 minutes.

Arterial Blood Gas and Chemistry Panels
Several small portable and, in some cases, hand-held instruments are available that measure panels or groups of commonly ordered stat tests such as blood gases and electrolytes. These analytes are normally maintained by the body in specific proportions within narrow ranges, and any uncorrected imbalance can quickly lead to death. Consequently, these tests are often ordered in emergency and critical care situations where immediate response is vital to the patient's survival.

COMMON POCT CHEMISTRY PANELS
Arterial Blood Gases
Arterial blood gases (ABGs) measured by POCT methods include **pH**, **partial pressure of carbon dioxide (pCO$_2$)**, and **partial pressure of oxygen (PO$_2$)**.

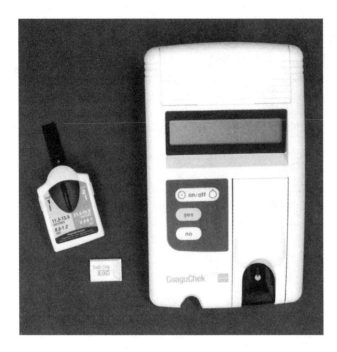

Figure 11-16   CoaguChek coagulation monitor. (Boehringer Mannheim Corp., Indianapolis, IN.)

The pH is a measure of the body's acid–base balance and is an indicator of a patient's metabolic and respiratory status. The normal range for arterial blood pH is 7.35 to 7.45. Below-normal pH is referred to as acidosis and above-normal pH is referred to as alkalosis.

The pCO_2 is a measure of the pressure exerted by dissolved CO_2 in the blood and is proportional to the pCO_2 in the alveoli and, therefore, an indicator of how well air is being exchanged between the blood and the lungs. CO_2 levels are maintained within normal limits by the rate and depth of respiration. An abnormal increase in pCO_2 is associated with hypoventilation and a decrease with hyperventilation.

The pO_2 is a measure of the pressure exerted by dissolved O_2 in the plasma and indicates the ability of the lungs to diffuse O_2 through the alveoli into the blood. It is used to evaluate the effectiveness of oxygen therapy.

Electrolytes

The most common electrolytes measured by POCT are **sodium (Na^+), potassium (K^+), chloride (Cl^-), bicarbonate ion (HCO_3^-),** and **ionized calcium (iCa^{++}).**

- *Sodium* is the most plentiful electrolyte in the blood. It plays a major role in maintaining osmotic pressure and acid–base balance and in transmitting nerve impulses. Reduced sodium levels are referred to as **hyponatremia**, and elevated levels are referred to as **hypernatremia**.
- *Potassium* is primarily concentrated within the cells, with very little found in the bones and blood. It is released into the blood when cells are damaged. Potassium plays a major role in nerve conduction, muscle function, acid–base balance, and osmotic pressure. It influences cardiac output by helping to control the rate and force

of heart contraction. Presence of a U wave on an electrocardiogram is indicative of potassium deficiency. Decreased blood potassium is called **hypokalemia**; increased blood potassium is called **hyperkalemia**.

- *Chloride* exists mainly in the extracellular spaces in the form of sodium chloride (NaCl) or hydrochloric acid. Chloride is responsible for maintaining cellular integrity by influencing osmotic pressure and acid–base and water balance. Chloride must be supplied along with potassium when correcting hypokalemia.

- *Bicarbonate ion* plays a role in transporting carbon dioxide (CO_2) to the lungs and in regulating blood pH. HCO_3^- is formed in the red blood cells and plasma from CO_2. Hydrogen ion (H^+) is released in the process, causing a decrease in pH, which means that the blood becomes more acid. HCO_3^- moves from the cells to the plasma and is carried to the lungs, where it re-enters the cells and releases CO_2 for removal through the walls of the alveoli. Removal of CO_2 by the lungs results in a decrease of H^+ ions and an increase in blood pH. Decreased ventilation (hypoventilation) results in higher CO_2 levels and production of more H^+ ions, which can lead to acidosis. Hyperventilation decreases CO_2 levels and can lead to alkalosis.

- *Ionized calcium* accounts for approximately 45% of the calcium in the blood; the rest is bound to protein and other substances. Only ionized calcium can be utilized by the body for such critical functions as muscular contraction, cardiac function, transmission of nerve impulses, and blood clotting.

POCT CHEMISTRY ANALYZERS

The hand-held i-STAT (Fig. 11-17) (i-STAT Corp., Princeton, NJ) measures blood gas values for pH, pCO_2, and O_2 and the electrolytes Na^+, K^+, Cl^-, and HCO_3^-. It can also measure BUN, glucose, and Hct values. Other instruments that measure blood gases and electrolytes are the AVL OPTI (AVL Scientific, Roswell, GA), the Nova Stat Profile Analyzer (Nova Biomedical, Waltham, MA), and the Gem Premier (Instrumentation Laboratories, Lexington, MA).

The small, portable IRMA (Fig. 11-18) (Diametrics Medical, Inc., St. Paul, MN) measures blood gas values for pH, pCO_2, and PO_2 and the electrolytes Na^+, K^+, and iCa^{++}. The IRMA system can also calculate other blood gas parameters such as HCO_3^- and O_2 saturation. A blood analysis is performed by a small cartridge that is inserted into the instrument. The cartridge automatically calibrates itself when it is inserted into the instrument. Once calibration is complete, a small sample of blood is injected into the system's sensor cartridge. The test is performed in less than 2 minutes. The cartridge is then removed from the instrument and discarded in a biohazard container. Results are displayed on a screen and a hard copy printout is generated.

Cardiac Troponin T

Cardiac troponin T (cardiac TnT) is a protein specific to heart muscle. Blood levels of cardiac TnT begin to rise within 4 hours of the onset of myocardial damage and may stay elevated for up to 14 days. Since cardiac TnT is specific for heart muscle, its measurement is a valuable tool in the diagnosis of acute myocardial infarction (AMI) or heart attack. It is also measured to monitor the effectiveness of thrombolytic therapy in heart attack patients.

A one-step, whole-blood bedside test for cardiac TnT, the CARDIAC T Rapid Assay (Fig. 11-19) (Boehringer Mannheim Corp., Indianapolis, IN), uses disposable test kits to provide cardiac TnT results in 1 to 20 minutes.

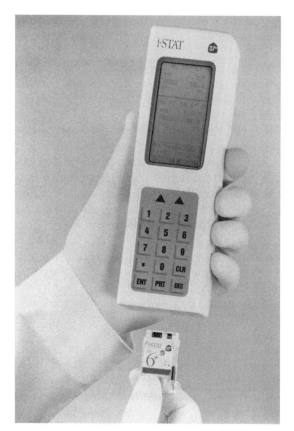

Figure 11-17   i-STAT instrument. (Courtesy i-STAT Corporation, Princeton, NJ.)

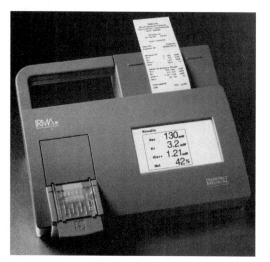

Figure 11-18   Portable IRMA (Immediate Response Mobil Analysis) blood chemistry analyzer. (Courtesy Diametrics Medical, Inc., St. Paul, MN.)

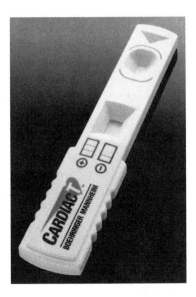

Figure 11-19 Cardiac T for performing Troponin T. (Courtesy Boehringer Mannheim Corp., Indianapolis, IN.)

Cholesterol

Total blood cholesterol levels can be obtained at the bedside using the Accu-Meter (Chem Trak, Inc., Sunnyvale, CA). The test requires a minimum of 40 μL of whole blood. Blood can be obtained by fingerstick or from heparinized venous samples. A quantitative result is obtained by visual evaluation of the height of a colored bar. The machine uses no instrumentation, which means preventive maintenance and calibration are unnecessary.

Electrocardiogram

An electrocardiogram (ECG or EKG) is a recording of the electrical impulses generated during heart contraction (Fig. 11-20). It is used to diagnose and monitor pathological heart conditions and disturbances in electrolyte balance, monitor cardiac drug

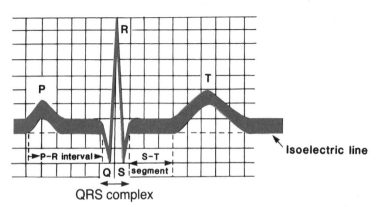

Figure 11-20 Normal ECG tracing showing one cardiac cycle (Jones SA, Weigel A, White RD, McSwain NE, Breiter M).

therapy, and evaluate implanted pacemaker and defibrillator function. Various types of ECG testing can be performed including resting ECG, continuous ambulatory ECG (Holter monitoring), and exercise ECG (stress test).

An ECG is performed by placing special electrodes on the patient's limbs and chest (Fig. 11-21). The electrodes are connected to an amplifier and a strip chart recorder. The electrical impulses generated during heart contraction are conducted through body fluids to the surface of the body, where they can be picked up by the electrodes. Because the impulses spread in several directions at the same time, 5 electrodes with 12 different views or leads are normally placed on the body to record a comprehensive picture of heart activity. The 12 leads are as follows:

Leads I, II, and III: Bipolar (positive and negative poles) limb leads that measure the difference in electrical activity between two selected limbs

Leads aVR, aVL, and aVF: Three unipolar, positive-pole only, augmented leads that measure electrical potential between the center of the heart and each limb

Leads V1 through V6: Six unipolar, positive-pole only, chest leads that measure electrical activity of the heart in the horizontal plane

An ECG is performed with the patient in a supine position. The skin is cleaned with alcohol to reduce skin oils before the electrodes are applied. When metal plates or suction

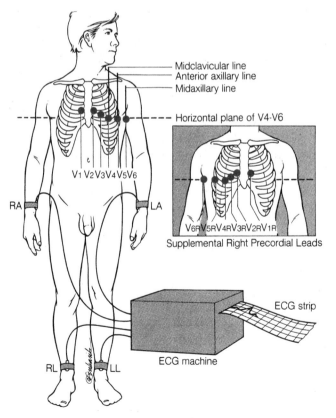

Figure 11-21 Twelve-lead ECG-electrode placement.

cups are used, electrode paste, gel, or saline pads are applied to the site first. Leads are placed anywhere on the four extremities and at specific sites on the chest (see Fig. 11-21).

Glucose

Ancillary blood glucose testing (ABGT), or bedside glucose testing, is one of the most common POCT procedures. It is also referred to as reflectance meter glucose (RMG) testing because of the method used to perform the test.

Glucose testing is most often performed to monitor glucose levels of patients with diabetes mellitus. Glucose levels are most commonly determined using small, portable, relatively inexpensive glucose analyzers such as the Glucometer II (Ames Division, Miles Laboratories, Elkhart, IN), Accu-check II (Boehringer Mannheim Diagnostics, Indianapolis, IN), ONE TOUCH II (Fig. 11-22) (Life Scan, Inc., Milpitas, CA), and the β-Glucose Analyzer (HemoCue, Inc., Mission Viejo, CA).

Most glucose analyzers utilize whole blood specimens obtained by routine skin puncture. Some analyzers will also accept heparinized venous specimens.

The Glucometer II, Accu-check II, and ONE TOUCH II require use of a special reagent test strip. The test strips come in airtight containers that must not be left open for more than a few moments. It is also important to protect the test strips from heat. The test strip container has a code number. The code number in the analyzer must be set to match the code number of the test strip container. To perform the test, a drop of blood is applied to the test strip, which has been inserted into the machine. The level of glucose in the blood is determined by the analyzer and the result appears on a screen.

The HemoCue β-Glucose Analyzer accepts arterial specimens as well as skin puncture and venous specimens. The test is performed using a microcuvette instead of a test strip.

NCCLS guidelines recommend that a phlebotomist receive institution authorization to perform ABGT only after completing formal training in ABGT procedures under the supervision of or sponsored by the particular health care institution.

Daily maintenance and quality control procedures must be performed and recorded before an ABGT analyzer is used. These procedures should be repeated if the unit is dropped, the battery is replaced, patient results are questioned, or functioning of the unit is questioned.

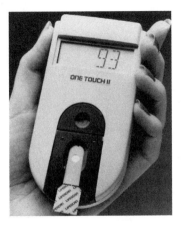

Figure 11-22   ONE TOUCH II® Blood Glucose Meter. (Courtesy of LifeScan Inc., Milpitas, CA.)

Hematocrit

The hematocrit (Hct), also called packed cell volume (PCV) is a measure of the volume of red blood cells in a patient's blood. It is calculated by centrifuging a specific volume of anticoagulated blood and determining the proportion of red blood cells compared to plasma. Blood is collected in special microhematocrit tubes. The tubes are sealed at one end with clay and placed in a special centrifuge. The results can often be calculated while the tube is still in the centrifuge by lining the tube up with a special chart that is part of the machine and reading the results from the chart. The result is expressed as a percentage.

The Hct is often performed in a physician's office labs (POLs), clinics, and blood donor stations to screen for anemia. It is also requested by physicians in the diagnosis and monitoring of patients with polycythemia.

Hemoglobin

Measurement of a patient's hemoglobin level is an important part of managing patients with anemia. A hand-held instrument called the HemoCue Hemoglobin System (Fig. 11-23) (HemoCue, Inc., Mission Viejo, CA) uses arterial, venous, or skin puncture specimens to determine hemoglobin levels. The sample is placed in a special microcuvette and inserted into the machine for a reading.

Occult Blood (Guaiac)

Detection of occult (hidden) blood in stool (feces) is an important tool in diagnosing and determining the location of a number of diseases of the digestive tract, including gastric ulcer and colon cancer.

Testing for occult blood in POCT settings involves the use of special kits containing cards on which small amounts of feces are placed (Fig. 11-24). The specimen can be collected and tested on-site or the cards sent home with the patient to collect and mail back to the lab. Another type of occult blood test that can be done on-site or sent home with a patient involves a special reagent-impregnated pad that is dropped into the toilet after a bowel movement. A color change on the pad is compared with a result chart.

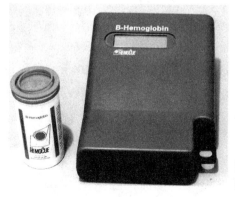

Figure 11-23 HemoCue hemoglobin system. (HemoCue, Inc., Mission Viejo, CA.)

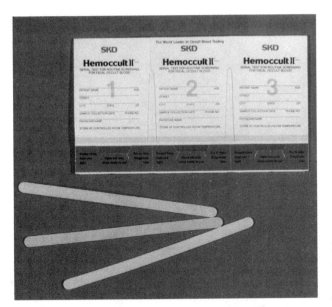

Figure 11-24 Hemoccult II occult blood collection cards. (SmithKline Diagnostics, Inc., San Jose, CA.)

PROCEDURE

Most tests for detecting fecal blood use substances that depend upon peroxidase content as an indication of hemoglobin content to cause a color change in the specimen being tested. For this reason, a patient's diet should be free of meat and vegetable sources of peroxidase, which may lead to false-positive results. Other sources of false-positive results may be certain drugs, vitamin C, alcohol, and aspirin.

Pregnancy Testing

Most rapid pregnancy tests detect the presence of **human chorionic gonadotropin (HCG)**, a hormone produced by the placenta that appears in both urine and serum beginning approximately 10 days after conception. Most rapid pregnancy testing is performed on urine. Peak urine levels of HCG occur at approximately 10 weeks of gestation.

A number of manufacturers supply urine pregnancy testing kits. Two examples are the Hybritech Icon II HCG urine assay (Fig. 11-25) (Hybritech, Inc., San Diego, CA) and the AccuStat (Boehringer Mannheim Corp., Indianapolis, IN). Each manufacturer's kit has unique reagents and timing and testing methods, and most test kits have a built-in control system. It is important to follow directions exactly.

Skin Tests

Although nurses most commonly perform skin testing, some laboratories do offer skin testing services, especially for outpatients. In addition, skin tests (especially for tuberculosis) are a part of employee screening programs. Skin tests do not involve the withdrawal of blood or body fluid; rather, they most often involve the intradermal

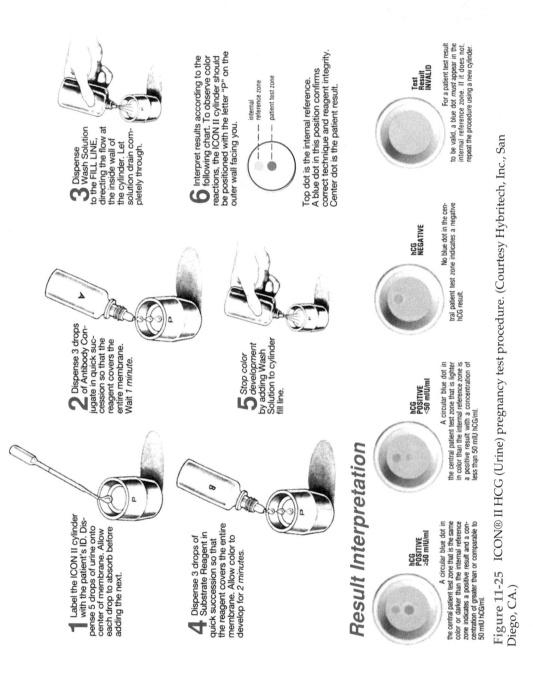

1 Label the ICON II cylinder with the patient's ID. Dispense 5 drops of urine onto center of membrane. Allow each drop to absorb before adding the next.

2 Dispense 3 drops of Antibody Conjugate in quick succession so that the reagent covers the entire membrane. Wait 1 *minute*.

3 Dispense Wash Solution to the FILL LINE, directing the flow at the inside wall of the cylinder. Let solution drain completely through.

4 Dispense 3 drops of Substrate Reagent in quick succession so that the reagent covers the entire membrane. Allow color to develop for 2 *minutes*.

5 *Stop color development* by adding Wash Solution to cylinder fill line.

6 Interpret results according to the following chart. To observe color reactions, the ICON II cylinder should be positioned with the letter "P" on the outer wall facing you.

internal reference zone
patient test zone

Top dot is the internal reference. A blue dot in this position confirms correct technique and reagent integrity. Center dot is the patient result.

Result Interpretation

hCG POSITIVE ≥50 mIU/ml

A circular blue dot in the central patient test zone that is the same color or darker than the internal reference zone indicates a positive result and a concentration of greater than or comparable to 50 mIU/hCG/ml.

hCG POSITIVE <50 mIU/ml

A circular blue dot in the central patient test zone that is lighter in color than the internal reference zone is a positive result with a concentration of less than 50 mIU hCG/ml.

hCG NEGATIVE

No blue dot in the central patient test zone indicates a negative hCG result.

Test Result INVALID

For a patient test result to be valid, a blue dot *must* appear in the internal reference zone. If it does not, repeat the procedure using a new cylinder.

Figure 11-25   ICON® II HCG (Urine) pregnancy test procedure. (Courtesy Hybritech, Inc., San Diego, CA.)

(within the skin) injection of an allergenic substance (substance that causes an allergic reaction) to determine whether the patient has come in contact with a specific allergen (most commonly an antigen) and developed antibodies against it. Many disease-producing microorganisms will function as allergens and stimulate an antibody response in susceptible individuals. Intradermal skin testing can be performed to determine a patient's immune status associated with such microorganisms.

TYPES OF SKIN TESTS
Common skin tests include the following:

Tuberculin (TB) Test: Also called PPD test because of the purified protein derivative used in testing; tests for tuberculosis. It is probably the most common skin test.

Schick Test: Tests for susceptibility to diphtheria.

Dick Test: Tests for susceptibility to scarlet fever caused by *Streptococcus pyogenes*.

Histoplasmosis (Histo) Test: Tests for past or present infection by the fungus *Histoplasma capsulatum*.

Coccidioidomycosis (Cocci) Test: Tests for an infectious fungus disease caused by *Coccidioides immitis*.

SKIN TEST PROCEDURE
1. A site is selected on the volar surface of the forearm, below the antecubital crease. Areas with scars, bruises, burns, rashes, excessive hair, or superficial veins should be avoided.
2. The site is cleaned with 70% isopropyl alcohol and allowed to dry.
3. 0.1 mL of diluted antigen is drawn into a tuberculin syringe using a ½-inch, 26- to 27-gauge needle.
4. The arm is held in the same manner as in venipuncture and the skin is stretched taut with the thumb.
5. The syringe is held at a very low angle (approximately 20 degrees) and the needle is slipped just under the skin.
6. The syringe plunger is pulled back slightly to make certain a vein has not been entered.
7. The contents of the syringe are slowly expelled, creating a distinct, pale elevation of the skin 6 to 10 mm in diameter, commonly called a bleb or wheal (Fig. 11-26).
8. The needle is removed and the arm remains extended until the site has time to close. Pressure is *not* applied to the site, nor is a bandage applied. (A bandage might absorb the fluid and also cause irritation, distorting test results.)
9. The reaction is read in 24 to 72 hours, depending upon the antigen tested.

INTERPRETATION
Interpretation of the test is based upon the presence or absence of erythema (redness) or induration (hardness).

Negative: Area (zone) of erythema and induration less than 5 mm in diameter (most tests).

Doubtful: Area of erythema and induration between 5 and 9 mm in diameter.

Positive: Area of erythema and induration 10 mm or greater in diameter.

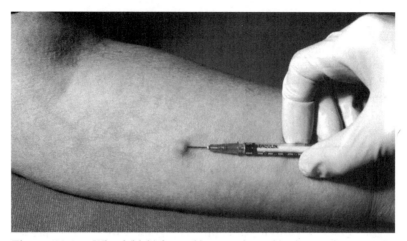

Figure 11-26   Wheal (bleb) formed by intradermal injection of antigen during skin test procedure.

Strep Testing

Numerous kits are available for direct detection of group A streptococci on throat swab specimens. Examples are the Abbott Test Pack Plus Strep A (Abbott Laboratories, Diagnostic Division, Abbott Park, IL), and the Strep A OIA (Optical Immuno Assay) (BIOSTAR, Boulder, CO) (Fig. 11-27). Performance of the test normally requires two steps. The first involves nitrous acid or enzymatic extraction of the swab; the second involves a latex agglutination or enzyme immunoassay method of antigen detection. Results are available in minutes.

Urinalysis

A routine urinalysis (UA) consists of a physical and chemical analysis of the specimen as well as a microscopic analysis if indicated. A microscopic analysis must be performed by a medical laboratory technician or technologist.

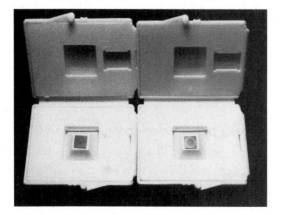

Figure 11-27   Two Strep A OIA test kits (BIOSTAR, Boulder, CO) showing test results: the kit on the left shows negative results and the kit on the right shows positive results.

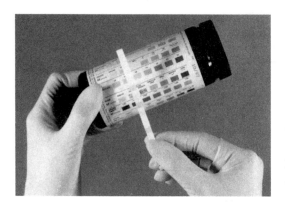

Figure 11-28 Technician comparing urine reagent strip with chart on reagent strip container.

Chemical composition is most commonly determined by use of an inert plastic reagent strip (Fig. 11-28) containing pads impregnated with reagents that test for the presence of bacteria, blood, bilirubin, glucose, leukocytes, protein, and urobilinogen, as well as measure pH and specific gravity. (Specific gravity can also be measured separately using an instrument called a refractometer.) A chemical reaction resulting in color changes to the strip takes place when the strip is dipped in urine. The results can be determined by comparing the strip visually against a code on the container or by inserting the strip into a machine called a reflectance photometer, which reads the strip and prints the results. Reflectance photometers include the Ames Clinitek 200+ (Miles, Inc., Elkhart, IN), the Chemstrip Urine Analyzer (Boehringer Mannheim Corp., Indianapolis, IN), and the Rapimat II/T (Behring Diagnostics, San Jose, CA).

To ensure the integrity of the strips, they should remain tightly capped in their original containers when not in use to protect them from the deteriorating effects of light, moisture, and chemical contamination. The containers should be protected from heat.

Study & Review Questions

1. When drawing a blood alcohol, it is acceptable to clean the arm with
   a. isopropanol.
   b. methanol.
   c. soap and water.
   d. tincture of iodine.

2. The most important part of blood culture collection is
   a. adequately filling two media vials.
   b. preparing the collection site. skin Antisepsis
   c. selecting the collection site.
   d. timing of the second set of cultures.

3. TDM peak concentration may be defined as the
   a. highest concentration of the drug during a dosing interval.
   b. lowest concentration of the drug during a dosing interval.
   c. maximum effectiveness of the drug.
   d. time when the amount of drug entering the body is equal to the amount leaving the body.

TDM - therapeutic drug monitoring

4. When performing a glucose tolerance test, the fasting specimen is drawn at 0815 and the patient finishes the glucose beverage at 0820. When should the 1 hour specimen be collected?
    a. 0915
    b. 0920
    c. 0945
    d. 0950

5. A bleeding time test detects
    a. abnormalities in drug metabolism.
    b. diabetes mellitus.
    c. platelet function disorders.
    d. septicemia.

6. Removing a unit of blood from a patient and not replacing it is used as a treatment for
    a. autologous donation.
    b. ABO Rh incompatibility.
    c. leukemia.
    d. polycythemia.

7. This test can determine whether a person produces antibodies to a particular antigen.
    a. Glucagon tolerance
    b. GTT
    c. Ionized calcium
    d. Skin test

8. Which of the following tests may require special chain of custody documentation when collected?
    a. Blood culture
    b. Crossmatch
    c. Drug screen
    d. TDM

9. What type of specimen is needed for a Guaiac test?
    a. Amniotic fluid
    b. Blood
    c. Feces
    d. Urine

10. The phlebotomist collects a blood specimen and wraps it in foil. Which of the following specimens could it have been?
    a. Bilirubin
    b. Cryoglobulin
    c. Glucose
    d. Protime

11. Which of the following specimens is collected in a trace–element-free tube?
    a. ABGs
    b. BUN
    c. Lead
    d. Occult blood

12. Common chemistry tests performed by POCT instruments include
    a. Hgb and Hct.
    b. Na and K.
    c. PT and PTT.
    d. T_4 and TSH.

13. A test that measures packed cell volume is
    a. ECG.
    b. hematocrit.
    c. hemoglobin.
    d. troponin T (TnT).

Suggested Laboratory Activities

1. Practice performing an ACT on a fellow student using a manual or automated method.

2. Perform ABO typing.

3. Practice proper site preparation and collection of blood cultures.

4. Run controls and perform glucose testing using a bedside glucose instrument.

5. Practice inflating a blood pressure cuff. Perform an ACT by simulating the incision, blotting, and timing.

6. Have manufacturers' representatives demonstrate various POCT instruments.

BIBLIOGRAPHY AND SUGGESTED READINGS

Bishop, M. L., Duben-Engelkirk, J. L., & Fody, E.P. (1996). *Clinical chemistry: Principles, procedures, correlations* (3rd ed.). Philadelphia: Lippincott-Raven Publishers.

Bishop, M. L., & Mass, D. (1989). *Clinical laboratory science: Strategies for practice*. Philadelphia: J. B. Lippincott.

Fischbach, F. (1996). *A manual of laboratory & diagnostic tests* (5th ed.). Philadelphia: Lippincott-Raven Publishers.

Lotspeich-Steininger, C. A., Stiene-Martin, E. A., & Koepke, J. A. (1992). *Clinical hematology: Principles, procedures, correlations*. Philadelphia: J. B. Lippincott.

National Committee for Clinical Laboratory Standards, AST2-P. (1994). *Point-of-care IVD testing: Proposed guideline*. Villanova, PA: NCCLS.

National Committee for Clinical Laboratory Standards, C30-A. (1994). *Ancillary blood glucose testing in acute and chronic care facilities*. Villanova, PA: NCCLS.

National Committee for Clinical Laboratory Standards, H-18A. (1990). *Procedures for the handling and processing of blood specimens: Approved guideline*. Villanova, PA: NCCLS.

National Committee for Clinical Laboratory Standards, H7-A. (1993). *Procedures for determining packed cell volume by the microhematocrit method. Second edition: Approved standard*. Villanova, PA: NCCLS.

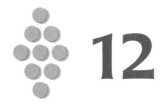

12

Arterial Blood Gases

KEY TERMS

Allen test	brachial artery	radial artery
arterial blood gases (ABGs)	collateral circulation	steady state
arteriospasm	femoral artery	thrombus (clot) formation

OBJECTIVES

Upon successful completion of this chapter, the reader will be able to:

1. State the primary reason for performing arterial punctures and identify the personnel who may be required to perform them.

2. Identify the sites that can be used for arterial puncture, the criteria used for selection of the site, and the advantages and disadvantages of each site.

3. List equipment and supplies needed for arterial puncture.

4. Describe patient assessment and preparation procedures, including the administering of local anesthetic, prior to performing arterial blood gases.

5. Describe how to perform the Allen test, define what constitutes a positive or negative result, and give the procedure to follow for either result.

6. Describe the procedure for collecting radial arterial blood gases, and the role of the phlebotomist in other site collections.

7. List complications associated with arterial puncture, identify factors that may affect the integrity of the blood gas sample, and describe the criteria for sample rejection.

INTRODUCTION

The composition of arterial blood is consistent throughout the body, whereas the composition of venous blood varies relative to the metabolic needs of the areas of the body it services. However, because arterial puncture is technically more difficult to perform and potentially more painful and hazardous to the patient than venipuncture, arterial specimens are not used for routine blood tests. The primary reason for performing arterial puncture is to obtain blood for evaluation of **arterial blood gases (ABGs)**. Arterial blood gas evaluation is used in the diagnosis and management of respiratory disease to provide valuable information about a patient's oxygenation, ventilation, and acid–base balance.

Unlike venipuncture procedures, which have been performed for centuries, arterial puncture has a relatively recent history. The first recorded human arterial puncture was performed in 1912. Although the first arterial sample used for blood gas analysis was obtained in 1919, routine blood gas analysis did not occur until after 1953 with the introduction of the Clark platinum electrode to measure oxygen pressure (pO_2).

PERSONNEL WHO PERFORM ARTERIAL PUNCTURE

Paramedical personnel (health care workers other than physicians) who may be required to perform ABGs include nurses, medical technologists and technicians, respiratory therapists, emergency medical technicians, and level II phlebotomists. According to NCCLS, all personnel who perform ABG procedures should be certified by their health care institution after successfully completing training involving theory, demonstration of technique, observation of the actual procedure, and performance of arterial puncture under the supervision of qualified personnel.

SITE SELECTION

Several different sites can be used for arterial puncture. The criteria for site selection include the presence of collateral circulation, how large and accessible the artery is, and the type of tissue surrounding the puncture site. The site chosen should not be inflamed, irritated, edematous, or in close proximity to a wound. In addition, *never* select a site in a limb with an A-V shunt or fistula. The following are sites commonly chosen for arterial puncture.

The Radial Artery

The first choice and most common site used for arterial puncture is the **radial artery,** located in the thumb side of the wrist (Fig. 12-1). Although smaller than arteries in other sites, the radial artery is readily accessible in most patients.

ADVANTAGES

The biggest advantage of using the radial artery is the presence of **collateral circulation**. Having collateral circulation means that the area is supplied with blood from more than one artery. Under normal circumstances, both the radial and the ulnar artery supply the hand with blood. If the radial artery were to be inadvertently damaged as a consequence of arterial puncture, the ulnar artery could supply blood to the hand. For this reason, the ulnar artery is never used for arterial puncture. Collateral circulation can be evaluated by an instrument called the Doppler ultrasonic flow indicator or by performing the modified Allen test. If collateral circulation is absent, the radial artery should not be punctured.

Another advantage of using the radial artery is that there is less chance of hematoma formation following the procedure, because the radial artery can be easily compressed over the ligaments and bone of the wrist.

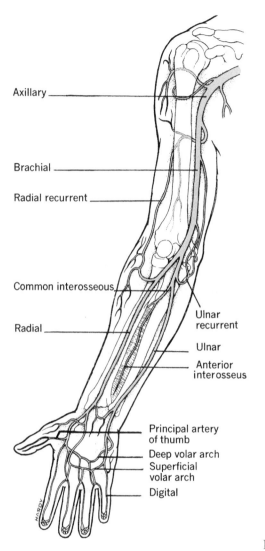

Axillary

Brachial

Radial recurrent

Common interosseous

Radial

Ulnar
recurrent

Ulnar

Anterior
interosseus

Principal artery
of thumb

Deep volar arch

Superficial
volar arch

Digital

Figure 12-1 Arteries of the arm and hand.

DISADVANTAGES

Disadvantages of using the radial artery include the fact that considerable skill is required to puncture it successfully owing to its small size, and that it may be difficult or impossible to locate on patients with low cardiac output.

The Brachial Artery

The **brachial artery** (see Fig. 12-1) is the second choice for arterial puncture. It is located in the medial anterior aspect of the antecubital fossa near the insertion of the biceps muscle.

ADVANTAGES

Advantages of the brachial artery are that it is large and easy to palpate and puncture. The brachial artery has adequate collateral circulation, though not as much as the radial artery.

DISADVANTAGES

There are a number of disadvantages to puncturing the brachial artery:

- It is deeper than the radial artery.
- It lies close to a large vein (the basilic) as well as the median nerve, both of which may be inadvertently punctured.
- Unlike the radial artery, there are no underlying ligaments or bone to support compression of the brachial artery, resulting in an increased risk of hematoma formation following the procedure.

The Femoral Artery

The **femoral artery** (Fig. 12-2) is the largest artery used for arterial puncture. It is located superficially in the groin, lateral to the pubis bone. Femoral puncture is performed primarily by physicians and specially trained emergency room personnel.

ADVANTAGES

The femoral artery is large and easily palpated and punctured. It is sometimes the only site where arterial sampling is possible, especially on patients with low cardiac output.

DISADVANTAGES

Disadvantages of femoral arterial puncture include poor collateral circulation, increased risk of infection owing to the location of the site, difficulty in achieving aseptic technique owing to the presence of pubic hair, and the possibility of dislodging plaque buildup from the inner artery walls of older patients. In addition, the femoral artery lies close to the femoral vein, which may be inadvertently punctured.

Because of the numerous disadvantages associated with femoral puncture, it is generally used only in emergency situations or when other sites are not available.

Other Sites

Other sites where arterial specimens may be obtained include the scalp and umbilical arteries in infants and the dorsalis pedis arteries of the adult. The phlebotomist is not trained to perform arterial punctures at these locations or to obtain specimens from cannulae, catheters, or other indwelling devices at these or any other locations.

EQUIPMENT AND SUPPLIES

The following equipment and supplies (Fig. 12-3) are needed to collect arterial blood gas specimens.

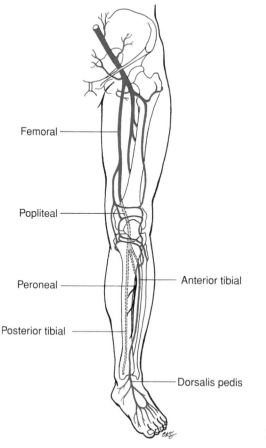

Femoral

Popliteal

Peroneal

Posterior tibial

Anterior tibial

Dorsalis pedis

Figure 12-2   Arteries of the leg.

Safety Equipment

Personal protective equipment (PPE) needed by the blood drawer when collecting ABG specimens includes a fluid-resistant lab coat, gown, or apron; gloves; and face protection because of the possibility of blood spray during arterial puncture. A puncture-resistant sharps container is needed to dispose of used needles and syringes.

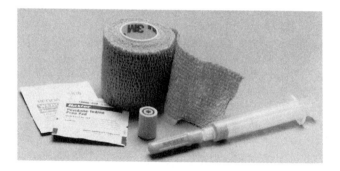

Figure 12-3   ABG Equipment.

Collection Equipment

1. Antiseptic solution for cleaning the site: NCCLS-recommended antiseptics are povidone–iodine or chlorhexidine.
2. Optional anesthetic solution: Local anesthetic solution such as 0.5% lidocaine may be used to numb the site.
3. Hypodermic needles: Needle gauge and length depends upon the site selected, the size of the artery selected, and the amount of blood needed. Needle sizes used include 20, 21, 22, 23, and 25 gauge, in lengths from ⅝ to 1½ inches. A 22-gauge, 1-inch is most commonly used for radial and brachial puncture; a 1½-inch needle is used for femoral puncture.
4. Syringes: ABGs are collected in 1- to 5-mL syringes, depending upon the amount of blood required. Special glass or plastic syringes are suitable. Heparin-containing syringes are available. Syringes most commonly contained in blood gas kits are prefilled with heparin and are designed to fill spontaneously upon arterial penetration. A 1- or 2-mL plastic syringe with a 25- or 26-gauge needle, ½- to ⅝-inch long is used for administration of anesthetic solution.
5. A small block of rubber or latex in which to insert the needle following specimen collection.
6. Luer tip cap: A Luer tip cap or other suitable device is used to cover the end of the syringe after needle removal in order to maintain anaerobic conditions within the specimen.
7. Lithium (or sodium) heparin: 1000 units/mL heparin solution is used to prevent the specimen from clotting.
8. **Coolant:** A coolant capable of maintaining a temperature of 1°C to 5°C is necessary to slow the metabolism of white blood cells, which consume oxygen. A container of ice water is most commonly used. The container should be large enough to allow the complete immersion of the barrel of the collection syringe.
9. Gauze: 2×2-inch gauze squares are used to hold pressure over the site until bleeding has stopped.
10. Identification materials: Labels and waterproof ink pens or makers are needed for specimen identification.
11. Oxygen analyzer: An oxygen measuring device is needed when patients are breathing oxygen-enriched gas mixtures instead of room air.

PREPARATION

General Instructions

As with any other test, a physician's order is needed before performing the test. The blood drawer must then properly identify the patient, explain the procedure, and obtain his or her consent. In addition it should be determined whether the patient is on anticoagulant therapy or allergic to the anesthetic.

Steady State

A patient's temperature and breathing pattern, as well as the concentration of oxygen inhaled, affect the amount of oxygen and carbon dioxide in the blood. Ideally, a patient should have been in a stable or **steady state** (*ie*, no exercise, suctioning, or respirator changes) for at least 30 minutes prior to obtaining blood gases.

Administration of Local Anesthetic

The advent of improved thin-wall needles has made the routine administration of anesthetic prior to arterial puncture unnecessary. However, it may be a reassuring option for some patients, especially children, who are fearful of the procedure. A fearful patient may respond by breath-holding, crying, or hyperventilation, all of which may affect blood gas results.

Allen Test

The **Allen test** (Fig. 12-4) may be used to assess collateral circulation prior to radial blood gas collection. The test is performed in the following manner:

1. Have the patient make a tight fist.
2. Using the middle and index fingers of both hands, apply pressure to the patient's wrist, compressing and occluding both the radial and ulnar arteries at the same time.
3. While maintaining pressure, have the patient open the hand slowly. The hand should appear blanched or drained of color.
4. Lower the patient's hand and release pressure on the ulnar artery.
5. The patient's hand should flush pink within 15 seconds.
6. Record the results on the request slip.

Positive Allen test.   The hand flushes pink within 15 seconds, indicating the presence of collateral circulation. If the Allen test is positive, proceed with ABG collection.

Negative Allen test.   The hand does not flush pink within 15 seconds, indicating the inability of the ulnar artery to adequately supply blood to the hand and therefore the absence of collateral circulation. If the Allen test is negative, the radial artery should not be used and another site should be selected.

PROCEDURE FOR RADIAL ABGs

1. Receive physician's order and note the time ABGs are to be drawn.
2. Assemble and transport equipment to the patient's bedside.
3. Identify the patient and explain the procedure.
4. Record the patient's temperature, respiratory rate, and breathing mixture (*eg*, room air) on the laboratory slip.
5. Wash hands and put on gloves.
6. Prepare the ABG syringe with heparin, if applicable, in the following manner:
    a. Check the syringe for free movement and attach a 20-gauge needle.
    b. Clean the top of the heparin bottle with alcohol.
    c. Draw 0.5 to 1 mL heparin into the syringe. Pull back on the plunger, rotating it at the same time to wet the entire barrel of the syringe.

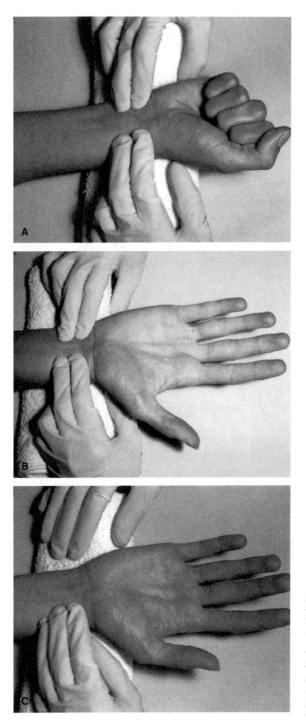

Figure 12-4   Allen test. (**A**) Occluding the radial and ulnar arteries by pressing with fingertips while the patient makes a fist. (**B**) Observing a blanched appearance to the hand when opened as both arteries are being pressed. (**C**) Releasing the ulnar artery and checking for the patient's hand to flush with color.

    d. With the syringe held vertically, expel the majority of the heparin.

    e. Replace the needle with the needle selected for arterial puncture.

7. (Optional) Prepare the anesthetic syringe in the following manner: After cleaning the top of the bottle, draw 0.5 mL anesthetic (*ie*, lidocaine) into a 1-mL syringe using a 25-gauge needle. Carefully replace the cap and leave the syringe in a horizontal position.

8. Position the patient's arm with the palm facing up. A rolled towel may be placed under the wrist for support.

9. Assess collateral circulation using the Allen test (see Fig. 12-4) or a Doppler ultrasonic flow indicator. If collateral circulation is present, continue with ABG collection. If collateral circulation is absent, choose another site.

10. With the palm still facing up, have the patient flex the wrist at a 30- to 45-degree angle to stretch and fix the soft tissues over the firm ligaments and bone.

11. Locate the radial artery on the thumb side of the wrist using the index and middle fingers of the left hand. Palpate the artery to determine its size, depth, and direction. *Never* use the thumb to palpate; it has a pulse, which can be misleading.

12. Prepare the site by cleaning first with alcohol and then with povidone–iodine. Prep the fingers used to palpate in the same manner. Allow the site to dry, being careful not to touch it with any unsterile object.

13. If local anesthetic is to be administered, infiltrate the skin over the selected site, entering the skin with the needle at an angle of approximately 10 degrees with the skin. Pull back slightly on the plunger to be certain a vein was not inadvertently penetrated. If blood appears in the syringe, withdraw the syringe, prepare a fresh syringe and needle, and repeat the procedure in a slightly different spot. If no blood appears in the syringe, slowly expel the contents into the skin, forming a raised wheal. Wait 1 to 2 minutes for the anesthetic to take effect before proceeding with arterial puncture. Note the lidocaine application on the request form.

14. Expel the remaining heparin from the ABG syringe, if applicable. Be careful not to draw air into the syringe. Hold the syringe in the dominant hand as if holding a dart. Relocate the artery with the index finger of the opposite hand.

15. Warn the patient. Insert the needle bevel up, into the skin at a 45-degree angle (femoral ABGs require a 90-degree angle) approximately 5 to 10 mm distal to the finger locating the artery. Direct the needle away from the hand with the bevel facing the blood flow (Fig. 12-5).

16. Slowly advance the needle, directing it toward the artery just under the finger. When the artery is pierced, a "flash" of blood will appear in the hub of the needle. When the flash appears, stop advancing the needle. The blood will continue to pump into the syringe. Do not pull back on the plunger. Hold the syringe very steady until the desired amount of blood has been collected.

17. If the artery is missed, slowly withdraw the needle until just the bevel is under the skin. Redirect the needle into the artery as above. Do not probe; probing is painful and may lead to hematoma or thrombus formation and damage to the artery.

18. After the desired amount of blood has been obtained, quickly withdraw the needle, immediately placing a clean, dry gauze over the site and applying firm pressure for a minimum of 5 minutes. Longer application of pressure is required for patients on anticoagulant therapy. *Never* allow the patient to apply the pressure. A patient may not apply pressure firmly enough.

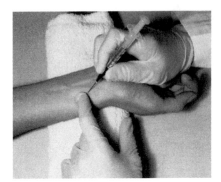

Figure 12-5   Performing an arterial puncture.

19. With your free hand, immediately eject any air bubbles from the specimen and embed the needle into the small latex cube (Fig. 12-6).
20. Gently mix the specimen by inversion or rolling.
21. Remove the needle, being careful not to introduce bubbles into the syringe. Discard needle in sharps container and replace the needle with the Luer cap.
22. Label the specimen and place in a bag or tray of crushed ice and water or other coolant.
23. After pressure has been applied to the site for 5 minutes, check the site for swelling or bruising. If none is noted, clean the povidone–iodine from the site with an alcohol prep pad, wait 2 minutes, and check the site again. Check the pulse distal to the site. If absent or faint, alert the patient's nurse to call the physician immediately. If the site appears normal, apply a pressure bandage.
24. Dispose of used equipment properly. Remove gloves and wash hands.
25. Thank the patient.
26. Deliver the specimen to the lab as soon as possible.

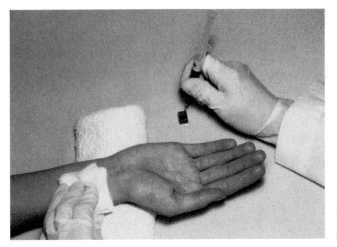

Figure 12-6   Embedding the point of the ABG needle in the latex cube while holding pressure over the patient's artery.

ABG COLLECTION FROM OTHER SITES

Collection of ABGs from other sites is similar to the procedure for radial ABGs. Because phlebotomists are not normally trained to collect specimens from these sites, specific procedures are not given in this text. Phlebotomists may, however, be asked to provide the equipment and assist in labeling and transporting specimens collected from these sites by others (*eg*, an emergency room physician).

COMPLICATIONS ASSOCIATED WITH ARTERIAL PUNCTURE

Discomfort. Some discomfort is generally associated with arterial puncture, even with use of a local anesthetic.

Infection. Proper antiseptic preparation of the site minimizes the chance of infection.

Hematoma. Because the blood is under considerable pressure in the arteries, blood is initially more apt to leak from an arterial puncture site than from a venipuncture site. However, arterial puncture sites tend to close more rapidly owing to the elastic nature of the arterial wall. Because this elasticity tends to decrease with age, the probability of hematoma formation is greater in older patients. The probability of hematoma formation is also greater in patients receiving anticoagulant therapy.

Arteriospasm. Irritation caused by needle penetration of the artery muscle can cause a reflex constriction of the artery or **arteriospasm**. The condition is transitory but may make it difficult to obtain a specimen.

Thrombus formation. Injury to the intima of the artery can lead to **thrombus (clot) formation**. A large thrombus can obstruct the flow of blood and impair circulation.

SAMPLING ERRORS

A number of factors can affect the integrity of a blood gas sample and lead to erroneous results.

Air bubbles. If air bubbles are not immediately or completely expelled from the sample, oxygen from the air bubbles can diffuse into the sample and CO_2 can escape from the sample, changing the results.

Delay in cooling or analysis. Blood cells continue to consume oxygen and nutrients and produce acids and carbon dioxide at room temperature. If the specimen remains at room temperature for more than 5 to 10 minutes, the pH, blood gas, and glucose values will change. Cooling to between 1° C to 5° C slows this metabolism and helps stabilize the specimen. Processing the specimen as soon after obtaining as possible will ensure the most accurate results.

Obtaining a venous sample by mistake.   Markedly inaccurate ABG values will result if a venous sample is obtained by mistake. Normal arterial blood is bright cherry red in color. However, it is sometimes difficult to distinguish between arterial and venous blood in poorly ventilated patients because their arterial blood may appear as dark as venous blood. The best way to be certain that a specimen is arterial is if the blood pulses into the syringe. In some instances, such as with low cardiac output, a specimen may need to be aspirated. In such cases it is hard to be certain that the specimen is truly arterial.

Use of improper anticoagulant.   Heparin is the acceptable anticoagulant for blood gases. Oxylates, EDTA, and citrates may alter results, especially pH.

Use of too much or too little anticoagulant.   Too much heparin can cause erroneous results owing to acidosis. Too little heparin can result in clotting of the specimen.

Improper mixing.   Inadequate or delayed mixing of the sample can lead to clotting, making the sample unacceptable for testing. Undetected microclots can lead to erroneous results.

Improper syringe.   Use only plastic syringes especially designed for ABG procedures. The use of regular plastic syringes will lead to erroneous values.

CRITERIA FOR SPECIMEN REJECTION

1. Inadequate volume of specimen for the test
2. Clotted specimen
3. Improper or absent labeling
4. Use of wrong syringe
5. Too long of a delay in delivering specimen to the lab
6. Specimen not on ice
7. Air bubbles in specimen

Study & Review Questions

1. Locations to obtain arterial blood gases are all of the following *except* the
   a. brachial artery.   c. femoral artery.
   b. ulnar artery.   d. radial artery.

2. The equipment used for ABGs includes all of the following *except*
   a. povidone–iodine.   c. a syringe.
   b. heparin.   d. a tourniquet.

3. The purpose of the Allen test is to determine
   a. blood pressure in the radial artery.   c. whether the patient is absorbing oxygen.
   b. the presence of collateral circulation   d. the coagulation time of the arteries.
      of the radial or ulnar arteries.

4. The angle of needle insertion for radial ABGs is
   a. 5 degrees.
   b. 15 degrees.
   c. 45 degrees.
   d. 75 degrees.

5. Which of the following complications are associated with ABGs?
   a. Hematoma
   b. Infection
   c. Arteriospasm
   d. All of the above

6. Which of the following will *not* produce erroneous ABG values?
   a. Cooling the specimen
   b. Improper mixing
   c. Air bubbles in the sample
   d. Too much heparin

Suggested Laboratory Activities

1. Identify the common sites for ABG collection and locate the radial, ulnar, and brachial pulses.

2. Perform the Allen test on a fellow student.

3. Identify and assemble the proper equipment for ABG collection.

4. Practice ABG technique on an artificial arm with a simulated pulse.

BIBLIOGRAPHY AND SUGGESTED READINGS

Burton, G. G., Hodgkin, J. E., & Ward, J. J. (1991). *Respiratory care: A guide to clinical practice* (3rd ed.). Philadelphia: J. B. Lippincott.
National Committee for Clinical Laboratory Standards, H11-A2. (May 1992). *Percutaneous collection of arterial blood for laboratory analysis*. Villanova, PA: NCCLS.

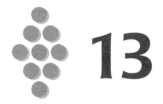

13

Nonblood Specimens and Tests

KEY TERMS

amniotic fluid
antibiotic susceptibility
body fluids
catheterized
cerebrospinal fluid (CSF)

clean-catch
culture and sensitivity (C&S)
midstream collection
nasopharyngeal (NP)
occult blood

semen analysis
suprapubic
sweat chloride
urinalysis (UA)
urinary tract infection (UTI)

OBJECTIVES

Upon successful completion of this chapter, the reader will be able to:

1. Describe nonblood specimen labeling and handling.
2. Name and describe the various urine tests, specimen types, and collection methods.
3. List the types of nonblood specimens, other than urine, and explain the principle behind the collection of each specimen.
4. Describe the collection and handling procedures associated with each nonblood specimen.
5. Describe the role of the phlebotomist in gastric analysis collection.
6. Differentiate between the throat culture collection procedure and the nasopharyngeal culture procedure.

INTRODUCTION

Although blood is the type of specimen most frequently analyzed in the medical laboratory, various other body fluids are also analyzed. The phlebotomist may be involved in obtaining the specimen (as in throat swab collection); test administration (as in sweat chloride collection); instruction (as in urine collection); processing (accessioning and preparing the specimen for testing); or merely labeling or transporting specimens to the lab.

NONBLOOD SPECIMEN LABELING AND HANDLING

As a minimum, nonblood specimens should be labeled with the same identifying information as blood specimens. Most institutions also require information on the type and/or source of the specimen. Before accepting specimens collected by other hospital personnel, the phlebotomist must check to see that the specimen is properly labeled. Universal precautions should be observed when handling nonblood specimens as many body fluids are potentially infectious.

TYPES OF NONBLOOD SPECIMENS

Urine

Urine is perhaps the most frequently analyzed nonblood body fluid. Analysis of urine can aid in the diagnosis and treatment of urinary tract infections and the detection of metabolic disease. Accuracy of results depends on the method of collection, type of container used, transportation, and handling of the specimen. Collection of urine specimens on hospitalized patients is usually handled by nursing personnel. Outpatient urine specimen collection, however, is often handled by a phlebotomist.

The phlebotomist must be able to explain procedures to the patient without causing him or her embarrassment. Verbal instructions must be followed by written instructions, preferably with illustrations. In outpatient areas, written instructions are often posted on the wall in the restroom designated for patient urine collections. The type of specimen preferred for many urine studies is the first urine voided (passed naturally from the bladder or urinated) in the morning because it is the most concentrated. However, the type of specimen and the method of urine collection varies and depends on the type of test ordered. The most common urine tests, types of urine specimens requested, and various collection methods follow.

COMMON URINE TESTS
Routine urinalysis

A routine **urinalysis (UA)** includes a physical, chemical, and microscopic analysis of the specimen. Physical characteristics noted include color, odor, transparency, and specific gravity or concentration. Chemical composition is most commonly determined by use of a plastic strip containing areas impregnated with reagents that test for the presence of bacteria, blood, white blood cells, protein, glucose, and other substances. The strip is dipped into the urine and compared to a color chart, usually found on the label of the reagent strip container. Special timing is involved in reading the results. The manner in which the results are to be reported is indicated on the reagent label. Most results are reported using the terms **trace**, 1+, 2+, and so on to indicate the degree of a positive result, and **negative** – (neg) when no reaction is noted. Machines are available that read the strips automatically (see the discussion of point-of-care testing in Chapter 11). The strip is used once and discarded.

Urine components such as cells, crystals, and microorganisms can be seen by microscopic examination of a sample of urine sediment obtained through centrifugation. A measured portion of urine is centrifuged in a special plastic tube. After centrifugation, the supernatant, or top portion of the specimen, is discarded and a drop of the remaining sediment is placed on a glass slide, covered with a small square of glass called a coverslip, and examined under the microscope by either a laboratory technician or technologist. There are also machines in the laboratory that perform this function.

Specimens for routine UA should be collected in clear, dry, chemically clean containers with tight-fitting lids. If a culture and sensitivity (C&S) are also ordered on the same specimen, the container should be sterile. Urine specimens should be transported to the lab promptly. Specimens for routine UA that cannot be transported or analyzed promptly can be held at room temperature and protected from light for up to 2 hours. Specimens held longer should be refrigerated. Specimens for which both a C&S and a UA are requested should be refrigerated if immediate processing is not possible.

A regular voided specimen is acceptable for routine urinalysis. However, to avoid contamination of the specimen by genital secretions, pubic hair, and bacteria surrounding the urinary opening, the ideal procedure for collecting a specimen for routine urinalysis is referred to as **midstream collection** (see Collection Methods for regular voided and midstream collection methods).

Urine culture and sensitivity

A urine **culture and sensitivity (C&S)** may be requested on a patient with symptoms of **urinary tract infection (UTI)**. A urine culture is performed by transferring a measured portion of urine onto a special nutrient medium. The medium is incubated for 18 to 24 hours and then checked for bacterial growth. If an organism is identified, a sensitivity or **antibiotic susceptibility** test is performed to determine which antibiotics will be effective against the organism.

Urine for C&S must be collected in a sterile container (Fig. 13-1), following midstream **clean-catch** (see Collection Methods) procedures to ensure that the specimen is free of contaminating matter from the external genital areas. Specimens for C&S and other microbiological studies should be transported to the lab and processed immediately. If a delay in transportation or processing is unavoidable the specimen should be refrigerated.

Urine cytology studies

Cytology studies are performed on urine to detect cancer, cytomegalovirus, and other viral and inflammatory diseases of the bladder and other structures of the urinary system. Because cells from the lining of the urinary tract are readily shed into the urine,

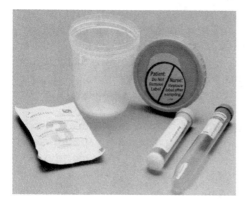

Figure 13-1   Becton Dickinson (Franklin Lakes, NJ) midstream urine collection sampling container and evacuated tubes for transporting and storing urine specimens.

a smear can be easily prepared from urinary sediment or filtrate. The smear is stained by the Papanicolaou (PAP) method and examined under a microscope for the presence of abnormal cells. A fresh, clean-catch specimen is required for the test. Ideally, the specimen should be examined as soon after collection as possible. If a delay is unavoidable, the specimen may be preserved by the addition of an equal volume of 50% alcohol.

Urine drug screening

Urine drug screening is performed to detect illicit recreational drug use, use of anabolic steroids to enhance performance in sports, and unwarranted use of prescription drugs; to monitor therapeutic drug use so as to minimize withdrawal symptoms; and to confirm a diagnosis of drug overdose. With the exception of alcohol, urine is preferred for drug screening since many drugs can be detected in urine but not blood.

Screening tests are normally performed in groups based on drug classifications (see Table 11-2). A random sample in a chemically clean, covered container is required for the test. Specimens containing blood cells or having a high or low urine pH (highly acid or alkaline) or a low specific gravity will yield erroneous results and will require recollection of the specimen. (For additional information see Forensic Specimens in Chapter 11.)

Other urine tests

Numerous chemistry tests, including electrophoresis, tests for heavy metals (*eg*, copper and lead), myoglobin clearance, creatinine clearance, and porphyrins, can be performed on urine specimens. Many of these tests require a pooled timed specimen such as a 24-hour collection.

TYPES OF URINE SPECIMENS
Random

Random urine specimens are collected at any time. They are used primarily for routine urinalysis and screening tests. Random refers only to the timing of the specimen and not the method of collection.

Timed collection

Some tests require individual urine specimens collected at specific times. Others require the collection and pooling of urine throughout a specific time period. Some of the most frequently encountered timed urine tests are as follows.

First morning (8-hour).   A **first morning** or **8-hour** urine specimen is usually collected immediately upon awakening in the morning after approximately 8 hours of sleep. This type of specimen normally has a higher specific gravity, which means that it is more concentrated than a random specimen. For this reason, 8-hour specimens are often requested to confirm results of random specimens and specimens with low specific gravity.

Tolerance tests.   Some **tolerance tests** require the collection of urine at specific times. The standard glucose tolerance test (GTT) requires individual urine specimens collected serially at specific times that correspond with the timing of blood collection, such as fasting, ½ hour, 1 hour, and so on. Timing of the specimens is important in the interpretation of test results. For this reason, the specimens must be collected as close to the requested time as possible, and the label of the specimen should include the time of collection and the type of specimen (*eg*, fasting, ½ hour).

Twenty-four hour urine collection. A **24-hour urine specimen** is collected to allow quantitative analysis of a urine analyte. Collection of all urine voided in the 24-hour period is critical. The best time to begin a 24-hour collection is when the patient wakes in the morning. Collection of the specimen requires a large, clean, usually wide-mouth container capable of holding several liters (Fig. 13-2). A special collection device that fits over the toilet and looks somewhat like an upside down hat is sometimes provided to the patient to make collection of the specimen easier. Some 24-hour specimens require the addition of a preservative prior to collection. Others must be kept refrigerated throughout collection. Information on proper handling of the specimen can be obtained by consulting the laboratory procedure manual. The label of the specimen, in addition to standard patient identification, must state that the specimen is a 24-hour specimen and, if applicable, the type of preservative added to the container and any precautions associated with it.

The procedure for a 24-hour urine collection is as follows:

24-HOUR URINE COLLECTION PROCEDURE

1. Void into toilet as usual after awakening; note the time and date on the specimen container label; and begin the timing.
2. Collect all urine voided for the next 24-hour period. Refrigerate the specimen throughout the collection period (except for urate testing). This can be accomplished by placing the specimen container in an ice chest placed in the bathtub, for example.
3. To prevent contamination of the specimen by fecal material, it is best to urinate *before* having a bowel movement rather than after.
4. At the end of the 24-hour period, void one last time and add this specimen to the collection container.
5. Put the container in a portable cooler and transport the specimen to the lab as soon as possible.

Fractional (double-voided)

A **fractional** or **double-voided** specimen is collected to compare the urine concentrations of an analyte to its concentration in the blood. It is most commonly used to test urine for glucose and ketones. The procedure requires the patient to collect a urine specimen, emptying the bladder in the process. The time is recorded and the specimen is tested for the analyte. In the mean time, the patient drinks approximately 200 mL of water. Urine is given time to accumulate in the bladder for a specified time, commonly

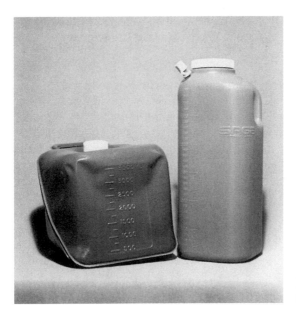

Figure 13-2 Two styles of 24-hour urine specimen collection containers.

30 minutes. At the end of the time period, another urine specimen is collected and tested for the analyte. Tolerance test urine specimens are also considered fractional specimens.

COLLECTION METHODS
Regular voided

A **regular voided** urine collection requires no special patient preparation and is collected by having the patient void (urinate) into a clean urine container.

Midstream

A **midstream** urine collection is performed to obtain a specimen that is free of genital secretions, pubic hair, and bacteria surrounding the urinary opening. To collect a midstream specimen, the patient voids the initial urine flow into the toilet. The urine flow is interrupted momentarily and then restarted, at which time a sufficient amount of urine is collected into a specimen container. The last of the urine flow is voided into the toilet.

Midstream clean catch

A **midstream clean-catch** urine is collected in a sterile container and yields a specimen that is suitable for microbial analysis or culture and sensitivity testing. Clean-catch procedures are necessary to ensure that the specimen is free of contaminating matter from the external genital areas. Special cleaning of the genital area is required before the specimen is collected. The cleaning methods vary somewhat depending upon whether the patient is male or female. A phlebotomist must be able to explain the proper procedure to both male and female patients, as follows:

CLEAN-CATCH PROCEDURES FOR MALE PATIENTS

1. Wash hands thoroughly.
2. Cleanse the end of the penis with sterile, soapy cotton balls (or special towelettes) beginning at the urethral opening and working away from it (the foreskin of an uncircumcised male must first be retracted).
3. Repeat the above procedure using two successive sterile, water-soaked cotton balls (or clean towelettes).
4. Void the first portion of urine into the toilet. Stop the urine flow momentarily, then resume the flow, and collect a portion of urine into the container. Be careful not to touch the inside or lip of the container with the hands or any other part of the body.
5. Void the remainder of urine into the toilet.
6. Cover the container with the sterile lid, touching only the *outside* surfaces of the lid and container.

CLEAN-CATCH PROCEDURES FOR FEMALE PATIENTS

1. Stand in a squatting position over the toilet.
2. Separate the folds of skin around the urinary opening. Cleanse the area around the opening with special towelettes (or sterile soapy cotton balls).
3. Cleanse the area again with clean towelettes (or water-soaked sterile cotton balls), wiping from front to back.
4. Void the first portion of urine into the toilet. Stop the urine flow momentarily, then resume the flow, and collect a portion of urine into the container, being careful not to touch the inside or lip of the container with the hands or any other part of the body.
5. Void the remainder of urine into the toilet.
6. Cover the specimen with the lid provided, touching only the *outside* surfaces of the lid and container.

Catheterized

A **catheterized** urine specimen is collected from a sterile catheter inserted through the urethra into the bladder. A catheterized specimen is collected when a patient is having trouble voiding or is already catheterized for other reasons. Catheterized specimens are sometimes collected on babies to obtain a specimen for C&S, on female patients to prevent vaginal contamination of the specimen, and on bedridden patients when serial specimen collections are needed.

Suprapubic

A **suprapubic** urine specimen is collected in a sterile syringe by inserting a needle directly into the urinary bladder and aspirating the urine directly from the bladder. The procedure normally requires use of local anesthetic and is performed by a physician. The specimen is then transferred into a sterile urine container or tube. If the patient has a suprapubic catheter, the specimen can be collected from the catheter by a nurse using a sterile needle and syringe. Suprapubic collection is used for samples for microbial analysis or cytology studies. It is sometimes used to obtain uncontaminated samples from infants and young children.

Pediatric urine collection

A plastic urine collection bag with hypoallergenic skin adhesive is used to collect a urine specimen from an infant or small child that is not yet potty trained. The patient's genital area is cleaned and dried before the bag is taped to the skin. The bag is placed around the vagina of a female and over the penis of a male. A diaper is placed over the collection bag. The patient is checked every 15 minutes until an adequate specimen is obtained. The bag is then removed, sealed, labeled, and sent to the lab as soon as possible. A 24-hour specimen can be obtained by using a special collection bag with a tube attached that allows the bag to be emptied periodically.

Other Nonblood Specimens

AMNIOTIC FLUID

Amniotic fluid is the normally clear, almost colorless–to–pale yellow fluid that surrounds a fetus in the uterus. It is obtained by transabdominal amniocentesis, a procedure that involves inserting a needle through the mother's abdominal wall into the uterus and extracting the fluid from within the membrane (amniotic sac) that contains the fetus. Amniotic fluid is normally sterile and must be collected in a sterile container. The specimen should be protected from light, and delivered to the laboratory ASAP. Specimens for chromosome analysis must be kept at room temperature; however, specimens for certain chemistry tests must be kept on ice.

Amniotic fluid is preferably collected after 15 weeks of gestation and is used for chromosome analysis to detect genetic defects and assess fetal development. It may also be collected on or near the patient's due date to determine the lung maturity of the fetus. This type of test is often ordered STAT when the fetus is in distress.

Chromosome analysis is performed on fetal cells removed from the fluid and cultured for 3 to 7 days. The fluid portion of the specimen is used for analysis of lung maturity and **alpha-fetoprotein (AFP)**, an antigen normally present in the human fetus that is also found in amniotic fluid and maternal serum. (AFP is also present in certain pathological conditions in males and nonpregnant females.) Abnormal AFP levels may indicate problems in fetal development such as neural tube defects. AFP testing is initially performed on maternal serum and abnormal results are confirmed by amniotic fluid AFP testing. Because normal AFP levels are different in each week of gestation, it is important that the gestational age of the fetus be included on the specimen label.

CEREBROSPINAL FLUID

Cerebrospinal fluid (CSF) is a clear, colorless liquid that circulates within the cavities surrounding the brain and spinal cord. CSF has many of the same constituents as blood plasma. CSF specimens are obtained by a physician, most often through lumbar (spinal) puncture. Common tests performed on spinal fluid include cell counts, glucose, chloride, and total protein. An increased white blood cell count in spinal fluid is most often associated with bacterial or viral meningitis. CSF is generally collected in three special sterile tubes labeled in order of collection. Laboratory protocol dictates which tests are to be performed on each particular tube, unless indicated by the physician. CSF should be delivered to the lab stat and analysis started immediately.

GASTRIC SECRETIONS/GASTRIC ANALYSIS

Gastric secretions are obtained by aspiration via a tube passed through the mouth or nose, down the throat, and into the stomach. Gastric specimens are collected in sterile containers.

A **gastric analysis test** examines gastric acid secretions to determine gastric function in terms of stomach acid production. A basal tube gastric analysis involves aspirating a sample of gastric secretions by means of a tube passed through the mouth and throat (oropharynx) or nose and throat (nasopharynx) into the stomach following a period of fasting. This sample is tested to determine acidity prior to stimulation. After this basal sample of gastric secretions has been collected, a gastric stimulant, most commonly histamine or pentagastrin, is administered intravenously and several more samples are collected at timed intervals. The role of the phlebotomist in gastric analysis testing is to assist in labeling specimens and to draw specimens for serum gastrin determinations.

OTHER BODY CAVITY FLUIDS

In addition to CSF and amniotic fluid, there are various other body cavity fluids which are commonly collected and analyzed. All body cavity fluids are collected in sterile containers. The type of fluid should be indicated on the specimen label. Commonly analyzed **body fluids** include:

Synovial fluid: aspirated from joint cavities

Pleural fluid: aspirated from the pleural cavity surrounding the lungs

Peritoneal fluid: aspirated from the abdominal cavity

Pericardial fluid: aspirated from the cavity surrounding the heart

---

NASOPHARYNGEAL CULTURE COLLECTION

Nasopharyngeal (NP) cultures are often collected to detect the presence of the microorganisms that cause diphtheria, meningitis, pertussis (whooping cough), and pneumonia. NP specimens are collected using a sterile Dacron or cotton-tipped flexible wire swab. The swab is inserted gently into the nose and passed into the nasopharynx. Once in the nasopharynx, the swab is gently rotated then carefully removed, placed into transport media, labeled, and transported to the lab.

SEMEN

Semen analysis is used to assess fertility and also to determine the effectiveness of sterilization following vasectomy. Semen specimens are collected in sterile containers similar to sterile urine containers. A semen specimen should *never* be collected in a condom. Condoms often contain **spermicides** (substances that kill sperm) and invalidate test results. Semen specimens should be kept warm and delivered to the lab immediately.

STOOL

Examination of **stool (feces)** is helpful in the evaluation of gastrointestinal disorders. Stool specimens can be evaluated for the presence of intestinal parasites and their eggs (ova and parasite, or O&P); checked for fat and urobilinogen content; cultured to detect the presence of pathogenic bacteria; and tested for the presence of **occult** (hidden) **blood** by means of the **guaiac** test.

Stool specimens are normally collected in clean, dry containers. They should be covered and sent to the laboratory immediately after collection. Special containers are available for ova and parasite collection (Fig. 13-3). Most specimens, especially those for detection of parasites, should be kept at body temperature (37° C). Large gallon containers, similar to paint cans, are used for 24-, 48-, and 72-hour stool collections for fat and urobilinogen; these specimens are refrigerated throughout the collection period.

Special test cards, such as Hematest (Miles Inc., Elkhart, IN) and Hemoccult (Smith-Kline Diagnostics, San Jose, CA), are often used by outpatients to collect stool specimens for occult blood. The patient is usually instructed to have a meat-free diet for 3 days prior to the test. Patients are then instructed to collect separate specimens for 3 successive days. Cards can be mailed or brought to the lab after collection.

SWEAT CHLORIDE

The chloride content in sweat is evaluated in the diagnosis of cystic fibrosis, primarily in children and adolescents under the age of 20. **Cystic fibrosis** is caused by a disorder of the exocrine glands, affecting primarily the lungs, liver, and pancreas. Children with cystic fibrosis have abnormally high levels (2 to 5 times normal) of chloride in their sweat.

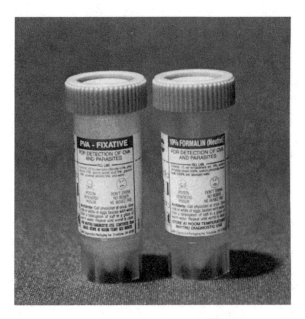

Figure 13-3 Ova and parasite specimen containers. (MML Diagnostic Packaging, Troutdale, OR).

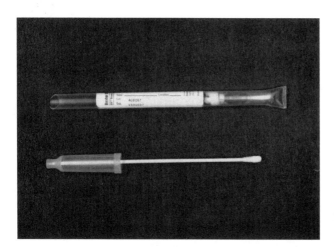

Figure 13-4 Throat swab and transport tube.

Lab evaluation of **sweat chloride** involves transporting pilocarpine (a sweat-stimulating drug) into the skin by means of electrical stimulation (**iontophoresis**) from electrodes placed on the skin. Sweat is collected, weighed to determine the volume, and analyzed for chloride content.

THROAT CULTURE COLLECTION

Throat cultures are most often collected to aid in the diagnosis of streptococcal (strep) infections. Throat specimens on inpatients are usually collected by nursing staff. However, it is not uncommon for a phlebotomist to be asked to collect a throat culture specimen on an outpatient. A throat culture is collected in the following manner using a culture kit containing a sterile polyester-tipped swab and covered transport tube containing transport media (Fig. 13-4).

THROAT CULTURE COLLECTION PROCEDURE

1. The patient is instructed to open his or her mouth wide while tilting the head back.
2. A small flashlight or other light source can be directed at the back of the throat to illuminate areas of inflammation. A tongue blade may be used to depress the tongue.
3. Both tonsils, the back of the throat, and any areas of ulceration, exudation, or inflammation should be brushed with the sterile swab, being careful not to touch the swab to the lips or tongue.
4. Because proper collection will often cause the patient to have a gag reflex or cough, the phlebotomist may wish to wear a mask or stand to the side of the patient.
5. When the specimen is collected, the swab is placed back into the collector tube. The ampule containing transport media is then crushed between the fingers and the swab embedded in the released media. The cover is secured and the specimen is properly labeled and sent to the lab immediately.

TISSUE SPECIMENS

Tissue specimens from biopsies may also be sent to the laboratory for processing. Most tissue specimens arrive at the laboratory in formalin or suitable solution and need only to be accessioned and sent to the proper department. However, with more biopsies being performed in outpatient situations, a phlebotomist in specimen processing may encounter specimens that have not yet been put into the proper solution. It is important for the phlebotomist to check the procedure manual to determine the proper handling for any unfamiliar specimen. (For example, tissues for genetic analysis should *not* be put in formalin.) Improper handling may ruin a specimen from a procedure that is, in all probability, expensive, uncomfortable for the patient, and not easily repeated.

Study & Review Questions

1. Additional information necessary on a nonblood specimen label includes the
   a. party to be charged.
   b. patient's age.
   c. physician.
   d. type of sample.

2. Which type of urine specimen is used to detect the presence of infection?
   a. 2-hour
   b. 24-hour
   c. Midstream
   d. Clean catch

3. Which nonblood specimen is most frequently analyzed in the lab?
   a. CSF
   b. Pleural fluid
   c. Synovial fluid
   d. Urine

4. Which of the following fluids comes from the lung area?
   a. Gastric
   b. Peritoneal
   c. Pleural
   d. Synovial

Suggested Laboratory Activities

1. Assemble, identify, and label the various containers used for nonblood specimens.

2. Practice proper patient instruction for 24-hour urine collection by role-playing with a fellow student.

3. Perform a reagent strip analysis on an actual urine specimen.

4. Collect a specimen for a throat culture from a fellow student.

BIBLIOGRAPHY AND SUGGESTED READINGS

Fischbach, F. (1996). *Laboratory diagnostic tests* (5th ed.). Philadelphia: J. B. Lippincott.

National Committee for Clinical Laboratory Standards, GP8-P. (1985). *Collection and transportation of single collection urine specimens.* Villanova, PA: NCCLS.

National Committee for Clinical Laboratory Standards, GP13-P. (1987). *Collection and preservation of timed urine specimens.* Villanova, PA: NCCLS.

National Committee for Clinical Laboratory Standards, GP16-A. (1995). *Routine urinalysis.* Villanova, PA: NCCLS.

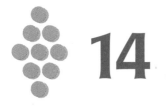

14

Quality Assurance and Specimen Handling

KEY TERMS

aerosol
aliquot
analyte
central processing
centrifugation
continuous quality
  improvement (CQI)

JCAHO
procedure manual
QA indicators
quality assurance (QA)
quality control (QC)

reference laboratory log book
threshold values
total quality management
  (TQM)
user manual

OBJECTIVES

Upon successful completion of this chapter, the reader should be able to:

1. List management techniques instituted by Dr. Deming and JCAHO and state the reasons for implementing such programs.
2. Define total quality management (TQM) and list major themes of TQM.
3. Define quality assurance (QA), list and describe the components of a quality assurance program, and differentiate quality control (QC) from QA.
4. List areas in phlebotomy subject to quality control and identify quality control procedures associated with each.
5. Describe specimen handling procedures for routine specimens, and special handling procedures for specimens that are light- or temperature-sensitive.
6. Identify time constraints and exceptions for delivery of specimens.
7. Identify OSHA-required protective equipment worn when processing specimens.
8. Describe the various steps involved in processing the different types of specimens and identify the criteria for specimen rejection.

QUALITY ASSURANCE IN HEALTH CARE

In the United States, an abundance of management tools and techniques have been offered for "getting the job done." All have promised to deliver more efficient and effective management. There were those that proved to be useful in the private, profit-making sector, whereas others were more successful in the not-for-profit, noncompetitive public sector. Very few were useful in both sectors. But beginning in 1988, **Total Quality Management (TQM)** made the jump from the private to the public sector with nods of approval and scowls of disgust from the observers on the sidelines. One of the leaders in TQM was Dr. W. Edwards Deming. Deming is credited with teaching post-World War II Japanese industrial leaders the quality control methods that led to their automobile and electronic triumphs of the 1970s and 1980s. As an engineer and physicist, Deming used statistics to analyze production processes and discover the source of product flaws. Deming's methods require that the workers actively participate in decisions to improve production continually, that is, a team effort with total involvement from all levels.

One of the key players in bringing **continuous quality improvement (CQI)** techniques to health care is the **Joint Commission on Accreditation of Healthcare Organizations (JCAHO)**, the foremost national accreditation body for hospitals. JCAHO is a voluntary, nongovernmental agency charged with, among other things, establishing standards for the operation of hospitals and other health-related facilities and services. In 1994, JCAHO required health care facilities to have an institution-wide total quality management/continuous quality improvement (TQM/CQI) plan in place. This meant that all departments of a health care facility were required to have ongoing evaluations of their activities and customer expectations. Current standards from JCAHO stress performance accountability for continuous quality improvement. In order to review health care performance, JCAHO developed the following list that focuses on desirable characteristics and degree of accomplishment to measure performance.

THE DIMENSIONS OF PERFORMANCE

I. *Doing the Right Thing*

- The **efficacy** of the procedure or treatment in relation to the patient's condition
  The degree to which the care of the patient has been shown to accomplish the desired or projected outcome(s)
- The **appropriateness** of a specific test, procedure, or service to meet the patient's needs
  The degree to which the care provided is relevant to the patient's clinical needs, given the current state of knowledge

II. *Doing the Right Thing Well*

- The **availability** of a needed test, procedure, treatment, or service to the patient who needs it
  The degree to which appropriate care is available to meet the patient's needs

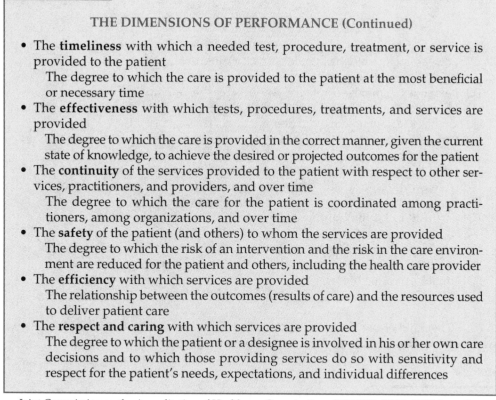

THE DIMENSIONS OF PERFORMANCE (Continued)

- The **timeliness** with which a needed test, procedure, treatment, or service is provided to the patient
  The degree to which the care is provided to the patient at the most beneficial or necessary time
- The **effectiveness** with which tests, procedures, treatments, and services are provided
  The degree to which the care is provided in the correct manner, given the current state of knowledge, to achieve the desired or projected outcomes for the patient
- The **continuity** of the services provided to the patient with respect to other services, practitioners, and providers, and over time
  The degree to which the care for the patient is coordinated among practitioners, among organizations, and over time
- The **safety** of the patient (and others) to whom the services are provided
  The degree to which the risk of an intervention and the risk in the care environment are reduced for the patient and others, including the health care provider
- The **efficiency** with which services are provided
  The relationship between the outcomes (results of care) and the resources used to deliver patient care
- The **respect and caring** with which services are provided
  The degree to which the patient or a designee is involved in his or her own care decisions and to which those providing services do so with sensitivity and respect for the patient's needs, expectations, and individual differences

Joint Commission on the Accreditation of Healthcare Organizations (JCAHO). (1996). 1996 Accreditation manual for hospitals. Oakbrook Terrace, IL: JCAHO.

TOTAL QUALITY MANAGEMENT

TQM stresses bringing about constant, gradual change in operations through improvement and innovation, rather than being satisfied with meeting a minimum standard. This is another way of saying that the health care facility makes a continuous effort to identify opportunities for improving services. The following box shows the 12 primary themes of TQM identified by Marchese (1991).

MAJOR THEMES OF TQM

TQM focuses on quality: the product or outcome must be the best.

TQM is customer-driven, which means that you must be able to identify explicitly who your customers are, identify their needs systematically, and commit to serving those needs.

TQM emphasizes continuous improvement: anything can be improved on.

(continued)

MAJOR THEMES OF TQM (Continued)

TQM concentrates on making processes work better: the aim is to identify those processes and enable the people who work in them to understand that work in relation to customer needs.

TQM extends the mindset: quality concerns reach in all directions.

TQM involves the discipline of information: if you're serious about quality, everybody has to know how they're doing.

TQM eliminates re-work: the aim of all this attention to work processes is to ferret out the scrap, waste, and complexity from a system.

TQM emphasizes teamwork: they are not the familiar committees, but are self-directed work groups with their own required competencies and protocols.

TQM empowers people who review their work processes.

TQM invests in training and recognition: it invests heavily in human resource development.

TQM requires vision: unlike the lofty piffle of mission statements, it urges compelling, down-to-earth language that gets all parties focused on the right things to do.

TQM requires leadership.

The number-one focus of TQM in the health care facility or in the phlebotomy area is that of assuring quality services to the customer.

QUALITY ASSURANCE IN PHLEBOTOMY

As members of the health care team, persons doing phlebotomy should understand the significance of their role in the medical environment and the reasons for assuring quality in their area of responsibility. Laboratory testing is an important part of patient diagnosis and medical care. Doctors rely on test results and assume that the process is carefully monitored from beginning to end with the quality remaining consistent. That is why it becomes necessary to set policies and procedures to ensure that sample procurement and handling are accurate. These established policies and procedures fall under an overall process called **quality assurance (QA).**

Quality Assurance Defined

Quality assurance is defined as a program that guarantees quality patient care by tracking outcomes through scheduled reviews in which areas of the hospital look at the appropriateness, applicability, and timeliness of patient care. Guidelines are developed for all processes used, and when these guidelines are formally adopted, they become the QA program. In the late 1980s, JCAHO developed a 10-step monitoring and evaluation process (p. 323) which can be used for assessing the appropriateness of care.

Identifying QA Indicators

One of the most important aspects of setting up a QA evaluation process is establishing indicators that monitor all aspects of patient care. These **QA indicators** must be measurable, well-defined, specific, objective, and clearly related to an important aspect

---

THE 10-STEP MONITORING AND EVALUATION PROCESS

1. Assign responsibility.
2. Delineate scope of care.
3. Identify important aspects of care.
4. Identify indicators related to these aspects of care.
5. Establish thresholds for evaluation related to the indicators.
6. Collect and organize data.
7. Evaluate care when thresholds are reached.
8. Take actions to improve care.
9. Assess the effectiveness of actions and document improvements.
10. Communicate relevant information to the organization-wide quality assurance program.

---

of care. Indicators can measure quality, adequacy, accuracy, timeliness, effectiveness, customer satisfaction, and so on. They are designed to look at areas of care that tend to cause problems. For example, an indicator on the quality assessment form shown in Figure 14-1 might be stated as follows: "Blood cultures will not exceed the national contamination rate." A contamination rate that increased beyond a preestablished threshold listed on the form would signify a problem.

Establishing Thresholds and Evaluating Data

Established levels or **threshold values** must be set for all clinical indicators. If this level of acceptable practice is reached, it may trigger intensive evaluation of the practice to see if there is an actual problem that needs to be corrected to improve care. During the evaluation phase, data are collected and organized. Data sources could include such information as patient records, laboratory results, incident reports, patient satisfaction reports, and direct patient observation. A corrective action plan is established if the data identify the outcome as a problem or opportunity for improvement. The action plan identifies who and what will change and when that change is expected to occur. Even when the problem appears to be corrected, monitoring and evaluation continue to insure that care is consistent and that quality continually improves.

The Process/Outcomes

TQM cannot be looked at only in terms of outcomes. For example, the number of times that a patient had to be redrawn because the improper tube was used for specimen collection is an outcome evaluation. Although it is important to know how often collection of a sample in the wrong tube occurs, this does not tell us what caused the outcome. All it gives us is a number. In order to solve the problem, we need to look at the whole process. This means following the total process, including what the requester did at the time he or she decided the test was needed, how it was ordered, and how the laboratory processed the request until the time the results were on the patient's chart and in the hands of the person that ordered them. To assure the same process is always followed, there must be controls and checks along the way.

QUALITY ASSESSMENT AND IMPROVEMENT TRACKING

CONFIDENTIAL A.R.S. 36-445

STANDARD OF CARE/SERVICE: _____

DEPARTMENTS/POPULATION: LABORATORY-MICROBIOLOGY/ALL PATIENTS
DATA SOURCE(S): _____ CULTURE WORKCARDS

IMPORTANT ASPECT OF CARE/SERVICE: LAB SVCS/BLOOD COLLECTION
DATA COLLECTOR: _____ P. BABINA
FREQUENCY REVIEW: _____ 3 MONTHS 100% SAMPLE
SIGNATURES: _____
METHODOLOGY: _____ RETROSPECTIVE
DIRECTOR: _____
TYPE: _____ OUTCOME
MEDICAL DIRECTOR: _____
PERSON RESPONSIBLE FOR:
VICE PRESIDENT/ADMINISTRATOR: _____
DATA ORGANIZATION: P. BABINA
ACTION PLAN: _____ J. BENSON
FOLLOW-UP: _____ J. BENSON
DATE MONITOR BEGAN: 1990
FOLLOW-UP: _____ 3RD QTR.

INDICATORS		THRESHOLD			CRITICAL ANALYSIS/ EVALUATION	ACTION PLAN
		EXP.	ACT.	PREV.		
Blood culture contamination rate will not exceed 3% from three groups of drawing personnel.		3%			N= 1385

Patient Centered Care draws a Nursing line draws are out of compliance but show improvement from January to March. | A communication has gone out to Nursing reminding to follow established protocols for drawing. Microbiology has implemented new protocol disallowing a line draw unless two consecutive venipunctures have failed or protocol is over-ridden by physician order.

PCC tecs have been reinserviced on proper technique. |
LAB	JAN FEB MAR	3%	1.1% 1.8% 1.7%			
PCC	JAN FEB MAR	3%	5.6% 4.8% 3.2%			
LINE DRAWS	JAN FEB MAR	3%	5.6% 7.9% 0.0%			

QICONFID

Figure 14-1 TQM form.

Quality Control Defined

Quality control (QC), a component of a QA program, is a form of procedure control. This means that if standards are followed during a given procedure, results will be consistent. Phlebotomy QC involves checking all the operational procedures to make certain they are performed correctly. In phlebotomy, it is the responsibility of the person who supervises the phlebotomist to oversee QA and insure that standards are being met. It is the responsibility of the person acquiring the blood sample to meet those standards at all times.

AREAS IN PHLEBOTOMY THAT ARE SUBJECT TO QUALITY CONTROL

Patient Preparation Procedures

Quality control actually starts before the specimen has been collected. To obtain an acceptable specimen, the patient must be prepared properly. In a hospital setting, this means the nurse should check a book of instruction called the laboratory **user manual** that has been given to the unit by the laboratory. The user manual describes preparation of the patient and special instructions for specimen collection. More concise pocket versions of this book are designed to be carried by the phlebotomist to assist in answering questions concerning unusual requests. Being informed and updated regularly helps the phlebotomist and specimen processors be well versed in testing protocol and better able to answer inquiries.

Specimen Collection Procedures

IDENTIFICATION

Patient identification (as described in Chap. 9) is the most important aspect of specimen collection. Methods are being continually improved to ensure correct patient identification. An example is the use of barcode readers and accompanying labels (Fig. 14-2), which can substantially reduce human error.

EQUIPMENT

Puncture devices.   Assuring the quality and sterility of every needle and lancet is essential for patient safety. All puncture devices come in sealed sterile containers and should be used only once. If the seal has been broken, the device should be put in a sharps container and a new one obtained. Manufacturing defects in needles, such as barbs and blunt tips, can be avoided before use by quickly inspecting the needle after unsheathing.

Evacuated tubes.   To maintain specimen integrity, the National Committee for Clinical Laboratory Standards (NCCLS) has established standards for evacuated tubes. Manufacturers print expiration dates on each tube for quality assurance. Outdated tubes should not be used because they may not fill completely, causing dilution of the sample, distortion of the cell components, and erroneous results. Anticoagulants may not work effectively in expired tubes, allowing small clots to form and thereby invalidating hematology and immunohematology test results. All new lots of evacuated tubes should be checked for adequate vacuum and additive, integrity of the stopper, ease of stopper removal, and tube strength during centrifugation. All control checks should be documented.

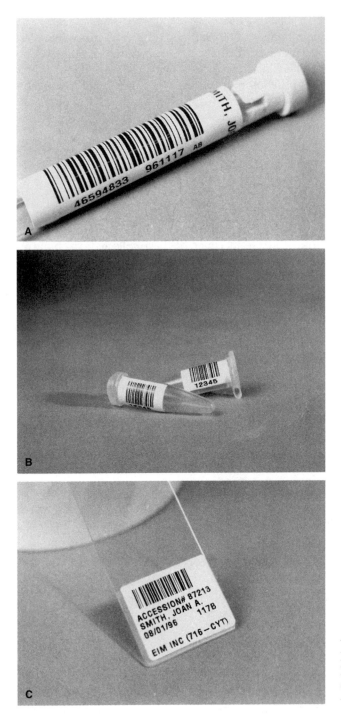

Figure 14-2 (**A**) Specimen tube with barcode label. (**B**) Microcollection container with barcode label. (**C**) Slide with barcode label. (Courtesy Electronic Imaging Materials, Inc., Keene, NH.)

LABELING

Labeling must be exact. Labeling requirements, as outlined in Chapter 9, should be strictly followed. Inaccuracies, such as transposed letters or missing information, will result in the specimen being discarded. With computer labels, the phlebotomist may be assured of correctly printed patient information, but this correct label must still be placed on the right patient's specimen.

TECHNIQUE

Proper phlebotomy techniques must be carefully taught by a professional who understands the importance of following standard procedures, as well as the reasons for using certain equipment or techniques. Incident reports, a form of QA documentation, are used to report inadequate technique or poor specimen quality. No matter how experienced phlebotomists may be, a periodic review of their techniques is necessary for QA.

COLLECTION PRIORITIES

Specimen collection priorities must be stressed. The importance of knowing how to recognize which specimen request is the most critical or has special collection criteria can save the patient unnecessary medication or additional testing, eg, renins or TDMs. It may even shorten the patient's stay in the hospital, because in many instances therapy is based on test values that are assumed to have been collected in the proper way at the right time.

CONTINUING EDUCATION

Continuing education is mandatory to maintain proficiency and consistency. It is usually the responsibility of the supervisor to present new methods and procedural changes to the phlebotomists on a regular basis. The phlebotomists must read laboratory literature or attend seminars to keep abreast of current practices outside of their institution. Continuing education is also necessary for phlebotomy recertification by agencies such as the National Certification Agency (NCA) and the American Society of Phlebotomy Technicians (ASPT).

Documentation

Different types of QA documents have been developed to record problems, standardize procedures, and inform nursing personnel of the importance of patient preparation.

THE USER MANUAL

As mentioned previously, the user manual is an example of a QA document. It typically contains in chart form the type of specimen required and minimum amount needed, special handling of the specimen, what the reference values for the test are, the days testing is available, and the normal turnaround time (TAT) (Fig. 14-3).

REFERENCE LABORATORY LOG BOOK

Test orders that cannot be performed on site are sent to another laboratory called a reference laboratory. All samples sent out must be logged in a **reference laboratory log book**, which includes patient identification, date sent out, and date the results were received. There is also a reference manual that explains how to handle specimens to be sent to a

| | | HEMATOLOGY | | |
TEST	TEST VOLUME	VACUTAINER COLOR (TOP)	NORMAL VALUES	NOTES
APT test	1 mL feces or gastric fluid	Plastic container	Negative	Suitable for grossly bloody specimens only
Acid hemolysin	0.4 mL (RBC) 2.5 mL serum	Lavender and red (non-Corvac)	0%–5%	
Acid phosphatase stain	3 mL blood	Green		
Acid phosphatase w/tartrate stain (TRAP)	3 mL blood	Green		
Alpha naphthol butyrate stain (nonspecific esterase)	3 mL blood	Green		
Blood smear— differential	.03 mL blood	Lavender or fingerstick	See individual tests	See page 27
Body fluid HCT	1 mL	Fluid		
Bone marrow				Schedule in advance (4-6281)
Coulter count	1 mL blood	Lavender or lavender microtainer	See page 27	Includes WBC, RBC, HGB, HCT, MCV, MCH, MCHC
Differential	1 mL blood	Lavender		See page 28
Eosinophil count	0.5 mL blood	Lavender	150–350 /uL	See page 28
Epinephrine/ endotoxin stimulation test				Schedule in advance (4-6281). Consultation form required
Fetal hemoglobin (APT) (qualitative)	1 mL feces or gastric fluid	Red Non-Corvac or plastic container	Negative	Suitable for grossly bloody specimens only

Figure 14-3   User manual. (Courtesy University Medical Center, Tucson, AZ.)

reference laboratory and how to complete requisitions and package samples for mailing or transporting.

LABORATORY PROCEDURE MANUAL

A complete **procedure manual** must be made available to all employees of the laboratory for standardization purposes. Accrediting agencies such as JCAHO demand that this manual be updated annually. A procedure manual states the laboratory policy and procedures that apply to each test or practice performed in the lab. Information provided includes the following:

- Purpose of the procedure
- Specimen type and collection method
- Equipment and supplies required
- Detailed step-by-step procedure
- Limitations and variables of the method
- Corrective actions
- Method validation
- Normal values and references

The manual will also include updates to procedures and notification of these changes to the nursing staff (Fig. 14-4). The procedure manual is a QA document that shows the intent of the lab to adhere to the national standards of good practice.

QUALITY ASSURANCE FORMS
Accreditation standards for agencies such as JCAHO require the facility to show documentation on all quality control checks.

Equipment check forms.   Special forms for recording equipment checks on tube additives, vacuum strength, and expiration dates are available for verification of new lot numbers. Refrigerator temperatures, which must be recorded daily, are often the responsibility of the phlebotomist. Control checks on the centrifuge require periodic documentation of the tachometer readings and maintenance performed.

Internal reports.   Confidential incident/occurrence reports must be filled out when a problem occurs. These forms identify the problem, state the consequence, and describe the corrective action. Incident reports are not limited to situations in which an injury occurred. For example, an incident form would be filled out when a tube of blood was mislabeled. Incident reports should state facts and not feelings. It is not the function of an incident report to place blame, but only to identify what took place and the corrective action taken so that such an event does not happen again.

SPECIMEN HANDLING

Proper handling throughout the collection process, including transportation and processing, is important for maintaining specimen integrity, as well as protecting the phlebotomist and others from accidental exposure to potentially infectious substances. Improper handling can render the most skillfully obtained specimen useless. However, the fact that a specimen has been improperly handled is not always easily discerned. To assure delivery of a quality specimen for analysis, it is imperative that the person doing phlebotomy be adequately instructed in this area. Policies and procedures should be established to cover specimen handling techniques. In addition, all specimens should be handled according to the standard precautions guidelines written by the Centers for

SAMARITAN HEALTH SYSTEM

July 6, 1995

TO: MEDICAL STAFF

FROM: JOSEPH J. FRANK, PH.D.
       CLINICAL CHEMIST
       GOOD SAMARITAN REGIONAL MEDICAL CENTER

RE: LD ISOENZYMES

In the interest of cost effective medical care, the Department of
Pathology is recommending that LD isoenzymes only be ordered on
those patients in which CK isoenzymes will have decreased
sensitivity (>24 hours post MI). In addition, a policy approved
by the Cardiology Committee limiting LD isoenzymes to one set
each 24 hours will be instituted.

Beginning Wednesday July 12, 1995, the laboratory will no longer
be performing LD isoenzymes by electrophoresis. The test will be
replaced by an immunoassay for the LD1 isoenzyme and a
calculation of the % LD1.

Reference Ranges:

        The likelihood of an acute myocardial infarction is
        high when one of the following criteria is met:

                LD Value   LD1 Value
                ≤250.........>102
                >250.........≥40% of LD Value

If CK isoenzymes are not positive, one must also rule out
hemolysis and renal infarct.

Good Samaritan Regional Medical Center ■ 1111 East McDowell Road ■ P.O. Box 2989 ■ Phoenix, AZ 85062 ■ 602-239-2000

Figure 14-4 Procedure manual update. (Courtesy Samaritan Health System,
Phoenix, AZ.)

Disease Control and Prevention (CDC) and enforced by the Occupational Safety and Health Administration (OSHA), as outlined in Chapter 6.

General Guidelines

Proper handling of specimens begins with the initiation of the test request and includes patient preparation, equipment selection, and "order of draw," all covered elsewhere in this text. This chapter deals with proper handling after the specimen is collected until it is deliver to the proper lab area for testing.

Handling of Routine Specimens

ADDITIVE TUBE MIXING

Additive tubes should be gently inverted 5 to 10 times as soon as they are drawn. Vigorous mixing may cause hemolysis and should be avoided. Potassium, magnesium, and certain enzyme tests are examples of tests that cannot be performed on hemolyzed specimens. Inadequate mixing may cause anticoagulant tubes to form clots, which may lead to erroneous results, especially for hematology studies. Inadequate mixing of gel separation tubes may prevent the additive from functioning properly and clotting may be incomplete. Nonadditive tubes do not require mixing.

TRANSPORTING SPECIMENS

Blood specimen tubes should be transported carefully so as not to break them or cause the blood to hemolyze. Tubes should be transported with the stopper up, which aids in clot formation of serum tubes; reduces agitation, which can cause hemolysis; and prevents contact of the contents of the tube with the tube stopper. Blood in contact with tube stoppers can be a source of contamination to the specimen and contributes to **aerosol** (a fine mist of the specimen) formation during stopper removal.

Nonblood specimens should be transported in leak-proof containers with adequately secured lids. Specimens transported through pneumatic tube systems should be protected from shock and sealed in zipper-type plastic bags to contain spills.

Specimens arriving in the lab from off-site locations should be transported as described earlier. In addition, special care should be taken to protect specimens from the effects of extreme heat or cold.

Specimens Requiring Special Handling

SPECIMENS REQUIRING PROTECTION FROM LIGHT

Some test components are broken down in the presence of light, causing falsely decreased values. The most common of these is bilirubin. Other tests sensitive to light include vitamin B_{12}, carotene, serum, and red cell folate, and urine specimens for porphyrins. Specimens can be easily protected from light by wrapping them in aluminum foil. Light-inhibiting, amber-colored microcollection containers are available for collection of bilirubin specimens from infants.

SPECIMENS THAT NEED TO BE CHILLED

Certain metabolic processes continue even after a specimen is drawn. Chilling the specimen slows down this process. Specimens requiring chilling should be completely immersed in a slurry of crushed ice and water. The use of large cubes of ice without water added prevents adequate cooling of the entire specimen. Placing the specimen in contact with a solid piece of ice can cause parts of the specimen to freeze, resulting in hemolysis and possible breakdown of analytes. (**Analyte** is a general term for a substance undergoing analysis.) Examples of specimens requiring chilling are blood gases, ammonia, lactic acid, renin, protime, partial thromboplastin time, and glucagon tests.

SPECIMENS THAT NEED TO BE KEPT WARM

Some specimens need to be transported at or near body temperature (37° C). Examples are specimens for cold agglutinins, cryoglobulin, and cryofibrinogen. Specimens that need to be kept warm should be transported in a 37° C heat block.

Some tests, such as the activated clotting time, require that the tube for the test be kept warm prior to drawing the blood for the test. Manual activated clotting time (ACT) methods require the tube to be kept in a 37° C heat block during performance of the test, as well as prior to the test procedure. Automated methods, such as the Hemochron® system (International Technidyne Corp., Edison, NJ), have a warming unit which is part of the machine.

Time Constraints for Specimen Delivery

All specimens should be transported to the lab promptly. Ideally, routine blood specimens should arrive at the lab within 45 minutes of collection and be centrifuged within 1 hour.

Guidelines recommended by NCCLS document H18-A set the maximum time limit for separating serum and plasma from the cells at 2 hours from time of collection. Less time is recommended for certain specimens, particularly potassium and cortisol specimens.

Prompt processing of specimens is easily achievable with an on-site lab, as in a hospital setting, but it is not always possible when specimens come to the lab from off-site locations, such as doctors' offices.

Specimens that cannot reach their destination within the allotted time period should be allowed to clot (if applicable), should be centrifuged, and the serum or plasma separated and transferred to a suitable container for transport.

If the specimens are drawn in serum separator tubes (SSTs) or plasma separator tubes (PSTs), they need only be centrifuged once they have clotted, if applicable (Fig. 14-5). Once centrifuged, the separator gel will prevent glycolysis for up to 24 hours. Applicable temperature requirements should be maintained until the specimens reach the laboratory.

Exceptions to the Preceding Guidelines

Specimens for glucose determination drawn in sodium fluoride tubes are stable for 24 hours at room temperature and up to 48 hours when refrigerated at 2° to 8° C. Hematology tests drawn in lavender stopper (EDTA) tubes are performed on whole blood specimens and should never be centrifuged. EDTA specimens are stable for 24 hours. However, it is important to make smears from EDTA blood within 1 hour of collection to preserve the integrity of the blood cells and prevent artifact formation due to prolonged contact with the anticoagulant. "Stat" or "medical emergency" specimens take priority over all other specimens and should be transported and processed immediately.

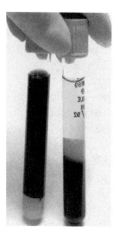

Figure 14-5   Hemogard SSTs: *Left*, prior to being centrifuged; *Right*, after being centrifuged.

SPECIMEN PROCESSING

Protective Equipment

OSHA regulations require the wearing of protective equipment when processing specimens. Protective equipment includes gloves, fully buttoned lab coats or aprons, and protective face gear such as mask and goggles with side shields or chin-length face shields.

Central Processing

Most laboratories have a specific area commonly called **central processing** (or specimen processing) where all specimens are received, triaged (prioritized), and prepared for testing. Here, the specimens are identified, logged (accessioned), and sorted by department and type of processing required. Specimens not requiring centrifugation, such as urine and hematology specimens, are then distributed to the proper department. Specimens for tests requiring serum or plasma must be centrifuged and labels generated for the tube (aliquot tubes) that will receive the serum or plasma obtained through centrifugation. **Aliquot** is defined as a portion of the specimen used for testing. Great care must be taken to match each specimen with the corresponding aliquot tube.

PLASMA SPECIMENS

Specimens for tests performed on plasma are collected in tubes containing anticoagulants and may be centrifuged immediately.

SERUM SPECIMENS

Specimens for tests performed on serum must be completely clotted prior to centrifugation. If clotting is not complete when the specimen is centrifuged, the resultant serum may clot and interfere with the performance of the test. Complete clotting normally takes around 30 to 45 minutes at room temperature. Specimens from patients on anticoagulant medication, such as heparin or dicumarol, as well as specimens from patients with high white blood counts, may take longer to clot. Chilled specimens may also take longer to clot. Serum separator tubes and other tubes containing clot-activating glass particles usually clot within 15 minutes. Thrombin tubes normally clot in 5 minutes. There are also several commercially available clot activators, which can be added to the tube after the specimen is drawn. Proper mixing of clot activator tubes will ensure proper clotting.

SPECIAL PRECAUTIONS FOR HANDLING SPECIMENS

Stoppers should remain on tubes awaiting **centrifugation**. Removing the stopper from a specimen can cause a loss of CO_2 and an increase of pH, leading to inaccurate results for tests such as pH, CO_2, and acid phosphatase. Leaving tubes unstoppered also exposes the specimen to possible contamination and evaporation. Evaporation leads to inaccurate results due to concentration of analytes. Sources of contamination can be as simple as a drop of sweat, which interferes with electrolyte results, or powder from gloves, which may interfere with calcium determinations (some powders contain calcium).

CENTRIFUGATION

Specimen preparation.   Once blood specimens have fully clotted, they may be centrifuged. A centrifuge is a machine that spins the blood at high revolutions per minute (rpms). The centrifugal force that this creates causes cells and plasma/serum to separate (Fig. 14-6). Tubes should remain stoppered during centrifugation to prevent contamination, evaporation, **aerosol** formation, and changes to pH.

If stoppers are removed to add separation devices, the tubes should be restoppered or covered with suitable closure devices. Use of applicator sticks to "rim" or release a clot is a potential source of contamination, as well as hemolysis; thus, the practice is no longer recommended.

Centrifuge operation.   It is imperative that equal-size tubes with equal volumes of specimen be placed opposite one another or "balanced" in the centrifuge. An unbalanced centrifuge may break specimen tubes, ruining specimens and causing the contents to form aerosols. The lid to the centrifuge should remain closed during operation and should not be opened until the machine has come to a complete stop without using the brake.

Centrifuge each specimen only once. Repeated centrifugation can cause hemolysis and analyte deterioration. In addition, once the serum or plasma has been removed, the volume ratio of plasma to cells changes. Because a centrifuge generates heat during operation, specimens requiring chilling should be processed in a temperature-controlled centrifuge.

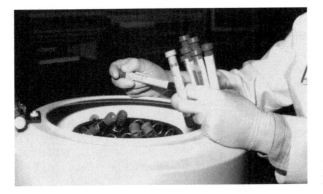

Figure 14-6 Specimen processor loading a centrifuge.

STOPPER REMOVAL

The stopper has to be removed to obtain the serum or plasma needed for testing. Stoppers can be removed using commercially available stopper removal devices. When not using such a device, the stoppers should first be covered with a 4 × 4–inch gauze or tissue to catch any aerosol that may be released. The stopper should be pulled straight up and off and not "popped." Becton Dickinson manufactures a different type of stopper for evacuated tubes. This tube stopper system is called Hemogard (Becton Dickinson, Franklin Lakes, NJ) (Fig. 14-7) and is designed to protect personnel from splatters and aerosols caused by blood that remains on the stopper or around the outer rim of the tube.

ALIQUOT PREPARATION

Serum or plasma should be transferred into the aliquot tubes using disposable pipets, such as the FILTER SAMPLE Dispense Filter (Porex Medical, Fairburn, GA). Pouring specimens into aliquot tubes is not recommended owing to the possibility of aerosol formation or splashing. OSHA's Final Rule for Occupational Exposure to Blood-borne Pathogens, published in December 1991, states "All procedures involving blood or potentially infectious materials shall be performed in such a manner as to minimize splashing, spraying, splattering, and generation of droplets of these substances." The Dispense Filter by Porex is considered such an engineering control because it is a closed system. After serum has been aspirated through the filtration system into the sampler, it can then be dispensed through a restricted opening in the transfer pipet into instrumentation or aliquot tubes if more than one department needs the same specimen (Fig. 14-8).

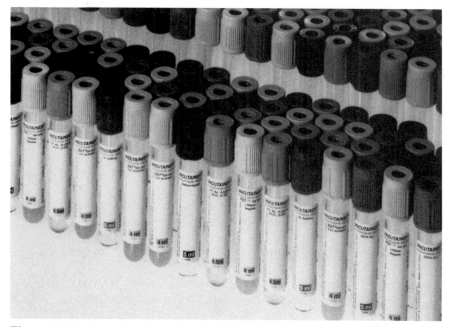

Figure 14-7   Examples of hemogard closure tubes. (Courtesy of Becton Dickinson, Franklin Lakes, NJ.)

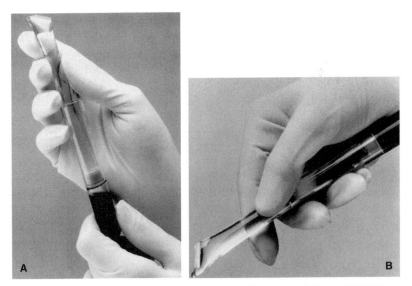

Figure 14-8   (**A**) Transferring serum into a self-contained Porex FILTER SAMPLE Dispense Filter; (**B**) Dispensing serum from a filter sampler. (Courtesy Porex Scientific, Fairburn, GA.)

After the serum or plasma is transferred into the aliquot tube, the tube is covered or capped and dispatched to the proper department.

CRITERIA FOR SPECIMEN REJECTION

Specimens received by the lab may be rejected for analysis for the following reasons:

1. Inadequate, inaccurate, or missing specimen identification (*eg*, a urine specimen that is not labeled).
2. Additive tubes containing an inadequate volume of blood (*eg*, a partially filled coagulation tube).
3. Hemolysis (*eg*, a hemolyzed specimen intended for potassium determination).
4. Wrong tube (*eg*, a CBC collected in a red top tube).
5. Outdated tube (*eg*, a CBC collected in a tube that expired the week before).
6. Improper handling (*eg*, a lavender top drawn for a CBC which has clots in it due to improper mixing).
7. Contaminated specimen (*eg*, a urine for culture and sensitivity in an unsterile container).
8. Insufficient specimen, referred to as "quantity not sufficient" (QNS) for the test ordered (*eg*, a specimen for an erythrocyte sedimentation rate submitted in a microtainer).
9. Collected at the wrong time (*eg*, a specimen for TDM collected before the drug has been given).

Study & Review Questions

1. Quality assurance programs are necessary
   a. because they are mandated by a regulatory agency.
   b. to receive third party reimbursements.
   c. for careful monitoring of patient care.
   d. all of the above.

2. What book describes in detail the steps to follow for specimen collection?
   a. Laboratory user manual
   b. OSHA safety manual
   c. Policy manual
   d. Quality control procedures

3. Which of the following specimens should be protected from light?
   a. BUN
   b. CBC
   c. Bilirubin
   d. Glucose

4. The machine used to separate the serum or plasma from blood samples is called
   a. an Autolet.
   b. a centrifuge.
   c. a glucometer.
   d. a hemostat.

5. After obtaining a renin level, the blood must be transported
   a. as "stat."
   b. away from light.
   c. in ice.
   d. at body temperature.

6. Contamination with perspiration could falsely elevate which blood levels?
   a. Amylase
   b. Calcium
   c. Chloride
   d. Magnesium

7. Which of the following instances would *not* be a reason for a specimen to be rejected for analysis?
   a. A CBC collected in a lavender top tube
   b. A specimen for potassium determination that is hemolyzed
   c. A protime specimen in a partially filled tube
   d. A specimen lacking an identification label

8. According to NCCLS guidelines, serum for analysis should not be in contact with cells for longer than
   a. 30 minutes.
   b. 60 minutes.
   c. 90 minutes.
   d. 120 minutes.

Suggested Laboratory Activities

1. Perform quality control checks on various pieces of lab equipment (*eg*, check tube volume).

2. Make a list of the types of specimens requiring special handling and practice proper specimen handling techniques.

3. Practice proper specimen processing techniques. Balance tubes in a centrifuge, demonstrate proper tube stopper removal, and prepare an aliquot tube.

4. Identify examples of specimens that may be rejected for testing.

5. Look up special handling instructions found in a reference laboratory manual for a list of "send out" tests supplied by your instructor.

BIBLIOGRAPHY AND SUGGESTED READINGS

Aguayo, A. (1990). *Dr. Deming: The American who taught the Japanese about quality.* New York: Simon & Schuster.

Bishop, M. L., Duben-Engelkirk, J. L., & Fody, E. P. (1992). *Clinical chemistry: Principles, procedures, correlations* (2nd ed.). Philadelphia: J. B. Lippincott.

British Deming Association. (1992). *UA perspective on Dr. Deming's theory of profound knowledge* (booklet number W1). Knoxville, TN: SPC Press.

Continuous quality improvement: An analysis of the new paradigm. (Sept/Oct 1992). *Healthcare, Journal for Healthcare Quality.*

Deming, W. E. (1982). *Out of the crisis.* Cambridge, MA: Massachusetts Institute of Technology.

Joint Commission on the Accreditation of Healthcare Organizations (JCAHO). (1996). *1996 Accreditation manual for hospitals.* Oakbrook Terrace, IL: JCAHO.

Marchese, T. (1991). TQM reaches the academy. *AAHE Bulletin 44*(3), 3–9.

National Committee for Clinical Laboratory Standards, H5-A2. (January 1985). *Procedures for the domestic handling and transporting of diagnostic specimens and etiologic agents* (2nd ed.). Villanova, PA: NCCLS.

National Committee for Clinical Laboratory Standards, H18-A. (December 1991). *Procedures for the handling and processing of blood specimens.* Villanova, PA: NCCLS.

National Committee for Clinical Laboratory Standards, H21-A. (December 1986). *Collection, transport and preparation of blood specimens for coagulation testing and performance of coagulation assays.* Villanova, PA: NCCLS.

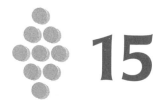

15

Communication and Computers

KEY TERMS

accession number	data	mnemonic	read only memory
barriers	empathy	networking	(ROM)
cathode ray tube	hardware	online	software
(CRT)	input	output	storage
central processing	kinesics	proxemics	tech code
unit (CPU)	kinesic slip	random access	
cursor	menu	memory (RAM)	

OBJECTIVES

Upon successful completion of this chapter, the reader should be able to:

1. Describe the basic concepts of communication.
2. List barriers in verbal communication.
3. Define active listening.
4. Define kinesics and proxemics and describe how they affect the communication process.
5. Describe the importance of appearance for phlebotomists.
6. Contrast normal communication with health care communication.
7. Describe proper telephone protocol in the laboratory.
8. Recognize computer classifications, define a computer network, and list advantages of networking computers.
9. Describe components and elements of a computer, identify general computer skills, and define associated computer terminology.
10. Trace the flow of specimens through the laboratory with an information management system.
11. List information found on a computer label.

INTRODUCTION

Phlebotomy is both a technical and a people-oriented profession. Many different types of people or customers interact with phlebotomists. Almost everyone agrees that the phlebotomist is the public relations agent for the laboratory. Customers expect quality service. Often, the customer's perception of the health care facility is derived from the employees they deal with on a one-to-one basis, such as a phlebotomist. If a phlebotomist lacks a good bedside manner (the ability to communicate empathically with the patient), he or she increases the chances of becoming part of a legal action should any difficulty arise while obtaining the specimen. Favorable impressions result when professionals respond properly to patient needs. This occurs when there is good communication between the health care provider and the patient.

COMMUNICATION DEFINED

Communication is a skill. Defined as the means by which information is exchanged or transmitted, communication is one of the most important processes that takes place in the health care system. This dynamic or constantly changing process involves three components: verbal skills, nonverbal skills, and the ability to listen.

Verbal Communication

Expression through the spoken word is the most obvious form of communication. Effective health care communication should be an interaction in which both participants are affected by the other. It involves a sender (speaker), a receiver (listener), and, when complete, a process called feedback. It is through feedback that the listener or receiver is given the chance to correct miscommunication caused by personal bias or barriers.

Normal human behavior sets up many **barriers** to accurate verbal communication. These biases or personalized filters are major obstructions to hearing and understanding what has been said, as illustrated in the feedback loop in Figure 15-1. Examples of listening barriers are language limitations, culture diversity, emotions, age, and physical disabilities such as hearing loss. To handle emotional barriers, such as an angry patient, the phlebotomist may try asking irrelevant questions, which will distract the patient from the procedure long enough to complete their venipuncture. To avoid creating suspicion and distrust in patients from other countries, the phlebotomist should be aware of cultural differences and avoid cliches that could be misunderstood.

Listening

It is more difficult to communicate than to speak because effective communication requires that the listener participate. It is always a two-way process. The ordinary person can absorb verbal messages at about 500 to 600 words per minute. The average speaking rate is only 125 to 150 words per minute. Therefore, the listener, in order not to be distracted, must use the extra time for active listening. Active listening means taking positive steps through feedback to ensure that the listener interprets what the speaker is saying exactly as the speaker intended. Listening forms the foundation for interpersonal communication and is particularly valuable in building rapport with

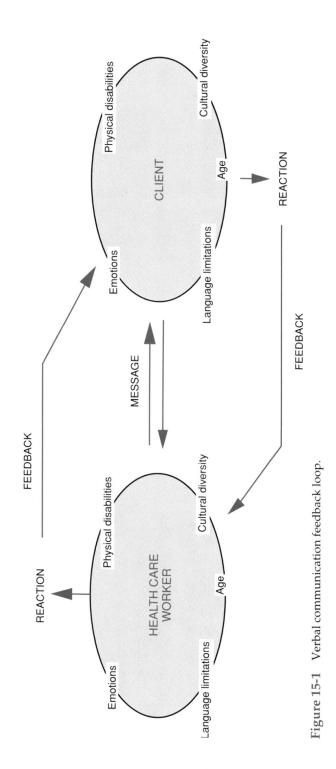

Figure 15-1 Verbal communication feedback loop.

patients. Phlebotomists should learn to watch the speaker, as well as listen, because non-verbal communication affects what they hear.

Nonverbal Communication

It has been stated that 80% of language is unspoken. Unlike verbal communication formed from words which are one-dimensional, nonverbal communication is multidimensional and involves the following elements.

KINESICS

The study of nonverbal communication is also called **kinesics**, and it includes characteristics of body motion and language such as facial expression, gestures, and eye contact. Figure 15-2 illustrates an exaggerated and simplified form of the six emotions that are most easily read by nonverbal facial cues. Body language, which most often is unintentional, plays a major role in communication because it is continuous and more reliable than verbal communication. In fact, if the verbal and nonverbal messages do not match, it is called a **kinesic slip**. When this happens, it has been shown that people tend to trust what they see rather than what they hear.

As health professionals, the phlebotomist can learn much about patients' feelings by observing nonverbal communication, which seldom lies. The patient's face often tells the health professional what the patient will not reveal verbally. For instance, when a patient

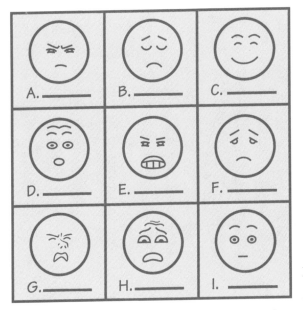

Can you match the above sketches with the correct affects?
(1) happy, (2) sad, (3) surprise, (4) fear, (5) anger, (6) disgust.

Answers: A-5, B-2, C-1, D-3, E-5, F-2, G-6, H-4, I-3.

Figure 15-2 Nonverbal facial cues. (Adapted from Northouse, P. G., & Northouse, L. L. (1992). *Health communication: Strategies for health care professionals* (2nd ed.) (p. 127). Reprinted by permission of Appleton & Lange, Stamford, CT.)

is anxious, nonverbal signs may include tight eyebrows, an intense frown, narrowed eyes, or a downcast mouth (see Fig. 15-2). Researchers have found that certain facial appearances, such as a smile, are universal expressions of emotion. Worldwide, we all recognize the meaning of a smile; however, strong cultural customs often dictate when it is used.

To communicate effectively with a person, it is important to establish good eye contact (Fig. 15-3). A patient or client may be made to feel unimportant and more like an object rather than a human being if no eye contact is established.

PROXEMICS

Proxemics is defined as the study of an individual's concept and use of space. This subtle but powerful part of nonverbal communication should be understood in order to relate better to the patient in a health care facility. Every individual carries around him or her an invisible "bubble," defined as personal territory. The size of this bubble depends on the individual's needs at the time. Naturally occurring territorial zones fall into four categories: intimate distance (a radius of 1 to 18 inches), personal distance (a radius of 1½ to 4 feet), social distance (a radius of 4 to 12 feet), and public distance (a radius of more than 12 feet). These "zones of comfort" are very obvious in human interaction. Entering personal or intimate zones is necessary in the health care setting, and if not carefully handled, the patient may feel threatened, insecure, or out of control. Fortunately, it is becoming more acceptable in certain instances to merge into each others' bubbles without discomfort, such as in the relationships of teacher and student or health care worker and client.

APPEARANCE

Most health care facilities have dress codes because it is understood that appearance makes a statement. The impression the phlebotomist makes as he or she approaches the patient sets the stage for future interaction. The right image portrays a trustworthy professional. Phlebotomists' physical appearance should communicate cleanliness and confidence. Lab coats, which completely cover the clothing underneath, should be clean and pressed. Shoes should be conservative and polished. Close attention should be paid

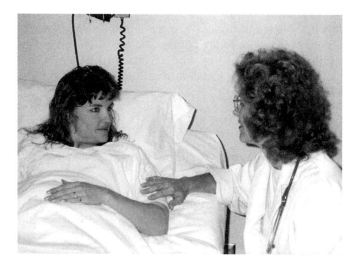

Figure 15-3 A health care worker communicates understanding through good eye contact.

to personal hygiene. Bathing and the use of deodorant should be a daily routine. Strong perfumes or colognes should be avoided. Hair and nails should be clean and look natural. Hair, if long, should be pulled back and fingernails should be short for safety's sake. Phlebotomists who deal with patients who are ill or irritable will find a confident and professional appearance helpful in doing their job.

TOUCH

Touching can take a variety of forms and convey many different meanings. For example, accidental touching could happen in a crowded elevator. Social touching could take place when a person grabs the arm of another while giving advice. Therapeutic touching is designed to aid in healing. This special type of nonverbal communication is a very important ingredient to the well-being of humans, and even more so in diseased (not at ease) humans. Numerous studies have shown the importance of touch in healing.

Because medicine is a contact profession, touching privileges are granted to and expected for health care workers under certain circumstances. Whether a patient or health care provider is comfortable with touching is based on his or her cultural background. Because touch is a necessary part of the phlebotomy procedure, it is important to realize that, as a phlebotomist, patients are often much more aware of your touch than you are of theirs; there may even be a risk of the patient questioning the appropriateness of touching. Generally speaking, patients respond favorably when touch portrays a thoughtful expression of caring.

COMMUNICATION IN HEALTH CARE

It is not easy for the patient/customer or the health professional to face disease and suffering every day. For many patients, being ill is a terrifying experience; having their blood drawn only contributes to their anxiety. Patients reach out for comfort and reassurance through conversation. Consequently, a phlebotomist must understand the unusual aspects of health care communication and its importance in comforting the patient.

Communication between the health professional and patient is more complicated than normal interaction. Not only is it often emotionally charged but it also involves, in many instances, other people who are very close to the patient and tend to be very critical of the way the patient is handled. Recognizing some of the elements in health care communication, such as empathy, control, trust, and confirmation, will aid the phlebotomist in successfully interacting with the patient.

Elements in Health Care Communication
EMPATHY

Defined as identifying with the feelings or thoughts of another person, **empathy** is an essential factor in interpersonal relations. It involves putting yourself in the place of another and attempting to feel like that person. Thoughtful and sensitive people generally have a high degree of empathy. Empathic health professionals help patients handle the stress of being in a health care institution. A health professional should communicate true feeling to the patient and seek to understand the other person's point of view. When a health professional recognizes the needs of the patient and allows the patient to express his or her emotions, this helps to validate the patient's feelings and gives the patient a very necessary sense of control.

CONTROL

An important element relating to communication in the health care setting is control. Feeling in control is essential to an individual's sense of well-being. People like to think that they can influence the way they respond to happenings in their lives. Many patients perceive themselves as unable to cope physically or mentally with events in a hospital because they feel fearful and powerless.

Consequently, a hospital is one of the few places where an individual gives up control over most of the personal tasks he or she normally performs. Due to this loss of control, the response of the patient is typically to act angry, which characterizes him or her as a "bad patient," or to act extremely codependent and agreeable, which characterizes him or her as a "good patient." The health care provider should be aware of the patient's feelings and learn ways to restore a sense of control to the patient. For instance, when a patient refuses to have his or her blood drawn, a phlebotomist should allow him or her to express that statement of control and even agree with the patient. If patients are allowed to exert that right, they will often change their mind and let the health care provider do the procedure, because then it is the *patient's* decision. Sharing control with the patient may be difficult and often time-consuming, but awareness of the patient's need is important. To allow patients more control of their environment actually improves their health.

TRUST

Another variable in the process of communication is trust. Trust, as defined in the health care setting, is the unquestioning belief by the patient that health professionals are performing their job responsibilities as well as they possible can. As is true with most professionals, health care providers tend to emphasize their technical expertise while completely ignoring the elements of interpersonal communication that are essential in a trusting relationship with the patient. Having blood drawn is just one of the situations in which the consumer must trust the health professional. Developing trust takes time and phlebotomists spend very little time with each patient. Consequently, during this limited interaction, the phlebotomist must do everything possible to win the patient's confidence by consistently appearing knowledgeable, honest, and sincere. Surveys have revealed that patients' trust and satisfaction are increased when one of their main caregivers, such as their nurse or PCT, is the one who also performs the phlebotomy.

CONFIRMATION

Confirmation deals with how health care providers respond to the patient during daily interactions. Confirming responses help the patient feel recognized as a person in spite of the depersonalizing environment of a hospital. The right response contributes to reducing the feelings of separation from loved ones while in a health care facility. Confirming responses, such as "Yes, I hear what you are saying," make the patient feel that his or her opinion is appreciated. For more clarification and a way of drawing out the patient's feelings, the health care provider could say, "Tell me more or help me to understand what you mean."

A familiar communication problem occurring in busy hospitals is the labeling of patients, for example, as "the burn case in room 322." Such communication is dehumanizing and is a subtle way of "disconfirming" patients. Each patient needs to be accepted as a unique individual with special needs. For instance, if the results of a blood test take a long time to get on the chart, a patient may feel uncertainty and needlessly think something is wrong. The patient needs confirmation by a caring health professional that the delay is a standard procedure and is expected for that particular test.

In summary, by recognizing the elements of empathy, control, trust, and confirmation, the phlebotomist can enhance communication with patients and assist in their recovery. Understanding these communication elements will help when used with other means of communication, such as the telephone.

TELEPHONE COMMUNICATION

The telephone is presently a fundamental part of communication. It is used 24 hours a day in the laboratory. To phlebotomists or laboratory clerks, it becomes just another source of stress, bringing additional work and uninvited demands on their time. The constant ringing and the interruption to the workflow often cause laboratory personnel to overlook the effect their style of telephone communication has on the caller. To maintain a professional image, proper protocol should be reviewed by every person given the responsibility of answering the phone. They should be taught how to answer, put someone on hold, and transfer calls properly.

Proper Telephone Protocol
To increase good communication, the telephone techniques shown in Table 15-1 should be followed.

Today, in many areas of health care, the telephone, a valued communication tool, is being replaced in part with a more objective and efficient means of communication: the computer.

COMMUNICATION THROUGH COMPUTERIZATION

As computers become more common in the United States, their use as an essential tool for the health care community increases. The computer can now be found throughout all departments of a hospital, group practice, or health maintenance organization. Various types of hardware and software are being used to manage **data** (information collected for analysis or computation), monitor patients' vital signs, and, most recently, aid in diagnosis. With the sophisticated support that computers provide in the health care context, we see health care and computer technology becoming increasingly interrelated. There is no doubt that today's health care providers will encounter a computer in their job environment, requiring computer literacy for people entering any area in health care. A person may be called "computer literate" if he or she can do the following:

1. Understand the computer and the functions it performs.
2. Perform basic operations in order to complete required tasks.
3. Demonstrate willingness to adapt to the changes that computers are making on the quality of life.

Table 15-1
Rules for Proper Telephone Technique

1. Answer promptly.	If the phone is allowed to ring too many times, the caller assumes the people working in the laboratory are inefficient or insensitive. When answering the phone, state your name and your department.
2. Be helpful.	When a phone rings, it is because someone needs something. Due to the nature of the health care business, the caller may be emotional and need a calm, pleasant voice on the other end to respond to the request. To assist the caller and facilitate the conversation, ask how you can be of help. Keep your statements and answers simple and to the point to avoid confusion.
3. Prioritize calls.	Callers should be informed if they are interrupting another call. Always ask if they can be put on hold in case it is an emergency that must be handled immediately. Coordinating several calls takes an organized person. Disconnecting a caller while transferring irritates the caller.
4. Be prepared to record information.	Documentation is necessary when answering the phone at work to ensure that accurate information is transmitted to the necessary person. Have a pencil and paper close to the phone. Listen carefully, which means clarifying, restating, and summarizing the information received.
5. Know the laboratory policies.	People who answer the telephone need to know the laboratory policies to avoid misinformation. Answers should be consistent. This helps to establish the laboratory's credibility, because a caller's perception of the lab involves more than accurate test results.
6. Diffuse hostile situations.	Some callers are angry because of lost results or errors in billing. Agreeing with a hostile caller will immediately diffuse the caller. After the caller has been calmed down, an inquiry can be handled.
7. Try to assist everyone.	It is possible to assist callers and show concern even if you are not actually answering their questions. Validate callers' requests by giving a response that tells them something can be done. Sincere interest in the caller will enhance communication and contribute to the good reputation of the laboratory.

Computer technology comes with its own vocabulary. The terms listed in Table 15-2 represent a few of the more common ones used in a computer-oriented health care environment.

Computer Classifications

Today's computers can be categorized according to type, function, and size. Size classifications include the microcomputer, minicomputer, mainframe, and supercomputer.

- **Microcomputer or personal computer (PC).** These computers are very popular with the general public and they serve a necessary function in business. They are easy to use and versatile. Microcomputers have been found in health care facilities for some time now because they are practical and inexpensive.
- **Minicomputer.** This classification is characterized by the amount of storage, the processing speeds, and the variety of equipment available, which all exceed the microcomputer. They are stand-alone computers that have the capability of maintaining a

Table 15-2
Common Computer Terminology

Accession number	A unique number generated when the test request is entered into the computer
CPU	Central processing unit
CRT	Cathode ray tube
Cursor	Flashing indicator on the CRT
Data	Information collected for analysis or computation
Hardware	Equipment used to process data
Input	Data that are entered into the CPU
LIMS	Laboratory information management system
Logging on	Entering as a user on the system via a password
Mainframe	A large CPU to which several terminals could be attached
Microcomputer	Personal computer used in the home or office
Minicomputer	A stand-alone computer with intermediate size and storage capacity
Mnemonic	Memory-aiding codes or abbreviations
On-line	The computer is operational
Output	Return of processed information to the user or other locations
Password	Secret word or phrase used to enter the system
Peripherals	All additional equipment attached to the CPU
Storage	A place for keeping data; outside the computer it is called secondary storage
RAM	Random access memory; temporary storage of data in the memory of the CPU
ROM	Read only memory; contains instructions for operation of the computer installed by the manufacturer
Software	Coded instructions required to control the hardware in the processing of data
Tech code	A unique code used to identify a person for purposes of tracking
Verify	To confirm or check for correctness of input

complete database system for processing patient accounts or laboratory information systems.

- **Mainframes.** This classification of computers has a more powerful central processing unit and more disk storage. These systems are capable of processing enormous amounts of information at very fast speeds, making them more appropriate for businesses such as insurance companies, banks, government agencies, and centralized hospital networks.
- **Supercomputers.** These computers, developed by companies such as Cray and Hitachi, are the largest of all systems. They are capable of processing more information at a greater speed, using highly complicated applications, than any other computer system in the world. Because of the heat generated by such speeds, they often require cooling that can be as elaborate as liquid nitrogen. Supercomputers are multimillion dollar expenditures and are, therefore, rarely encountered. Presently, they are being used in national defense and research in health care and for the development of artificial intelligence, a concept that will undoubtedly be used extensively in health care.

Computer Networks

A computer network is a group of microcomputers that are all linked for the purpose of sharing resources. In a computer network, individual stations are called *nodes*. The network interconnection allows all the computers to have access to each other's information or to a large database of information at a remote site through a special node called a server, as shown in Figure 15-4. They can be connected by coaxial cables, optical fibers, or standard telephone lines. These systems are also known as local area networks (LANs).

Networking can take the form of simple interoffice connections or complex systems between several organizations in different cities or across continents. A good example of a large and complex system is the Internet, where computers all over the world (through the use of telephone lines, fiber optics, and satellite connections) can access multiple sites and unlimited information (Fig. 15-5). The advantage of networking for businesses, such as health care institutions, is its efficiency. Along with reducing costs, it can speed up processing and increase productivity because of the convenience of immediate access. For example, a medical complex can purchase one word processing program for their network system and then all of the different users can have access to it. Additionally, information can be distributed to any number of users immediately, saving time and the expense of duplicating.

Computer Components

Whether operating a small microcomputer or interacting with a supercomputer, the user will employ the three basic components of any system. All computers must have a means to **input** information, a way to process information, and a method to output information.

INPUT

There are several ways to input or move information into a computer. The most common form used is a keyboard, much like a typewriter keyboard with additional keys for computer functions. Other methods of input include the light pen designed to read information on a computer screen and scanners programmed to read barcodes.

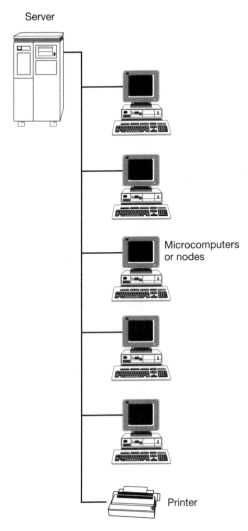

Server

Microcomputers
or nodes

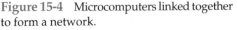
Printer

Figure 15-4   Microcomputers linked together
to form a network.

PROCESS

After information has been input, it is processed through a unit called the **central processing unit (CPU)**. This CPU, made up of many electrical components and microchips, has three elements as shown in Fig. 15-6. The communications and control unit manages or oversees the processing and completion of each task required by the operator. The arithmetic and logic unit (ALU) performs mathematical processes and makes decisions based on logical comparisons of input data. The third element, memory, may be of two types: **random access memory (RAM)** and **read only memory (ROM)**. **RAM** serves as temporary storage for data that will be lost when the computer is shut off. If the information needs to be kept for a later date, the operator must transfer it to a hard disk or diskettes. **ROM** storage is installed by the manufacturer; its purpose is to instruct the computer on how to begin the necessary operation requested by the user. Because ROM has characteristics of both hardware and software, the term "firmware" has been applied to it to lessen confusion.

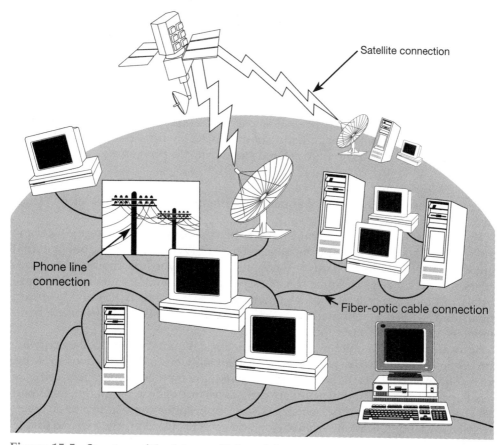

Figure 15-5 Structure of the Internet. (Adapted from Carey, P., & Ambrosia, A. (1995). *The internet*. Cambridge, MA: Course Technology.)

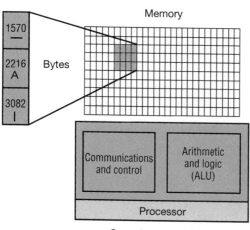

Figure 15-6 The three elements of the central processing unit, showing memory bytes (characters of data) represented by blocks that have been assigned a unique location in RAM. (Adapted from Trainor, D., & Krasnewich, D. (1994). *Computers!* New York: McGraw-Hill.)

OUTPUT

Output describes the return of processed information to the user or to someone in another location. Just as there are several ways to input information, there are several means by which processed data can be received. One of the most common ways is through a printer. When data are printed on paper, it is said to be "hard copy." Another output device is the monitor or **cathode ray tube (CRT),** which looks like a television screen and displays data as they are entered and during the processing.

Elements of the Computer

There are three elements that make up computer systems. These elements are called hardware, software, and storage.

Hardware is the equipment that is used to process data and includes the CPU and peripherals (all additional equipment attached to the CPU) used for the input or output of information. Examples of hardware peripherals are keyboards, monitors, bar code readers, scanners, tablets, facsimile machines, printers, and modems (devices that transfer data to other computers over telephone lines). A monitor (CRT) and keyboard combination is called a "terminal" (Fig. 15-7); these are necessary peripherals for minicomputers, mainframes, and supercomputers.

Software is the programming (coded instructions) required to control the hardware in processing of data. Two basic types exist: systems software and applications software. Systems software controls the normal operation of the computer. Applications software refers to programs prepared by software companies or in-house programmers to perform specific tasks required by users. Software applications come in five basic types: spreadsheets, communication systems, database systems, word processing, and graphics. Packages that perform more than one application, such as word processing, spreadsheet, and database, are called integrated software. The advantage of integrating applications is that it allows the different functions to be merged easily in one document.

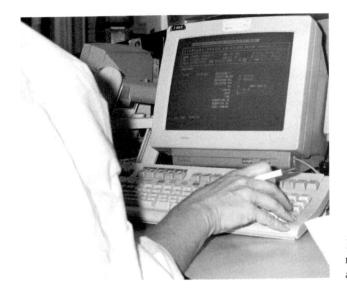

Figure 15-7 A computer terminal in the specimen-processing area of the laboratory.

Storage of information outside the CPU is necessary because RAM, as mentioned previously, is limited temporary storage which will be lost when the computer is turned off. Storage outside the CPU is called secondary storage. Examples of permanent secondary storage devices for documents and programs are diskettes, external hard drives, magnetic tapes, cartridges, and compact disks (CDs).

Computers and the Laboratory

As discussed previously, computers are accurate processors of information at incredible speeds. For this reason, computer systems in health care are considered more efficient and cost effective than relying on manual methods. Systems have been designed that will manage patient data and interface with automated analyzers and the main hospital information system. Competition between companies that sell lab information management systems (LIMS) is based on the ease of input, the format of output, and the availability of customized software. Extensive research goes into selecting the right computer system for specific laboratory needs. After selecting a vendor, it will take several months to bring a system **online** (make it operational). Usually one or two people are put in charge of the system's daily operation; they are called "system managers." These individuals have the responsibility to train other personnel in the laboratory and keep them updated as changes are made to the software. They must readily develop troubleshooting skills as they solve day-to-day problems that develop after the system is installed.

Today's health care facility may be totally integrated (connected) through networking of computers and a common software system. This means that patient demographics can be accumulated in a central database and shared with ancillary services such as radiology, dietary, pharmacy, and the laboratory, thus facilitating diagnosis and contributing to quality care of the patient. In the future, a totally integrated system will have an "electronic chart" and may make a paperless facility possible. With the emphasis on cost efficiency and total patient care, system integration has become a necessity to survive in the immediate health care environment.

General Computer Skills

General skills that the phlebotomist will learn, regardless of the LIMS that is used, are as follows:

- *Logging on.* Each person that is allowed on a system is given a password. This password uniquely identifies each person who is trying to "log on" (become a system user). Most systems require a username to be entered before the password. When the log-on sequence is completed, a **menu** will be displayed listing the options the user may choose from.
- *Cursor movement.* After logging on, a flashing indicator on the screen, called the **cursor**, indicates the starting point for input. When entering patient information in a LIMS, the cursor will automatically reset itself at the correct point for data input after the Enter key has been pressed.
- *Entering data.* Once the necessary information has been input, the Enter key must be pressed for information to be processed. If an error in spelling or selection is made, it can easily be deleted by back spacing before pressing the Enter key. If the wrong information is entered, however, it is still possible to correct errors.

- *Correcting errors*. This procedure is necessary to correct mistakes that are detected after the Enter key has been pressed. The procedure to delete errors is program dependent and must be learned with each system. Some LIMS programs use order verification, an additional step in the process, to allow a review of the information before it is accepted.
- *Verifying orders*. After all patient information has been entered, it will appear on the monitor screen as a complete order. At this point, the user can review the information again and can choose to modify, delete, or accept it. When all orders have been entered, the user can request an inquiry of the orders as still another check.
- *Inquiry about orders*. Requesting order inquiry allows the user to retrieve any or all of the test orders associated with a patient.
- *Deleting orders*. If, after entering an order, a user finds that it is not correct, he or she can request the computer delete or reject it. The command "delete" can also be used when an order is cancelled.

Laboratory Information Management Systems

The objectives of LIMS are to file results efficiently, accumulate statistics to determine workload, generate report forms, and monitor quality assurance in the laboratory. There are several types of systems on the market at this time (*eg*, Cerner, CHC, and Sunquest). Each type of information system allows users to define their own parameters for terms and conditions that make the system unique to that facility. Several programs within the system allow the users to do specific tasks, seemingly at the same time, such as (1) admit patients, (2) request test orders, (3) print labels, (4) enter results, and (5) inquire about results.

TECH CODE

In laboratory settings, users are given a **tech code** and a password. Passwords are used to gain access to the system. Passwords should be kept strictly confidential as the security associated with each password determines what system functions can be accessed. Passwords are also logged with every transaction on the system, allowing the system manager to identify the person performing each transaction. Tech codes, on the other hand, are used to further identify each person entering data into the system, mainly for the purpose of accruing workload. Tech codes do not need to be confidential. Often, phlebotomists do not verify their own collections. Rather, a data entry clerk may verify all collections and must have access to the list of tech codes so that he or she can associate the proper phlebotomist with each draw.

MNEMONIC CODES

The LIMS uses **mnemonic** (memory-aiding) codes, often in the form of abbreviations, to request the appropriate program or function necessary to enter data. For example, in the Sunquest Laboratory Information System, a phlebotomist would type the mnemonic RE (requisition entry) at the function prompt. This requisition entry program can be called by many different names, but it is basically the same procedure for any of the systems. During this data entry phase, an **accession number** is given to each requested order. This number is generated by the LIMS when the specimen request is entered into the computer and will be identified with the specimen as long as it is in the laboratory.

To create labels and collection lists for the phlebotomist to use in collecting the appropriate samples, it is necessary to use another program mnemonic, CLR (collection labels and reports). After collection has been accomplished, the phlebotomist returns to the laboratory and verifies the collection through another program, CLV (collection list verification). Other programs in the lab system that the phlebotomist might use are I (inquiry) to search for lab orders or results and DIS (discharge) to remove a patient from the system.

One of the mnemonic codes used in identifying tube types is always printed whenever a label is generated. For example, if the code on the label reads 5.0 mL LAV, the phlebotomist knows that a complete blood count is ordered and a lavender tube is required. This demonstrates one of the benefits of computerized label generation; the label aids the phlebotomist in acquiring the proper specimen in a timely fashion (Fig. 15-8).

The steps and program mnemonics Sunquest LIMS uses for processing a typical specimen, from arrival in the lab through reporting of results, are shown in Figure 15-9.

Figure 15-8 A computerized label generated when the requisition order is entered. (Courtesy Cerner Corp., Kansas City, MO.)

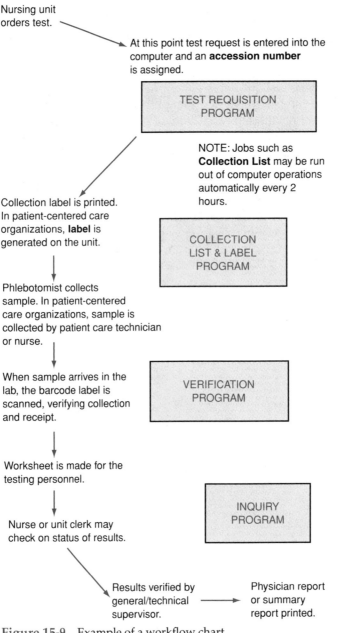

Nursing unit
orders test.

At this point test request is entered into the
computer and an **accession number**
is assigned.

TEST REQUISITION
PROGRAM

NOTE: Jobs such as
Collection List may be run
out of computer operations
automatically every 2
hours.

Collection label is printed.
In patient-centered care
organizations, **label** is
generated on the unit.

COLLECTION
LIST & LABEL
PROGRAM

Phlebotomist collects
sample. In patient-centered
care organizations, sample is
collected by patient care technician
or nurse.

When sample arrives in the
lab, the barcode label is
scanned, verifying collection
and receipt.

VERIFICATION
PROGRAM

Worksheet is made for the
testing personnel.

INQUIRY
PROGRAM

Nurse or unit clerk may
check on status of results.

Results verified by
general/technical
supervisor.

Physician report
or summary
report printed.

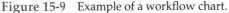

Figure 15-9   Example of a workflow chart.

Laboratory Computerization in the Future

Current trends in health care indicate that clinical laboratory operations will continue to decentralize and point-of-care testing will increase. The need for complete networking becomes even more apparent as remote laboratory testing facilities proliferate. Large reference laboratories, totally separate from the hospital, will need to download results from automated instruments into patient charts or centralized databases. Barcode label systems for the identification of patients and their samples, medication, and supplies will decrease the risk of human error. Hardware will improve with voice-activators that can be worn around a person's neck; optical scanners that will fit the hand; and sensors that read vitals signs, which will be displayed on the goggles of the health care worker.

Study & Review Questions

1. Which of the following is an example of proxemics?
   a. Eye contact
   b. Zone of comfort
   c. Facial expressions
   d. Personal hygiene

2. Which of the following is *not* one of the major elements in health care communication?
   a. Confirmation
   b. Empathy
   c. Deliberation
   d. Trust

3. The best way to handle a "bad" patient is to
   a. refuse to collect specimens from the patient.
   b. help the patient to feel in control of the situation.
   c. tell the patient that you will report him or her to your superiors.
   d. talk sharply to the patient and let him or her know that you are the one in control.

4. Which of the following is proper telephone protocol?
   a. Wait for the phone to ring three or four times so as not to appear anxious.
   b. Do not identify yourself in case there are problems later.
   c. Be careful of the tone of voice used and keep answers simple.
   d. Listen carefully; do not take notes because it takes too much time.

5. A computer, such as the Macintosh, often found in the home is called a
   a. mainframe.
   b. microcomputer.
   c. minicomputer.
   d. supercomputer.

6. Peripherals on a computer include all of the following *except* a
   a. bar code reader.
   b. scanner.
   c. modem.
   d. CPU.

7. To log on to most computer systems requires the use of
   a. an accession number.
   b. a bar code reader.
   c. a modem.
   d. a password.

8. Mnemonics are
   a. memory-aiding codes.
   b. hardware.
   c. programs.
   d. questions.

Suggested Laboratory Activities

1. Practice verbal and nonverbal communication by role-playing with a fellow student.

2. Practice proper telephone communication skills.

3. Practice working with a computer.

4. Using a simulated hospital computer system, practice admitting patients, requesting tests, and verifying test collection.

5. Identify the coded information on a computer label.

BIBLIOGRAPHY AND SUGGESTED READINGS

Chambers, D. W., & Abrams, R. G. (1986). *Dental communication.* Stamford, CT: Appleton-Century-Crofts.

Cronbach, L. J. (1963). *Educational psychology* (2nd ed.). New York: Harcourt, Brace and World.

Egan, G. (1970). *Encounter: Group process for interpersonal growth.* CA: Wadsworth.

Fast, J. (1977). *The body language of sex, power and aggression.* New York: M. Evans and Co.

Montagu, A. (1986). *Touching: The human significance of the skin.* (3rd ed.). New York: Harper & Row.

Northouse, P. G., & Northouse, L. L. (1992). *Health communication: Strategies for health professionals* (2nd ed.). Stamford, CT: Appleton & Lange.

Purtilo, R. (1984). *Health professional/patient interaction* (3rd ed.). Philadelphia: W. B. Saunders.

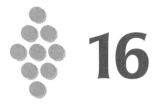

16

Laboratory Mathematics

KEY TERMS

blood volume	Fahrenheit (F)	meter	military time
Celsius (C)	gram	metric system	Roman numeral
centigrade	liter		

OBJECTIVES

Upon successful completion of this chapter, the reader will be able to:

1. Name basic metric units and prefixes.
2. Convert English units to metric units and vice versa.
3. Describe how to convert larger metric units to smaller units and vice versa.
4. Define military time and convert 12-hour time to 24-hour time.
5. Convert Fahrenheit temperature to Celsius temperature and vice versa.
6. Convert Roman numerals to Arabic (common) numbers.
7. Calculate percentages and describe how to prepare a 10% dilution.
8. Calculate adult and infant blood volumes.

INTRODUCTION

Aside from basic proficiency in addition, subtraction, multiplication, and division, it is helpful to the phlebotomist to understand systems of measurement, associated terminology, and calculations commonly encountered in the medical laboratory.

THE METRIC SYSTEM

The **metric system** is the system of measurement used in the health care industry. The metric system derives its name from its fundamental unit of distance, the **meter**

(M or m). In the metric system, the meter is the basic unit of linear measure, the **gram** (G or g) is the basic unit of weight, and the **liter** (L or l) is the basic unit of volume.

The metric system is a **decimal system** (a system based on the number 10). In a decimal system, units larger or smaller than the basic units are arrived at by multiplying or dividing by 10 or powers of 10.

In the metric system, prefixes added to the basic units indicate larger or smaller units. Prefixes are the same whether or not the units are meters, grams, or liters. Table 16-1 shows prefixes commonly used in the medical laboratory.

Basic metric units (grams, meters, liters) can be converted to larger units by moving the decimal point to the *left* according to the appropriate multiple. The multiple is the value of the exponent. The exponent is a number that indicates how many times a number is multiplied by itself. For example, a kilogram is 1,000 or $10 \times 10 \times 10$ or 10^3 grams. The multiple, determined by the exponent, is three.

Example: Convert 100 grams to kilograms.

From Table 16-1 we determine that 1 kg is equal to 1,000 or 10^3 g. The multiple is three. Therefore, to convert 100 grams to kilograms, move the decimal point three places to the left:

100 g = 100.0 = 0.1 kg

To convert basic metric units to smaller units, move the decimal point to the *right* the appropriate multiple.

Example: Convert 100 grams to milligrams.

From Table 16-1, we see that 1 mg is equal to 10^{-3} g. The multiple is a minus three. We therefore move the decimal point three spaces to the right:

100 g = 100.000 = 100,000 mg

Metric units other than basic units can be converted to larger units by moving the decimal point to the *left* according to the appropriate multiple, determined by subtracting the value of the exponent of the desired unit from the value of the exponent of the existing unit.

Example: Convert 200 milligrams to kilograms.

Table 16-1
Commonly Used Measurement Prefixes

| | | Unit of Measure | | |
		meter (m)	*gram (g)*	*liter (l)*
Prefix	*Multiple*			
kilo- (k)	1,000 (10^3)	km	kg	kL
deci- (d)	1/10 (10^{-1})	dm	dg	dL
centi- (c)	1/100 (10^{-2})	cm	cg	cL
milli- (m)	1/1,000 (10^{-3})	mm	mg	mL
micro- (μ)	1/1,000,000 (10^{-6})	μm	μg	μL

From Table 16-1, we determine that 1 mg is 10^{-3} and 1 kg is 10^3. The desired unit is kilograms; therefore, subtract -3 from 3:

$$3 - (-3) = 3 + 3 = 6$$

We are going from a smaller unit to a larger unit, so the decimal point moves to the left.

200 mg = 000200. = 0.0002 kg

Metric units other than basic units can be converted to smaller units by moving the decimal point to the *right* according to the appropriate multiple, determined by subtracting the value of the exponent of the desired unit from the value of the exponent of the existing unit.

Example: Convert 25 centimeters to micrometers.

From Table 16-1, we determine that 1 cm is 10^{-2} and 1 µm is 10^{-6}. The desired unit is micrometers; therefore subtract -6 from -2:

$$-2 - (-6) = -2 + 6 = 4$$

We are going from a larger unit to a smaller unit, so the decimal point moves to the right.

25 cm = 25.0000 = 250,000 µm

It is often necessary to convert our English system of units to metric units. Table 16-2 lists English units and their metric equivalents commonly encountered in the health care setting.

To convert from English units to metric units, multiply by the factor listed. Metric units can be converted back to English units by dividing by the same factor or multiplying by the factor in the metric conversion chart.

Example: Convert 200 pounds to kilograms.

Table 16-2
English–Metric Equivalents

	English		*Metric*
Distance	yard (yd)	=	0.9 meters (m)
	inch (in)	=	2.54 centimeters (cm)
Weight	pound (lb)	=	0.454 kilograms (kg) or 454 grams (g)
	ounce (oz)	=	28 grams (g)
Volume	quart (qt)	=	0.95 liters (L)
	fluid ounce (fl oz)	=	30 milliliters (mL)
	tablespoon (tbsp)	=	15 millimeters (mL)
	teaspoon (tsp)	=	5 milliliters (mL)

1 pound is equal to 0.454 kg.

Therefore, multiply 200 × .454 to arrive at 90.8 kg.

Table 16-3 shows the common equivalents for converting metric units to English units.

To convert metric units to English units, multiply by the factor listed. To convert English units back to metric, divide by the same factor or multiply by the factor in the English unit conversion chart.

Example: Convert 15 mL to teaspoons.

1.0 mL is equal to ⅕ tsp.

Therefore, multiply 15 × ⅕ to arrive at ¹⁵⁄₅ or 3 tsp (or 15 × 0.2 = 3.0 tsp).

MILITARY TIME

Most hospitals use **military** (or European) **time**, which is based on a clock with 24 numbers instead of 12 (Fig. 16-1). Twenty-four-hour time eliminates the need for designating AM or PM. Each time is expressed by four digits. The first two digits represent hours, and the second two digits represent minutes. Twenty-four-hour time begins at midnight (0000) and ends at 2359. One AM is 0100, 2 AM is 0200, and so on. Noon is 1200; 1 PM is 1300.

To convert regular (12-hour) time to 24-hour time, *add* 12 hours to the time from 1 PM on.

Example: 1:00 PM becomes 1:00 + 12 hours = 1300 hours.

5:30 PM becomes 5:30 + 12 hours = 1730 hours.

To convert 24-hour time to 12-hour time, *subtract* 12 hours after 1 PM.

Example: 1300 hours becomes 1300 − 12 hours = 1:00 PM.

Table 16-3
Metric–English Equivalents

	Metric		English
Distance	meter (m)	=	3.3 feet / 39.37 inches
	centimeter (cm)	=	0.4 inches
	millimeter (mm)	=	0.04 inches
Weight	gram (g)	=	.0022 pounds
	kilogram (kg)	=	2.2 pounds
Volume	liter (L)	=	1.06 quarts
	milliliter (mL)	=	.03 fluid ounces
	milliliter (mL)	=	.20 or 1/5 tsp

Note: A milliliter (mL) is approximately equal to a cubic centimeter (cc) and the two terms are often used interchangeably.

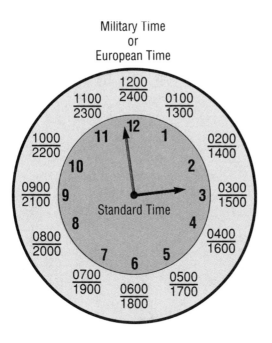

Military Time
or
European Time

Figure 16-1 Clock showing 24-hour (military) time.

TEMPERATURE MEASUREMENT

Two different temperature scales (Fig. 16-2) are used in the health care setting. The **Fahrenheit (F)** scale is used to measure body temperature, whereas the **Celsius (C)**, also known as the **centigrade**, scale is used to measure temperatures in the laboratory.

- Fahrenheit: The freezing point of water is 32° F, and the boiling point is 212° F. Normal body temperature expressed in Fahrenheit is 98.6° F.
- Celsius/centigrade: The freezing point of water is zero (0° C) and the boiling point is 100° C. Normal body temperature expressed in the Celsius scale is 37° C.

The following formulas can be used to convert from one temperature scale to the other:

Celsius temperature = ⅝ (°F − 32)
Fahrenheit temperature = ⅝ (°C + 32)

ROMAN NUMERALS

In the **Roman numeral** system, letters represent numbers. Roman numerals may be encountered in procedure outlines, in physician's orders or prescriptions, and in the identification of values or substances such as coagulation factors.

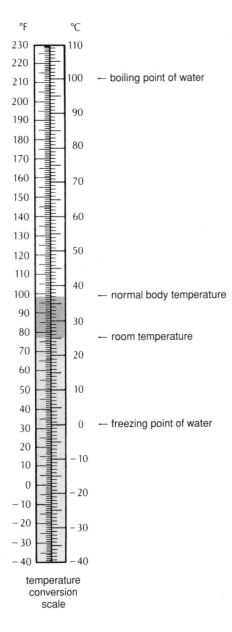

°F   °C

— boiling point of water

— normal body temperature

— room temperature

— freezing point of water

temperature
conversion
scale

Figure 16-2 Thermometer showing both Fahrenheit and Celsius degrees. (Memmler RL, Cohen BJ, Wood DL.)

The basic Roman numeral system consists of the following seven capital (or lowercase) letters:

I (i) = 1
V (v) = 5
X (x) = 10
L (l) = 50

C (c) = 100
D (d) = 500
M (m) = 1,000

Guidelines for Interpreting Roman Numerals

1. When numerals of the same value follow in sequence, the values should be added. There should never be more than three of the same numeral in a sequence.

   Example: III = 1 + 1 + 1 = 3

   XX = 10 + 10 = 20

2. When a lower-value numeral precedes a numeral with a higher value, the lower value should be subtracted from the higher value. Numerals V, L, and D are never subtracted. No more than one lower-value number should precede a higher-value number.

   Example: IV = 5 − 1 = 4

   IX = 10 − 1 = 9

3. When a numeral is followed by one or more numerals of lower value, the values should be added.

   Example: XI = 10 + 1 = 11

   VII = 5 +1 + 1 = 7

4. When a lower-value numeral comes between two higher-value numerals, it is subtracted from the numeral following it.

   Example: XIX = 10 + 10 − 1 = 19

   XXIV = 10 + 10 + 5 − 1 = 24

5. Roman numerals are written from left to right in order of decreasing value (except for numerals that are to be subtracted from subsequent numerals).

   Example: XXVII = 10 + 10 + 5 + 1 + 1 = 27

   MCMXCII = 1,000 + (1,000 − 100) + (100 − 10) + 1 + 1 = 1992

6. A line over a Roman numeral means multiply the numeral by 1,000.

   Example: $\overline{V}$ = V × 1,000 = 5,000

PERCENT

Percent means per 100 and is represented by the symbol %.

Two values are involved when a number is expressed as a percentage. They are the number itself, and 100.

Example: 10% means 10 per 100 or 10 parts in a total of 100 parts.

To change a fraction to a percentage, multiply by 100 and add a percent sign to the result.

Example: Change ¾ to a percentage.

$$¾ \times {}^{100}\!/_{1} = {}^{300}\!/_{4} = 4\overline{)300}^{\,75} = 75\%$$

DILUTIONS

The concentration of laboratory reagents is often expressed as a percentage. For example, a solution of 70% isopropyl alcohol is used in skin cleansing prior to blood collection.

A 10% dilution of bleach (5.25% sodium hypochlorite) is used to disinfect countertops and other surfaces.

A 10% dilution of bleach means that there are 10 parts of bleach in a solution containing a total of 100 parts. The above dilution can also be expressed as a ratio, showing the relationship between the part of the solution and the total solution. A 10% solution is also a 1:10 solution or one part bleach in a total of 10 parts solution. A dilution of 10 parts in a total of 100 parts is the same as 1 part in a total of 100 parts, or a 1:10 (1 to10) dilution.

A 10% dilution of bleach can be prepared by adding 10 mL bleach to 90 mL water, resulting in a total of 100 mL of bleach solution. The same percentage dilution would result from adding 1 mL bleach to 9 mL water or 20 mL bleach to 180 mL water, and so on.

BLOOD VOLUME

Blood volume in adults is generally stated as 5.0 quarts or 4.75 liters (L). Because people are not the same size, common sense tells us that they should not all have 5 quarts of blood. Actual blood volume is based on weight. Blood volume can be calculated for any size person from infant to adult, as long as the weight of the person is known.

Adult Blood Volume

Adult blood volume is 70 mL per kg of weight.

Example: Calculate the amount of blood volume for a man who weighs 250 lb.

---

1. Change the weight in pounds to kilograms.

   Because 1 lb = .454 kg, you need to multiply 250 lb by .454 to arrive at 113.5 kg.

2. Next, multiply the number of kilograms by 70 because there are 70 mL of blood for each kg of weight.

   113.5 kg × 70 mL/kg = 7,945 mL

3. Because blood volume is reported in liters rather than milliliters, divide the total number of mL by 1,000 (1 liter = 1000 mL).

   Blood volume = 7,945 mL/1,000 mL = 7.945 L or 7.9 L

Infant Blood Volume

     It is very important to be able to estimate the blood volume of an infant, especially if that infant is in an intensive care unit where blood samples may be taken several times a day. A very small infant can become anemic if not monitored closely. Removal of more than 10% of an infant's blood volume in a short amount of time can lead to serious consequences including cardiac arrest.

     An infant's blood volume is 100 mL per kg.

Example: Calculate the blood volume of a baby who weighs 5.5 lb.

---

1. Change the weight from pounds to kilograms using the same formula as for adults.

    5.5 lb × .454 = 2.5 kg

2. Multiply 2.5 kg by 100 for total blood volume in milliliters.

    2.5 kg × 100 = 250 mL

3. Change blood volume in mL/kg to liters.

    250 mL/1,000 mL = 0.25 L

Study & Review Questions

1. An RBC is approximately 7 micrometers in diameter. What is its size in centimeters?

2. A PPD test reaction measures 12.5 millimeters in diameter. How many inches is this?

3. Your requisition says that a specimen must be drawn at 1530. What time would that be in standard time?

4. A specimen must be transported at body temperature (98.6° F). The thermometer in the heat block reads 30° C. Is the heat block warm enough to transport the specimen?

5. Your book says that Factor VIII is the antihemophilic factor. What common (Arabic) number is this factor?

6. Your test paper shows that you correctly answered 45 out of a total of 50 questions. What is your grade expressed as a percent?

7. How would you prepare 500 mL of a 1:10 dilution of bleach?

8. Calculate the blood volume of an infant weighing 4 lb 12 oz.

Suggested Laboratory Activities

1. Practice converting English units to metric units.

2. Fill one of each of the various sizes of tubes with water using a teaspoon, tablespoon, and so on, and record the results.

3. Practice converting 12-hour time to 24-hour time and vice versa.

4. Compare a centigrade thermometer with a Fahrenheit thermometer. Record the actual temperature of the classroom or lab in both Fahrenheit and centigrade.

5. Prepare a 1:10 dilution of bleach.

6. Perform the calculations needed to determine an infant's and an adult's blood volume.

BIBLIOGRAPHY AND SUGGESTED READINGS

Bishop, M. L., Duben-Engelkirk, J. L., & Fody, E. P. (1996). *Clinical chemistry: Principles, procedures, correlations* (2nd ed.). Philadelphia: Lippincott-Raven Publishers.

Campbell, J., & Campbell, J. (1984). *Laboratory mathematics: Medical and biological applications* (3rd ed.). St. Louis: Mosby-Year Book Publishers.

Hayden, J., & Davis, T. (1996). *Fundamental mathematics for health careers* (3rd ed.). New York: Delmar Publishers.

Highers, M., & Forrester, R. (1987). *Mathematics for the allied health professions.* East Norwalk, CT: Appleton & Lange.

Glossary

AAAHP: American Association of Allied Health Professionals, Inc. Organization that approves phlebotomy programs, certifies phlebotomy personnel, and provides continuing education in phlebotomy.

ABO blood group system: A genetically determined blood group system that recognizes four blood types: A, B, AB, and 0, based on the presence or absence of the A and B antigens on the red blood cells.

accepting assignment: When a provider agrees to accept a fixed amount from an insurer as payment in full for a given service.

accession number: A unique number given to each test request.

accreditation: The process by which a professional or governmental agency evaluates an educational institution according to accepted criteria or standards to assure that graduates are qualified for professional employment.

activated coagulation time (ACT): Also referred to as activated clotting time, this procedure tests the activity of the intrinsic coagulation factors and is used to monitor heparin therapy.

additive: Any substance such as an anticoagulant, antiglycolytic agent, separator gel, cell preservative, or clot activator added to a blood collection tube. Additives do not include tube or closure coatings.

aerobic: With oxygen.

aerosol: A substance released in the form of a fine mist.

agglutinate: Clump together.

agglutination: An antigen–antibody reaction that causes clumping (such as seen when antibodies attach to antigens on the surface of the RBCs of a different blood type).

agglutinins: Antibodies present in the plasma of a person's blood that will react against and agglutinate RBCs carrying antigens of a different blood type.

agranulocytes: WBCs lacking easily visible granules.

airborne precautions: Precautions to follow in addition to standard precautions for patients known or suspected to be infected with microorganisms transmitted by airborne droplet nuclei. Anyone entering the room of a patient with airborne precautions must wear an N95 respirator.

albumin: A plasma protein manufactured by the liver that functions to help regulate osmotic pressure of the blood.

aliquot: A portion of a sample used for testing.

Allen test: A test performed to ascertain collateral blood flow to the hand prior to performing radial ABCs.

alveoli: Thin-walled, sac-like chambers in the lungs where the exchange of O_2 and CO_2 takes place between the air and blood.

ambulatory care: Care provided outside of inpatient institutions, or "care for the walking client."

amniotic fluid: The liquid in the amniotic sac that surrounds and cushions the fetus.

AMT: American Medical Technologists. Organization that approves phlebotomy programs, certifies phlebotomy personnel, and provides continuing education in phlebotomy.

anabolism: The process by which the body converts simple compounds into complex substances needed for the cellular activities of the body.

anaerobic: Without oxygen.

analyte: A general term for a substance undergoing analysis.

anatomic position: A way of referring to the body or body parts when the patient is standing erect, arms at the side, with palms and eyes facing forward.

ancillary blood glucose testing (ABGT): Instant or "rapid" glucose testing commonly performed using small, portable glucose analyzers. Also called bedside glucose testing.

anemia: An abnormal reduction in the number of RBCs in the circulating blood.

aneurysm: A localized dilatation or bulging in the wall of a blood vessel, usually an artery.

antecubital fossa: The area of the arm located anterior to and below the bend of the elbow, where the major veins for venipuncture are located.

antecubital veins: Major superficial arm veins located in the antecubital fossa.

anterior: Also called ventral, refers to the front.

antibody: Protein substance manufactured by the body as a response to a foreign protein or antigen and directed against it.

antibiotic susceptibility: Procedure to determine the ability of an antibiotic to slow or stop the growth of a specific microorganism.

anticoagulant: A substance that prevents blood from clotting.

antigen: A substance that causes the formation of antibodies that are directed against it.

antiglycolytic agent: A substance that inhibits the metabolism of glucose by the cells of the blood. The most common antiglycolytic agents are sodium fluoride and lithium iodoacetate.

antimicrobial therapy: Use of chemical substances to kill or stop the growth of microorganisms.

antiseptics: Germicidal solutions that are used to clean the skin prior to venipuncture or skin puncture.

anuclear: Without a nucleus.

aorta: The largest artery in the body, arising from the left ventricle of the heart and approximately 1 inch (2.5 cm) in diameter.

approval: A process similar to accreditation.

ARD: Antimicrobial Removal Device. A bottle containing a resin that removes antimicrobials and antibiotics from the blood.

arrhythmia: An irregularity in the heart rate, rhythm, or beat.

arterial blood gases (ABGs):   Evaluation of arterial blood to provide valuable information about a patient's oxygenation, ventilation, and acid–base balance, which is needed for the diagnosis and management of respiratory disease.

arterialized: Arterial composition of the specimen was increased by warming the collection site to increase arterial blood flow prior to specimen collection.

arteries: Thick-walled vessels that carry blood away from the heart.

arterioles: The smallest branches of arteries.

arteriosclerosis: A disease that involves thickening, hardening, and the loss of elasticity of artery walls.

arteriospasm: Involuntary contraction of an artery.

ASAP: As soon as possible.

ASCLS: The American Society for Clinical Laboratory Sciences. Organization that provides continuing education in phlebotomy.

ASCP: American Society of Clinical Pathologists. Certifying agency and professional organization for laboratory personnel.

ASMT: American Society for Medical Technology. Professional organization for laboratory personnel.

ASPT: American Society for Phlebotomy Technicians. Certifying agency and professional organization for phlebotomists.

assault: An intentional threat or movement that could make a person feel in danger of harmful physical contact.

atherosclerosis: A form of arteriosclerosis involving changes in the intima of the artery due to an accumulation of lipid material.

atria: The upper chambers on each side of the heart which receive blood before it enters the ventricles.

atrioventricular (AV) node: A structure located in the lower right atrium of the heart that slows conduction of the electrical pulse generated by the sinoatrial node, creating a slight delay before electrical impulses are carried to the ventricles.

atrioventricular valves: Valves at the entrance of the ventricles.

autologous donation: The process by which a person donates blood for his or her own use.

AV bundle (bundle of His): A group of cardiac muscle fibers that form part of the electrical impulse-conducting system of the heart.

A-V shunt: Arterial–venous passage artificially constructed to divert blood flow.

avascular: Containing no blood vessels.

bacteremia: Bacteria in the blood.

bactericidal: Kills bacteria.

bacteriostatic: Prevents or inhibits the growth of bacteria.

barriers: Anything, such as personal bias or cultural diversity, that interferes with communication.

basal state: Metabolic state early in the morning, while the body is still at rest, and approximately 12 hours after the last intake of food, exercise, or activity.

basilic vein: The large vein on the inner side of the arm in the antecubital fossa. The third-choice vein for venipuncture.

basophils: The least numerous of the WBCs, comprising less than 1% of the WBC population. The granules of basophils are large, stain dark blue, and often obscure the nucleus.

battery: Intentional, unconsented-to physical contact with one person by another person.

bedside manner: Behavior by a phlebotomist that puts the patient at ease while the phlebotomist performs his or her duties.

bevel: The point of the needle that has been cut on a slant for ease of entry.

biconcave: Indented from both sides.

biohazard: Anything that is potentially harmful to the environment and man.

bleeding time (BT): The time required for blood to stop flowing from a standardized incision. The BT is dependent on platelet plug formation in the capillaries, and is measured to determine platelet and vascular function.

bloodborne pathogen: A term applied to any infectious microorganism present in the blood and other body fluids and tissues.

bloodborne pathogen standard: OSHA's regulations for all employees with occupational exposure to pathogens found in the blood.

blood pressure: A measure of the force exerted by the blood on the walls of blood vessels.

blood smear: A drop of blood spread into a thin film on a microscope slide. Also called a blood slide.

blood volume: An individual's calculated amount of blood based on the individual's body weight. In adults it is calculated on 70 mL of blood per kilogram of body weight, and in infants, on 100–110 mL per kilogram of body weight.

B-lymphocytes: WBCs that give rise to plasma cells which produce antibodies.

body cavities: Large hollow spaces that house various organs of the body.

body plane: A flat surface determined by making a real or imaginary cut through a body in the normal anatomic position.

body substance isolation (BSI): Recently proposed modification of routine patient care practices augmented by elements of disease-specific precautions for bloodborne pathogens. Used for all patients.

brachial artery: Main artery of the arm, which is located in the medial anterior aspect of the antecubital fossa near the insertion of the biceps muscle.

bradycardia: A slow heart rate, less than 60 beats per minute.

breach of confidentiality: An unauthorized release of information concerning a patient.

bundle of His: Part of the electrical conduction system of the heart. It is located between the ventricles, and conducts impulses from the AV junction to the right and left bundle branches.

butterfly needle: *See* winged infusion set.

calcaneus: Heel bone.

calcium (Ca): A mineral needed for proper bone and teeth formation, nerve conduction, and muscle contraction, and essential to the clotting process.

cannula: A temporary surgical connection between an artery and a vein, used for dialysis and blood drawing.

CAP: College for American Pathologists.

capillaries: Tiny vessels, one cell layer thick, that connect the arterioles and venules and allow the exchange of oxygen and nutrients between the cells and the blood.

capillary action: Process by which blood is drawn up, by contact only, into a small tube.

capillary blood gases: Blood gas determinations performed on arterialized capillary (skin puncture) specimens.

capitation: A method of reimbursement in which the provider is paid an established fee for each patient in a panel or group of assigned patients.

Caraway tubes: Disposable, glass microcollection tubes.

carbaminohemoglobin (HbCO$_2$): Hemoglobin combined with CO_2.

cardiac cycle: One complete contraction and subsequent relaxation of the heart, with each cycle lasting approximately 0.8 seconds.

cardiac output: The volume of blood pumped by the heart in 1 minute: approximately 5 liters per minute.

cardiopulmonary resuscitation (CPR): Revival of heart and lung activity after they have stopped functioning.

catabolism: The process by which complex substances in food are broken down into simple substances.

catheter: A tube passed through the body for injecting or withdrawing fluids from body cavities or blood vessels.

catheterized specimen: A urine specimen collected from a sterile catheter inserted through the urethra into the bladder.

causative agent: In infection control, the pathogen responsible for causing an infection.

CDC: Centers for Disease Control and Prevention. A division of the U.S. Public Health Service that investigates diseases that have epidemic potential.

Celsius: A temperature scale on which melting point is 0 degrees and boiling point is 100 degrees. Normal body temperature expressed in Celsius (or Centigrade) is 37 degrees. Also known as the Centigrade scale.

Centigrade: *See* Celsius.

central processing: Also called specimen processing, where all specimens are received and prepared for testing.

centrifugation: A process of separating substances of different densities, such as blood and urine, by using a centrifuge (a machine that spins substances at high speeds).

cephalic vein: The second-choice vein for venipuncture, located in the lateral aspect of the arm in the antecubital fossa.

cerebrospinal fluid (CSF): A clear, colorless liquid that circulates in the cavities surrounding the brain and spinal cord, which has many of the same constituents as blood plasma.

certification: A process that indicates the completion of defined academic and training requirements, and the attainment of a satisfactory score on a national examination.

chain of custody: Special protocol for forensic specimens that must be strictly followed; requires documentation that the specimen is accounted for at all times.

chain of infection: A series of related events that leads to infection.

Chordae tendineae: Thin threads of tissue which attach the AV valves to the walls of the ventricles.

circulatory system: Also called the cardiovascular system. Consists of the heart, blood, and blood vessels, along with the lymph, lymph vessels, and nodes (lymphatic system).

civil law: The law of private rights between persons or parties.

clay sealant: Special clay used to seal one or both ends of microcollection tubes after specimen collection.

clean-catch: Method of obtaining a urine sample so that it is free of contaminating matter from the external genital areas.

CLIA '88: Clinical Laboratory Improvement Amendments, signed into federal law in 1988, mandating that all laboratories be regulated using the same standards—regardless of their location, type, or size.

clot activator: Clot-enhancing substance, such as siliceous earth, silica, or celite.

coagulation: Blood-clotting process.

coinsurance: A percentage of the bill in an indemnity plan; in HMOs, this copayment is a fee that is required at the time of service for an office visit.

cold agglutinin: An antibody that attaches to red blood cells and causes them to clump together or agglutinate at temperatures below body temperature.

collapsed vein: An abnormal retraction of the vessel walls.

collateral circulation: A process that allows tissue to be supplied with blood from an accessory vessel.

combining form: A word root, along with a combining vowel, that can be attached to a suffix or another word root.

combining vowel: A vowel (usually an "o") that joins a word root to a suffix, or to another word root, to ease pronunciation.

compatibility: Able to be mixed together with favorable results, such as in blood transfusions.

concentric circles: Beginning from the center and moving outward in ever-widening even circles.

contact precautions: Precautions used in addition to standard precautions when a patient is known or suspected to be infected or colonized with epidemiologically important microorganisms that can be transmitted by direct contact with the patient, or indirect contact with surfaces or patient-care items.

continuing education units (CEUs):   Credits given for workshops and seminars, offered to continually upgrade skills and knowledge.

coring: Removal of a portion of the skin or vein.

coronary arteries: The first branches off of the aorta, just beyond the aortic semilunar valve, which supply blood to the heart muscle.

cost shifting: Term used to describe how providers attempt to make up for reduced reimbursements from government-paid programs by charging more to other payers.

CPU: Central Processing Unit. Handles input/output, *ie,* manipulation and calculation of data.

CQI: Continuous Quality Improvement. An ongoing commitment by all levels of the administrative structure of an organization to improve all aspects of that organization. The objective of CQI in a health care facility is to enhance patient care and improve patient outcomes.

crossmatch: A compatibility test performed before a unit of blood is determined to be suitable for transfusion.

CRT: Cathode Ray Tube. Monitor or screen for displaying computer output.

culture & sensitivity (C&S):   The process by which organisms are grown on media and identified, and an antibiotic susceptibility (sensitivity) test is performed to determine which antibiotics will be effective against the organism.

cursor: A flashing marker on the CRT that indicates where the next key stroke will appear.

cyanotic: Pertaining to cyanosis or blue-gray discoloration of the skin due to lack of oxygen.

data: Information collected for analysis or computation.

decimal system: System based on the number 10. In a decimal system, units larger or smaller than the basic units are arrived at by multiplying or dividing by 10 or powers of 10.

dermis: Corium or true skin; a layer composed of elastic and fibrous connective tissue.

diabetes insipidus: A condition characterized by increased thirst and increased urine production, caused by inadequate secretion of ADH.

diabetes mellitus: A condition in which there is impaired carbohydrate, fat, and protein metabolism due to a deficiency of insulin.

diagnostic-related groups (DRGs):   A system of disease classification used to determine PPS rates for reimbursement purposes.

diastole: The relaxation phase of the cardiac cycle.

diastolic pressure: The pressure on the arteries during relaxation of the ventricles;

averages 80 mm Hg, and is an estimate of systemic vascular resistance.

differential: Determination of the number and characteristics of cells on a smear by staining and examining the cells under a microscope.

discard tube: Also called "clear tube." A tube used to collect and discard approximately 5 mL of blood, to prevent IV or tissue fluid contamination of a specimen.

disinfectants: A solution containing an agent intended to kill or irreversibly inactivate microorganisms (but not necessarily their spores). Disinfectants are used on surfaces and instruments, and generally are not safe for use on human skin.

distal: Farthest from the center of the body, origin, or point of attachment.

diurnal (daily) variations: Normal fluctuations throughout the day.

dorsal: Posterior or pertaining to the back.

dorsal cavities: Internal spaces located in the back of the body.

droplet precautions: Precautions used in addition to Standard Precautions for patients known or suspected to be infected with microorganisms transmitted by droplets (particles larger than 5 μ in size), generated when a patient talks, coughs, or sneezes, and during certain procedures.

edema: An accumulation of fluid in the tissues.

electrocardiogram (EKG or ECG): An actual record of the electrical currents that correspond to each event in the heart muscle contraction.

electrolytes: Substances, such as potassium or sodium, that conduct electricity when dissolved in water.

electrical safety: Rules related to the safe use of electrical equipment.

embolism: Obstruction of a blood vessel by an embolus.

embolus: A blood clot, part of a blood clot, or other mass of undissolved matter circulating in the blood stream.

empathy: Objective insight into the emotions and feelings of another person.

endocardium: A thin membrane lining the heart that is continuous with the lining of the blood vessels.

engineering controls: One of the primary methods used to control the transmission of HBV, HIV, and other blood-borne pathogens by removing or isolating the hazard, or isolating the worker from exposure.

entitlements: A right earned by individuals through employment, such as Social Security or Worker's Compensation.

epicardium: The thin outer layer of the heart, continuous with the lining of the pericardium.

epidermis: The outermost and thinnest layer of the skin.

Environmental Protection Agency (EPA): The federal agency that regulates the disposal of waste.

eosinophils (eos): Granular leukocytes whose granules are beadlike and stain bright orange-red with the eosin acid stain.

erythema: Redness.

erythrocyte: A mature, anuclear, biconcave, disk-shaped blood cell that is responsible for transporting oxygen to the cells of the body, and transporting carbon dioxide away from the cells. Also called red blood cell (RBC).

erythropoietin: Hormone secreted by the kidneys which stimulates red blood cell production.

essentials: Educational standards set forth by accrediting agencies.

ethanol: Ethyl or grain alcohol when referred to as part of a blood alcohol test.

evacuated tubes: Premeasured vacuum tubes that receive the patient's blood during the venipuncture procedure.

expressed consent: Consent expressed verbally or in writing, used for proposed treatment involving surgery, experimental drugs, or high-risk procedures. The written form must be signed by the person providing the treatment and the patient, and be witnessed by a third party. If consent is given verbally, the treatment provider should make an entry in the patient's chart of what was discussed with the patient.

external respiration: The process by which O_2 from the air enters the bloodstream in the lungs, and CO_2 leaves the bloodstream and is breathed into the air from the lungs.

extrinsic pathway: A coagulation pathway initiated by the release of thromboplastin (factor III) from injured tissue and the activation of factor VII (proconvertin).

extravascular: Outside the bloodstream.

Fahrenheit: A scale used to measure body temperatures, based on the freezing point (32 degrees) and the boiling point (212 degrees) of water.

fasting: Abstinence from eating or drinking, except water, for approximately 12 hours prior to collection of the specimen.

feather: The thinnest area of a blood smear where the differential is performed.

femoral artery: Major systemic artery located superficially in the groin, lateral to the pubis bone.

fibrin: A filamentous protein formed by the action of thrombin on fibrinogen.

fibrin degradation products (FDP): Small fragments of partially digested fibrin found in the bloodstream.

fibrinogen: Also called factor I; a protein found in plasma that is essential for clotting of blood.

fibrinolysis: Process initiated by the activation of the clotting mechanism that releases substances that lead to the dissolution of the fibrin clot.

fistula: A tube passing from a cavity or vessel to a free surface or another cavity. Also the term used to describe an artificial joining of an artery and a vein.

flanges: Extensions on the sides of an evacuated tube holder that aid in tube placement and removal.

flea: Small metal bar that is inserted into the tube after collection of a capillary blood gas specimen to aid in mixing the anticoagulant by means of a magnet.

floor book: Also called User Manual; a manual of instruction provided to the unit by the laboratory which describes preparation of the patient and special instructions for specimen collection.

fomite: Any substance that adheres to and transmits infectious material.

forensic specimen: Specimen collected for legal reasons.

fraud: A type of deceitful practice or willful plan resorted to with the intent to deprive another person of rights, or in some manner to cause that person injury.

frontal plane: Also called coronal plane; divides the body vertically into front and back portions.

FUO: Fever of unknown origin.

gastric analysis: A laboratory test that examines gastric acid secretions to determine gastric function in terms of stomach acid production.

gatekeeper: The primary care physician in a managed care plan, such as an HMO or PPO, who acts as the patient advocate in advising and coordinating the patient's health care needs.

gauge: A standard for measuring the diameter of the lumen of a needle.

germicide: An agent that kills pathogenic microorganisms.

glucose: Blood sugar.

glucose monitoring: A means of observing and recording blood sugar for the purpose of maintaining a normal level.

glucose tolerance test (GTT): A test used to diagnose carbohydrate metabolism problems.

glycolysis: Normal body reaction in which glucose is hydrolyzed or broken down by an enzyme.

gram: The basic unit of weight in the metric system; approximately equal to a cubic centimeter or milliliter of water.

granulocytes: WBCs with easily visible granules.

great saphenous vein: The longest vein in the body, located in the leg.

guaiac test: Also called occult blood; tests for blood in stool.

hardware: CPU, monitor, and all peripherals, such as barcode readers, modems, and joysticks.

HazCom: The abbreviation for the Hazardous Communication Standard, enacted in 1986 by OSHA, that requires employers to maintain documentation on all hazardous materials.

health maintenance organization (HMO): Group practice that is reimbursed on a prepaid, rather than a fee-for-service, basis.

hematocrit (Hct):   Percentage by volume of red blood cells in whole blood.

hematoma: A swelling or mass of blood (usually clotted) caused by blood leaking from a blood vessel during or following venipuncture or arterial puncture.

hemochromatosis: A disease characterized by excess iron deposits in the tissues.

hemoconcentration: A condition in which the plasma portion of the blood filters into the tissues, causing an increase in nonfilterable blood components such as RBCs, enzymes, iron, and calcium.

hemoglobin (Hb or Hgb):   An iron protein pigment found in red blood cells that carries O_2 and CO_2 in the blood stream.

hemolysis: The destruction of RBCs and the liberation of hemoglobin into the fluid portion of the specimen, causing the serum or plasma to be pink (slight hemolysis) to red (gross hemolysis) in color.

hemostasis: Process by which the body stops the leakage of blood from the vascular system.

hemostatic plug: Fibrin clot.

heparin lock: A special winged needle set that can be left in a patient's vein for up to 48 hours, used to administer medication and draw blood.

hepatitis: Inflammation of the liver, from toxic or viral origin.

Hepatitis B Virus (HBV):   The virus that causes Hepatitis B.

homeostasis: A "steady state" condition in which the body maintains its internal environment in a state of equilibrium or balance.

Hospital Infection Control Practices Advisory Committee (HICPAC):   Federal organization, established in 1991, that advises the CDC on updating guidelines regarding prevention of nosocomial infection.

human chorionic gonadotropin (HCG):   A hormone produced by the placenta that appears in both urine and serum, beginning approximately 10 days after conception.

Human Immunodeficiency Virus (HIV):   The virus that causes acquired immunodeficiency syndrome (AIDS).

hyperglycemia: Condition in which the blood sugar (glucose) is increased, as in diabetes mellitus.

hypoglycemia: A condition in which the blood sugar (glucose) is abnormally low, as in hyperinsulinism.

ID band: Identification bracelet.

identification cards: ID cards given to clinic patients, from which specimen labels can be imprinted using an Address-o-graph machine.

immunoglobulins: Antibodies that are released into the blood stream, where they circulate and attack foreign cells.

implied consent: Consent implied by actions of the patient. For example, if a phlebotomist explains that he or she is there to collect a blood specimen, and the patient holds out his arm, consent is assumed.

indemnity insurance: When the insurance company agrees to pay the health care provider a set amount of money.

induration: Hardness.

indwelling line: Tubing inserted into a main vein or artery, used primarily for administering fluids and medications.

infection: Invasion of a body by a pathogenic microorganism, resulting in injurious effects or disease.

inferior: Also referred to as caudal; beneath, lower, or toward the feet.

inflammation: Tissue reaction to injury, such as redness or swelling.

informed consent: Agreement by the patient to medical treatment after having received adequate information about the procedure, risks, and consequences.

inpatient care: Care performed in a health care setting where patients stay overnight.

input: Data that is entered into the CPU.

intravascular: Within the vascular system.

intrinsic pathway: A coagulation pathway involving coagulation factors circulating within the bloodstream, initiated with activation of Factor XII.

integumentary system: The skin and its appendages, including the hair and nails; also referred to as the largest organ of the body.

internal respiration: The process by which O_2 leaves the bloodstream and enters the cells, and CO_2 from the cells enters the bloodstream.

interstitial fluid: Fluid found between cells, or in spaces within an organ or tissue.

intracellular fluid: Fluid found within cell membranes.

iontophoresis: Introduction of various ions into the skin by electrical stimulation from electrodes placed on the skin.

ischemia: Temporary lack of blood flow to the heart due to obstruction.

isolation procedure: An infection-control procedure that separates patients with certain transmissible infections or diseases from other patients.

invasion of privacy: The violation of one's right to be left alone and to live without being subject to unwarranted or undesired publicity; includes the publishing or releasing of private information without the subject's permission.

Ivy Bleeding Time: A bleeding time test modified by Ivy in 1941; performed on the volar (inner) surface of the forearm using a blood pressure cuff to maintain constant pressure.

JCAHO: Joint Commission on Accreditation of Healthcare Organizations. A voluntary, nongovernmental agency charged with, among other things, establishing standards for the operation of hospitals and other health-related facilities and services.

keloid: Fibrous tissue growth at scar area of the skin.

kinesics: The study of body motion or language, such as facial expressions, gestures, and eye contact.

kinesic slip: When nonverbal messages don't match verbal messages.

lancet: A sterile, disposable, sharp-pointed instrument used to pierce the skin to obtain droplets of blood used for testing.

lateral: Toward the side.

leukemia: An increase in WBCs characterized by the presence of a large number of abnormal forms.

leukocytosis: An abnormal increase in WBCs in the circulating blood.

leukopenia: An abnormal decrease of WBCs in the circulating blood.

leukocyte: Also called white blood cell (WBC); round cell containing a nucleus whose main function is to combat infection and remove disintegrating tissue.

licensure: A process similar to certification, but offered by a governmental agency, granted through examination to a person who can meet the requirements for education and experience in that field.

lipemic: Cloudy serum or plasma caused by increased lipid content in the blood.

liter: The basic unit of volume in the metric system, which is equivalent to 1,000 mL.

local: Restricted to one place or part.

Luer adapter: In the Luer-Lok system, a device for connecting the syringe to the needle; when locked into place it gives a secure fit.

lumen: The internal space of a vessel or tube.

lymphocyte: A nongranular leukocyte; the second most numerous of the WBCs, comprising approximately 15% to 30% of the WBC population.

lymphostasis: A stoppage of lymph flow caused by lymph node removal.

lysis: Rupturing of red blood cells.

malpractice: A claim of improper treatment or negligence brought against a professional person by means of a civil lawsuit.

managed care: A variety of financial and organizational methods used to control the delivery of health care, ie, a predetermined monthly payment for providing services to patients is set up with physicians, hospitals, and other health care agencies. Consequently, the financial risk lies with the provider and not the insurer.

material safety data sheets (MSDS): Required written information on all products with a hazardous warning on the label.

medial: Toward the midline or middle.

median cubital vein: The vein located in the middle of the antecubital fossa area of the arm. The first-choice vein for venipuncture.

median cutaneous nerve: A major motor and sensory nerve in the arm that lies along the path of the brachial artery and in the vicinity of the basilic vein.

Medicaid: A program funded by the state and federal governments for providing medical care to the poor.

medical emergency (med emerg): Designation replacing "stat" for requesting tests that are needed in critical or "life or death" situations.

medical record number: The unique number given to a patient for purposes of identification.

Medicare: A federally funded program, enacted in 1965, that provides health care to people over the age of 65 and to the disabled, regardless of financial status.

megakaryocyte: A large cell that is formed in the bone marrow and is the precursor to platelet cells.

menu: A listing on the computer screen of options from which the user selects the program or process he or she needs.

meter: The basic unit of linear measurement in the metric system; equal to 39.37 inches.

metric system: A decimal system of weights and measures based on the basic meter, gram, and liter units.

metabolism: The sum of all the chemical reactions necessary to sustain life.

microbes: Microscopic organisms, or organisms not visible to the naked eye.

microcollection containers or tubes: Small plastic containers or tubes, often referred to as "bullets" because of their size and shape, that are primarily used to collect skin puncture blood specimens.

microhematocrit tubes: Disposable, narrow-bore glass or plastic tubes that fill by capillary action and are primarily used for hematocrit (packed cell volume) determinations on micro samples.

midstream collection: Specimen obtained during the middle of the urination rather than the beginning or end.

military time: Also called European time; based on a clock with 24 numbers instead of 12, eliminating the need for designating AM or PM.

milliliter (mL): A unit of volume measurement which is approximately equal to a cubic centimeter (cc); the two terms are often used interchangeably.

mnemonics: Memory-aiding codes, such as the abbreviations used to request the appropriate computer program or function necessary to process data.

monocytes (monos): The largest of the leukocytes, comprising from 1% to 7% of the WBC population.

modes of transmission: The route by which an organism is transferred from one host to another.

myocardial infarction (MI): Heart attack or death of heart muscle due to obstruction of the coronary artery.

myocardium: The thick, muscle layer of the heart.

NAACLS: National Accrediting Agency for Clinical Laboratory Sciences.

nasopharyngeal (NP) culture: A sample collected using a special NP swab, inserted gently through the nose into the nasopharynx area, to detect the presence of microorganisms such as those which cause diphtheria, meningitis, whooping cough, and pneumonia.

Natelson tubes: Microcollection tubes that are approximately 47 mm in length, and that fill by capillary action to a capacity of approximately 250 μ.

NCA: National Certification Agency. Certifies all levels of clinical laboratory personnel.

NCCLS: National Committee for Clinical Laboratory Standards. A national nonprofit organization, formed by representatives from the profession, industry, and government, that develops guidelines and sets standards for all areas of the laboratory.

needle sheath: Covering or cap of a needle.

negligence: The violation of a duty to exercise reasonable skill and care in performing a task.

neutrophils: Normally the most numerous of the WBCs; averaging 65% of the total WBC count, with granules that are fine in texture and that stain lavender.

newborn screening: Tests performed on neonates (newborns) to check for the presence of genetic or inherited diseases, such as phenylketonuria (PKU), hypothyroidism, galactosemia, homocystinuria, maple syrup urine disease, and sickle cell.

noninvasive: Not penetrating the skin.

nosocomial: Pertaining to a hospital or place of care for the sick.

nosocomial infection: An infection acquired in a health care institution.

occlusion: Obstruction.

occult blood: *See* guaiac test.

occupational exposure: An anticipated skin, eye, mucous membrane, or parenteral contact with blood or other potentially infectious materials that may result from the performance of the employee's duties.

on-line: When a computer system is operational.

order of draw: The special sequence in which multiple specimen tubes are collected during a draw or filled from a syringe; designed to reduce interference in specimen testing caused by carryover of additives between tubes, and to minimize the effects of tissue thromboplastin on coagulation specimens.

OSHA: Occupational Safety and Health Administration; a U.S. government agency that regulates the safety and health of workers.

osteochondritis: Inflammation of the bone and cartilage.

osteomyelitis: Inflammation of the bone (especially the bone marrow) caused by bacterial infection.

outpatient care: *See* ambulatory care.

output: Any data that flows from the CPU to peripherals.

ova & parasite (O & P): A stool sample for diagnosis of intestinal parasites.

oxyhemoglobin (HbO$_2$): Hemoglobin combined with O$_2$.

palmar surface: Palm side of the hand.

palpate: To examine by feel or touch.

parenteral: Any route other than the alimentary (digestive tract), ie, intramuscular, intravenous, or subcutaneous.

patency: State of being freely open, as in a patient's veins.

paternity test: A test to determine the probability that a specific individual fathered a particular child.

pathogen: An organism or substance capable of causing disease.

pathogenic: Capable of causing disease.

patient identification: The process by which a health care worker verifies the fact that a patient is the same as the one described on a requisition or work order.

Patient's Bill of Rights: The rights or privileges a patient has while in a hospital or other health care facility that are clearly defined in a document originally published in 1975 by the American Hospital Association.

peak level: Drug level collected when the highest serum concentration of the drug is anticipated, around 15–30 minutes after administration of the drug.

pediatric tubes: Small evacuated tubes designed to be used on small veins.

percutaneous: Delivered through the skin.

pericardial fluid: Fluid aspirated from the cavity surrounding the heart.

pericardium: A thin, fluid-filled sac surrounding the heart.

peritoneal fluid: Fluid aspirated from the abdominal cavity.

personal protective equipment (PPE): Disposable gloves, lab coats or aprons, and/or protective face gear, such as masks and goggles with side shields, required by OSHA to be worn when handling body fluids.

petechiae: Small, nonraised red spots which appear on a patient's skin under certain conditions, such as when a tourniquet is applied.

phagocytosis: A process by which bacteria and antigens are surrounded and engulfed by WBCs.

phlebitis: Inflammation of a vein.

phenylketonuria (PKU): A hereditary disease caused by the inability of the body to metabolize phenylalanine due to a defective enzyme. Mental retardation results if not treated early.

phlebotomy: The procedure for withdrawing blood from the body.

plasma: A clear, pale yellow fluid that is nearly 90% water (H$_2$O).

plantar surface: Bottom or sole of the foot.

platelet adhesion: The process by which platelets stick to injured surfaces.

platelet aggregation: The process by which platelets degranulate and stick to one another.

platelet plug formation: Platelet aggregation and adhesion to a blood vessel following an injury.

pleural fluid: Fluid aspirated from the pleural cavity which surrounds the lungs.

point-of-care testing: Testing done at the patient's bedside or virtually anywhere the patient happens to be, using portable or hand-carried instruments.

polycythemia: A disease characterized by an over-production of red blood cells.

polymorphonuclear (PMN): A term used to describe a type of WBC whose nucleus has several lobes or segments.

posterior: Also called dorsal, refers to the back.

postprandial (PP): After a meal.

potassium (K): A mineral that is essential for normal muscle activity and the conduction of nerve impulses.

pneumatic tube system: A unidirectional, continuously operating vacuum system that transfers specimens in plexiglass carriers from the patient units to the laboratory.

PPD: Purified protein derivative. *See* tuberculin test.

Preferred Provider Organization (PPO): An independent group of doctors and hospitals that offer their services to employers at discounted rates.

prefix: A word part that precedes a word root and modifies its meaning.

pre-op: Before an operation or surgery.

primary care: A type of service that originates with the family physician who offers the initial consult and related treatment.

primary hemostasis: First part of the coagulation process, which involves formation of a platelet plug.

procedural manual: A document required by JCAHO that states in detail the step-by-step procedure for each test or practice performed in the laboratory.

professionalism: The conduct and qualities that characterize a professional person.

prone: Lying horizontal, with the face down; the opposite of supine. Also denotes the hand with the palm down.

Prospective Payment System (PPS): A program begun in 1983 to standardize the Medicare/Medicaid payments made to hospitals by reimbursing hospitals a set amount for each patient procedure.

prothrombin: Protein in circulating blood, called factor II, that is involved in coagulation.

proxemics: The study of an individual's concept and use of space.

proximal: Nearest to the center of the body, origin, or point of attachment.

psychoneuroimmunology (PNI): A new field of medicine that deals with the study of interactions among the brain, the endocrine system, and the immune system.

pulmonary circulation: The system that carries blood from the heart to the lungs to remove carbon dioxide, and returns oxygenated blood to the heart.

pulse: A measurement of pressure created as the ventricles contract and blood is forced out of the heart and through the arteries.

pumping: Vigorous opening and closing of the fist.

QA Indicator: A monitor for all aspects of patient care; indicators must be measurable and cover high-volume procedures and high-risk situations.

quality assurance: A complete program that guarantees quality client care by tracking outcomes through scheduled audits in which the hospital looks at the appropriateness, applicability, and timeliness of patient care.

quality control (QC): A form of procedural control that is a component of a quality assurance program.

quantity not sufficient (QNS): Insufficient amount of substance required for testing.

radial artery: An artery located on the thumb side of the wrist, which is usually the first-choice, and therefore most common, site for arterial puncture.

random access memory (RAM): Temporary storage of data in the CPU that will be lost when power is discontinued, unless transferred to permanent storage.

read only memory (ROM): Firmware installed by the manufacturer. Its purpose is to instruct the CPU on how to begin the necessary operations requested by the user.

reciprocity: Granting of corresponding privileges, such as a state recognizing another state's license.

reference laboratory: An off-site laboratory to which specimens are referred for testing procedures not routinely done in-house.

reference laboratory log book: A manual for recording information including patient ID, date sent out, and date results were received for specimens sent to a reference laboratory.

reference laboratory manual: Information on ordering, handling, packaging, and transporting specimens sent to a reference laboratory.

reference values: Normal values for lab tests, usually established using basal state specimens.

reflux: A backward flow of blood into the patient's veins from the collection tube during the venipuncture procedure.

resheathing: To recap or replace the sheath on a needle.

respondeat superior: A Latin phrase which means "let the master respond." It is another way of saying that employers must answer for damages their employees cause within the scope of employment.

reticulocytes: Immature RBCs in the blood stream that contain nuclear remnants.

Rh antigen: A substance that, when present on the surface of RBCs, causes the formation of antibodies that interact specifically with it.

Rh immunoglobulins: A substance that, if given before as well as shortly after an Rh-negative mother delivers an Rh-positive baby, will prevent sensitization by destroying any Rh factor in the mother's bloodstream.

risk management: A department in organizations that identifies risk, and oversees the protection of employees, employers, and patients from the chance of injury or loss associated with the risk.

roman numeral: A letter used to represent a number.

sagittal plane: Divides the body vertically into right and left portions.

sclerosed: Hard, cordlike, and lacking resilience.

secondary care: Health care beyond primary care which until recently was considered inpatient service.

secondary hemostasis: Second stage of coagulation that involves formation of a tougher "fibrin" clot formed of RBCs, platelets, and fibrin.

semen analysis: Laboratory test used to assess fertility and to determine the effectiveness of sterilization following vasectomy.

semilunar valves: The crescent-shaped valves that control blood exiting the ventricles of the heart.

septicemia: Blood poisoning or pathogenic bacteria in the blood.

serum: A clear, pale yellow fluid that remains after blood clots and is separated. It has the same composition as plasma, except it does not contain fibrinogen.

service insurance: When the insurance company agrees to provide health care services in place of money to the patient.

sexually transmitted diseases (STDs): Diseases such as syphilis, gonorrhea, and genital herpes, which are usually transmitted by sexual contact.

sharps container: Special puncture-resistant, leak-proof, disposable containers used to dispose of used needles, lancets and other sharp objects.

sinoatrial (SA) node: A node, also called the pacemaker, located in the upper wall of the right atrium, which generates an electrical impulse that initiates contraction of the heart.

skin antisepsis: Destruction or inhibition of multiplication of microorganisms on the skin through use of antiseptics or germicides.

skin puncture: Collecting blood after puncturing the skin with a lancet or similar skin puncture device.

skin test: Intradermal injection of an allergenic substance to determine whether a patient has come in contact with a specific allergen (antigen) and developed antibodies against it.

sodium (Na): An extracellular ion in the blood plasma that helps maintain fluid balance.

software: Programs; for example, word processing, graphics, and games.

solutes: Dissolved substances.

sphygmomanometer: Blood pressure cuff.

standard of care: A prevailing set of standards set by licensing and regulatory agencies.

standard precautions: Guidelines recommended by the CDC and HICPAC to minimize the risk and spread of infection in hospitals. Standard precautions apply to blood, *all* body fluids (including all secretions and excretions except sweat, whether or not they contain visible blood), nonintact skin, and mucous membranes. The guidelines replace universal precautions and are to be used for the care of all patients.

STAT (stat):   A term derived from the Latin word "statim," meaning immediately.

statute of limitations: A time limit for filing a lawsuit after an alleged injury has occurred.

steady state: A stable condition; no exercise, suctioning, or respirator changes, for at least 30 minutes prior to obtaining blood gases.

subcutaneous layer: A layer of connective and adipose tissue that connects the skin to the surface of muscles.

suffix: The end of a word (word ending), that follows a word root and either changes the meaning of the word root or adds to it.

superior: Also referred to as cranial: higher, above, or toward the head.

supine: Lying on the back, face upward.

systemic: Affecting the entire body.

suprapubic aspiration: Collection of a urine specimen by inserting a needle into the urinary bladder and aspirating the urine directly from the bladder.

susceptible host: A person who has little resistance to an infectious disease.

sweat chloride: A test that uses iontophoresis to stimulate sweat production to evaluate chloride content in sweat. The test is used to diagnose cystic fibrosis, primarily in children and adolescents under the age of 20.

sweeps: Hospital rounds which occur at regular intervals throughout the day.

synovial fluid: Fluid aspirated from joint cavities.

syncope: Fainting.

systemic: Affecting the entire body.

systemic circulation: The system that carries oxygenated blood from the heart, along with nutrients, to all the cells of the body, and then returns to the heart carrying waste products from cellular metabolism.

systole: The contraction phase of the cardiac cycle.

systolic pressure: The pressure in the arteries during contraction of the ventricles, usually around 120 mm Hg.

tech code: Code given to computer users that uniquely identifies each user within the laboratory, and is recorded with all entries on the system.

tertiary care: Highly complex services and therapy that are performed on an inpatient basis, requiring the patient to stay overnight or longer.

test requisition: The form on which a test is ordered and sent to the lab.

therapeutic drug monitoring (TDM):   Process used by the physician to determine an effective drug dosage and to manage individual patient drug treatment.

therapeutic phlebotomy: The withdrawal of a large volume of blood as a treatment for certain medical conditions, such as polycythemia and hemochromatosis. It is performed in a manner similar to collecting blood from donors.

third party payer: A fiscal intermediary; most often an insurance company that pools individual contributions for a common group objective, eg, protection from financial disaster.

thixotropic gel: An inert (nonreacting) synthetic substance that prevents blood cells from continuing to metabolize substances in the serum or plasma by forming a physical barrier between the cellular portion of a specimen and the serum or plasma portion, once the specimen is centrifuged.

threshold values: Acceptable level for a quality assurance indicator.

thrombin: An enzyme formed from prothrombin that reacts with fibrinogen to form fibrin during the clotting process.

thrombocytes: Also known as platelets; the smallest of the formed elements in the bloodstream.

thrombocytopenia: Decreased platelets.

thrombocytosis: Increased platelets.

thrombophlebitis: Inflammation of a vein, particularly in the lower extremities, along with thrombus formation.

thrombus: Blood clot in a blood vessel.

T-lymphocytes: Specialized WBCs that play an important role in immunity by directly attacking infected cells.

tolerance test: A test of the body's ability to absorb and utilize a particular substance.

tort: A civil wrong or other breach of contract, ie, negligence or battery.

Total Quality Management (TQM): An institution-wide plan to assure quality care, mandated by JCAHO to be instituted by 1994, requiring all departments in the hospital to have ongoing evaluations that focus on quality of process rather than outcome.

trace elements: Metals or minerals, including aluminum, arsenic, copper, lead, iron and zinc, normally found in minute amounts.

transfusion reaction: A response to an incompatible blood transfusion resulting in antigen/antibody reactions that cause agglutination or lysis of the RBCs.

transmission-based precautions: Precautions in addition to Standard Precautions to be followed for patients known or suspected to be infected or colonized with highly transmissible or epidemiologically significant pathogens. There are three transmission-based precautions: airborne, droplet, and contact.

transport media: The medium or agent used to carry infective material to a laboratory for culturing.

transverse plane: Divides the body horizontally into upper and lower portions, often called a cross section.

trough level: Drug level collected when the lowest serum concentration of the drug is expected, usually immediately prior to administration of the next scheduled dose.

tube additive: Any substance placed within a tube other than the coating of the tube or tube stopper (closure).

tuberculin (TB) test: Tuberculosis test also called PPD test. *See* PPD.

tuberculosis (TB): Infectious airborne disease affecting the respiratory system, caused by the bacteria *Mycobacterium tuberculosis.*

tunica adventitia: The outer layer of blood vessels, made up of connective tissue, which is thicker in arteries than in veins.

tunica intima: The inner layer or lining of blood vessels, made up of a single layer of endothelial cells.

tunica media: The middle layer of blood vessels, made up of smooth muscle tissue, which is much thicker in arteries than in veins.

turn-around time (TAT): Specified amount of time for sample to be drawn and processed, and for test results to be sent to the floor or unit.

Typenex ID band: A special three-part identification bracelet for a blood recipient that contains the same information and unique ID number for client confirmation on all three parts.

universal precautions: A set of rules established by the CDC, and adopted by OSHA, to control infection from body fluids in the health care setting.

user manual: A manual containing specimen collection information, including the type of specimen required, minimum amount needed, special handling, reference values for the test, when testing is available, and the normal turnaround time (TAT).

urinalysis: Laboratory test that includes physical examination, and chemical and microscopic analysis of urine.

UTI: Urinary tract infection.

vascular access device (VAD): Tubing inserted into a main vein or artery, used primarily for administering fluids and medications, monitoring pressures, and drawing blood. It is also called an indwelling line.

vasoconstriction: Constriction of a blood vessel to decrease the flow of blood to an area.

vector transmission: The transfer of the causative organisms of disease to a susceptible individual by an insect, arthropod or animal.

vehicle transmission: The transmission of an infective microbe to a susceptible individual through contaminated food, water or drugs. Includes the transmission of hepatitis and HIV through blood transfusion.

veins: Vessels that return blood to the heart.

vena cava: The largest vein in the body.

venesection: Slicing a vein in the forearm and collecting the specimen in a cup or bowl.

venipuncture: Collection of blood by penetrating a vein with a needle, syringe, or other collection apparatus.

venous stasis: Stagnation or stoppage of the normal blood flow.

ventral: Anterior or pertaining to the front.

ventral cavities: Internal space located in the front of the body.

ventricles: Lower chambers of the heart. Also known as the delivering chambers of the heart, because they pump blood into the arteries.

venules: The smallest veins at the junction of the capillaries.

vicarious liability: Institutions are liable for injury occurring as a result of negligent acts committed by independent contractors they have hired.

virulence: The degree to which an organism is capable of causing disease.

virulent: Infectious or capable of overcoming the defensive mechanism of the host.

whorls: Circular pattern of a fingerprint formed by the ridges and grooves of the papillary dermis.

winged infusion set (butterfly):   A $\frac{1}{2}$- to $\frac{3}{4}$-inch stainless steel needle connected to a 5- to 12-inch length of tubing. It is called a butterfly because of its wing-shaped plastic extensions, which are used for gripping the needle.

word root: Foundation of all medical terms.

zones of comfort: In communication, the different distances around a person which are comfortable for intimate, personal, social, and public discourse.

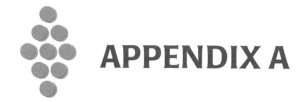

APPENDIX A

Answers To Study and Review Questions

Chapter 1
1. a
2. d
3. a
4. b
5. d
6. c
7. c
8. b

Chapter 2
1. c
2. a
3. a
4. d
5. b
6. a
7. d
8. c

Chapter 3
1. a
2. a
3. c
4. a
5. d
6. b
7. d
8. a

Chapter 4
1. b
2. c
3. c
4. d
5. d
6. d
7. c
8. d
9. b
10. c

Chapter 5
1. c
2. a
3. d
4. a
5. b
6. c
7. b
8. d
9. a
10. b

Chapter 6
1. c
2. d
3. a
4. b

5. a
6. c
7. d

Chapter 7
1. d
2. c
3. b
4. d
5. b
6. c

Chapter 8
1. a
2. b
3. c
4. c
5. c
6. d
7. b
8. d

Chapter 9
1. c
2. a
3. b
4. b
5. a
6. a

7. b
8. a
9. c
10. d
11. d
12. a

Chapter 10
1. d
2. c
3. b
4. d
5. c
6. b
7. a
8. b

Chapter 11
1. c
2. b
3. a
4. b
5. c
6. d
7. d
8. c
9. c
10. a
11. c

12. b
13. b

Chapter 12
1. b
2. d
3. b
4. c
5. d
6. a

Chapter 13
1. d
2. d

3. d
4. c

Chapter 14
1. d
2. a
3. c
4. b
5. c
6. c
7. a
8. d

Chapter 15
1. b

2. c
3. b
4. c
5. b
6. d
7. d
8. a

Chapter 16
1. 0.0007 centimeters
2. 0.5 inches
3. 3:30 PM
4. No
5. Factor 8

6. 90%
7. Add 50 mL bleach to 450 mL water
8. 216 mL or 0.216 L

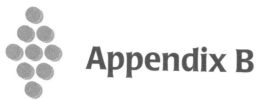

Appendix B

Conversational Phrases in English and Spanish

The following remarks or sentences are designed to assist the phlebotomist when conversing with a patient who speaks only Spanish. Before approaching the patient, these basic phrases should be said aloud several times to a person who could correct the pronunciation, if necessary. If these phrases are said incorrectly, the meanings could be changed enough to insult or bewilder the patient.

Hello

¡Hola!
(Ō-lah)

Good morning

Buenos días
(BWĀ-nōs DĒ-ahs)

Good afternoon

Buenas tardes
(BWĀ-nahs TAHR-dās)

Good evening

Buenas noches
(BWĀ-nahs NŌ-chās)

I am from the laboratory

Soy del laboratorio
(soy dāl lah-bō-rah-tō-RĒ-ō)

My name is

Me llamo
(mā YAH-mō)

I am here to take a blood sample

Estoy aquí para tomarle una prueba de sangre
(ās-TOY ah-KĒ PAHR-ah tō-MAHR-lā UN-ah prū-Ā-bah dā SAHN-grā)

What is your name?

¿Cual es so nombre?
(kwahl ās sō NŌM-brā?)
OR ¿Como se llama?
(CŌ-mō sā YAH-mah?)

May I see your wristband?	¿Me permite ver su identificación? (mā pār-MĒ-tā vār sū ē-dān-tē-fē-cah-sē-ŌN?)
Mr. or Sir	Señor (sā-NYOR)
Mrs. or Madame	Señora (sā-NYŌ-rah)
Ms. or Miss	Señorita (sā-nyō-RĒ-tah)
Okay	Muy bien (MŪ-ē byān)
You are the person I need	Usted es la persona que necesito (ūs-TĒD ās lah pār-SŌN-ah kā na-sā-SĒ-tō)
I am going to put a tourniquet on your arm	le voy a poner un torniquete en su brazo (lā voy ah pō-NĀR ūn tor-nē-KĀ-tā ān sū BRAH-sō)
Please	Por favor (por fah-VOR)
close your hand	cierra su mano (SYĀ-rah sū MAH-nō)
open your hand	abra su mano (AH-brah sū MAH-nō)
straighten your arm	ponga derecho su brazo (PŌN-gah dā-RĀ-chō sū BRAH-sō) OR estire su brazo (ās-tĒ-rā sū BRAH-sō)
bend your arm	doble su brazo (DŌ-blā sū BRAH-sō)
relax	relajese (rā-lah CHĀ-sā) NOTE: the "ch" in this word is pronounced gutturally
sit there	sientese aquí (syān-TĀ-sā ah-KĒ)
Your doctor ordered this	Su doctor ordeno esto (sū dōc-TOR or-DĀ-nō ĀS-tō)
You need to ask your doctor	Necesita preguntarle a su doctor (nā-sā-SĒ-tah prā-gūn-TAHR-lā ah sū dōc-TOR)

Have you eaten?	¿La comido? (lah cō-MĒ-dō)
It will hurt a little	le dolerá un poco (lā dō-lā-RAH ūm PŌ-kō)
I will get the nurse	Buscaré a la enfermera (būs-cah-RĀ ah lah ām-fār-MĀ-rah)
Thank you	¡Gracias! (GRAH-syahs)
Have a good day	Qué le vaya bien (kā lā VĪ-yah byān)
Someone will be back in a few minutes	Alguien regresará en un momento (ahl-GWĒ-ān rā-grā-sah-RAH ān ūm mō-MĀN-tō)

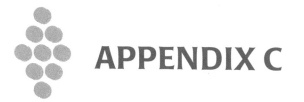

APPENDIX C

A Patient's Bill of Rights

Introduction

The American Hospital Association presents *A Patient's Bill of Rights* with the expectation that observance of these rights will contribute to more effective patient care and greater satisfaction for the patient, his physician, and the hospital organization. Further, the Association presents these rights in the expectation that they will be supported by the hospital on behalf of its patients, as an integral part of the healing process. It is recognized that a personal relationship between the physician and the patient is essential for the provision of proper medical care. The traditional physician–patient relationship takes on a new dimension when care is rendered within an organizational structure. Legal precedent has established that the institution itself also has a responsibility to the patient. It is in recognition of these factors that these rights are affirmed.

Bill of Rights

1. The patient has the right to considerate and respectful care.
2. The patient has the right to obtain from his physician complete current information concerning his diagnosis, treatment, and prognosis in terms the patient can be reasonably expected to understand. When it is not medically advisable to give such information to the patient, the information should be made available to an appropriate person in his behalf. He has the right to know, by name, the physician responsible for coordinating his care. Refer to physician, if question
3. The patient has the right to receive from his physician information necessary to give informed consent prior to the start of any procedure and/or treatment. Except in emergencies, such information for informed consent should include but not necessarily be limited to the specific procedure and/or treatment, the medically significant risks involved, and the probable duration of incapacitation. Where medically significant alternatives for care or treatment exist, or when the patient requests information concerning medical alternatives, the patient has the right to such information. The patient also has the right to know the name of the person responsible for the procedures and/or treatment.
4. The patient has the right to refuse treatment to the extent permitted by law and to be informed of the medical consequences of his action.
5. The patient has the right to every consideration of his privacy concerning his own medical care program. Case discussion, consultation, examination, and treatment are confidential and should be conducted discreetly. Those not directly involved in his care must have the permission of the patient to be present.
6. The patient has the right to expect that all communications and records pertaining to his care should be treated as confidential.

7. The patient has the right to expect that, within its capacity, a hospital must make reasonable response to the request of a patient for services. The hospital must provide evaluation, service and/or referral as indicated by the urgency of the case. When medically permissible, a patient may be transferred to another facility only after he has received complete information and explanation concerning the needs for and alternatives to such a transfer. The institution to which the patient is to be transferred must first have accepted the patient for transfer.
8. The patient has the right to obtain information as to any relationship of his hospital to other health care and educational institutions insofar as his care is concerned. The patient has the right to obtain information as to the existence of any professional relationships among individuals, by name, who are treating him.
9. The patient has the right to be advised if the hospital proposes to engage in or perform human experimentation affecting his care or treatment. The patient has the right to refuse to participate in such research projects.
10. The patient has the right to expect reasonable continuity of care. He has the right to know, in advance, what appointment times and physicians are available and where. The patient has the right to expect that the hospital will provide a mechanism whereby he is informed by his physician or a delegate of the physician of the patient's continuing health care requirements following discharge.
11. The patient has the right to examine and receive and explanation of his bill, regardless of source of payment.
12. The patient has the right to know what hospital rules and regulations apply to his conduct as a patient.

Conclusion

No catalog of rights can guarantee for the patient the kind of treatment he has a right to expect. A hospital has many functions to perform, including the prevention and treatment of disease, the education of both health professionals and patients, and the conduct of clinical research. All these activities must be conducted with an overriding concern for the patient, and, above all, the recognition of his dignity as a human being. Success in achieving this recognition assures success in the defense of the rights of the patient.

Reaffirmed by the Institutional Practices Committee in 1990. *A Patient's Bill of Rights* was first adopted by the American Hospital Association in 1973. © 1990 by the American Hospital Association. Used with permission.

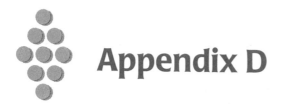

Appendix D

Listing of Departments and Tests

Department	Tube Type
Chemistry	Red—nonadditive (do not mix) SST—inert gel & silica Green—sodium heparin 　　　　 lithium heparin 　　　　 ammonia heparin Gray—sodium fluoride & potassium oxalate Royal blue—free of trace element, can be: red, green, or lavendar label

The following list of tests should be collected.

Test	Abbreviation	Special Considerations	Clinical Correlation
Acid phosphatase		Freeze serum; draw before rectal examination or biopsy	Cancer of the prostate
Alanine transferase	ALT (SGPT)		Evaluate hepatic disease
Alcohol	ETOH	Use non-alcohol germicidal solution to cleanse skin; chain-of-custody required if for legal purposes	Intoxication
Aldosterone		Refrigerate serum	Overproduction of this hormone
Alkaline phosphatase	Alk phos or ALP	Refrigerate serum	Liver function

Test	Abbreviation	Special Considerations	Clinical Correlation
Alpha-fetoprotein		Avoid hemolysis; do not freeze; can be performed on amniotic fluid	Fetal abnormalities, adult hepatic carcinomas
Aluminum	Al	Avoid all sources of external contamination; use stainless steel needle and royal blue tube; no additive	Dialysis
Ammonia	NH_4	Green-top tube placed immediately on ice; centrifuge within 15 minutes without removing stopper; separate plasma and freeze	Liver function
Amylase		Avoid hemolysis & lipemia	Acute pancreatitis
Asparate transferase	AST (SGOT)		Acute & chronic liver disease
Bilirubin, total & direct	Bili	Wrap in foil to protect from light; refrigerate	Liver function, erythroblastosis
Blood urea nitrogen	BUN		Kidney function
Calcitonin		Overnight fasting preferred, freeze serum immediately	Thyroid function
Carbon monoxide (carboxyhemoglobin)	CO level	Fill lavender tube completely	Carboxyhemoglobin intoxication
Carcinogenic antigen	Ca 125	Refrigerate; freeze if testing is delayed	Tumor marker primarily for ovarian carcinoma
Calcium, ionized	Ca	Allow blood to clot for 20 minutes; centrifuge with cap on; do not pour over; refrigerate	Bone cancer, nephritis, multiple myeloma
Carcinoembryonic antigen	CEA	Refrigerate serum	Indicator of tumors
Carotene		Wrap in aluminum foil to protect from light and freeze	Carotenemia
Chemistry panel	Chem-6, -8, -12 or chem panel basic	Fasting 8–12 hours is required	A designated number of tests covering a certain body system
Cholesterol	Chol		Evaluates risk of coronary heart disease (CHD)
Chromium	Cr level	Royal blue—no additive; metal-free	Associated with diabetes and aspartame toxicity
Copper	Cu level	Royal blue—no additive; separate immediately	Wilson's disease or nephrotic syndrome

Test	Abbreviation	Special Considerations	Clinical Correlation
Cortisol, timed		Refrigerate serum; clearly note time drawn	Cushing's syndrome
Creatine kinase	CK	Refrigerate serum	Muscular dystrophy and trauma to skeletal muscle
Creatine kinase isoenzymes	CK isoenzymes	Refrigerate serum	Organ differentiation
Creatinine			Kidney function
Cyclosporin		Whole blood or serum refrigerated; NOTE: use same type of specimen each time analyte is measured	Immunosuppressive drug for organ transplants
Cryoglobulin		Draw and process at room temperature; should be fasting	Multiple myeloma, leukemia, certain forms of pneumonia
Drug monitoring:			
Amikacin		Do not use gel barrier tube; centrifuge & separate within one hour	Broad-spectrum antibiotic
Carbamazepine (Tegretol)		Do not use gel barrier tube	Mood-stabilizing drug in bipolar affective disorder
Digoxin (Lanoxin)		Do not use gel barrier tube	Heart stimulant
Dilantin (Phenytoin)		Do not use gel barrier tube	Treatment of epilepsy
Gentamicin		Do not use gel barrier tube	Broad-spectrum antibiotic
Lithium		Do not use gel barrier tube, should be drawn 8–12 hours after dose administered	Manic–depression medication
Phenobarbitol (barbiturates)		Do not use gel barrier tube	Anticonvulsant for seizures
Salicylates (aspirin)		Do not use gel barrier tube	Evaluation of therapy
Theophylline		Do not use gel barrier tube	Asthma medication
Tobramycin		Do not use gel barrier tube	Broad-spectrum antibiotic
Vancomycin		Do not use gel barrier tube	Broad-spectrum antibiotic
Electrolytes	Na+, K+, Cl^-, CO_2, lytes	Avoid hemolysis	Fluid balance, cardiotoxicity, heart failure, edema

Test	Abbreviation	Special Considerations	Clinical Correlation
Ferritin		Refrigerate serum	Hemachromatosis, iron deficiency
Gamma-glutamyl transpeptidase	GGTP		Liver function
Gastrin		Overnight fasting is required; separate serum from cells within one hour after collection; freeze serum	Stomach disorders
Glucose	FBS—fasting blood sugar RBS—random blood sugar	Separate from cells within one hour or use gray-top tube	Diabetes, hypoglycemia
Glycosylated hemoglobin	Hgb A_{1C}	Lavender tube	Monitoring diabetes mellitus
Glucose-6-phosphate dehydrogenase	G-6-PD	Lavender tube; do not freeze	Drug-induced anemias
Hemoglobin electrophoresis		Refrigerate; whole blood; do not spin	Hemoglobinopathies and thalassemia
HLA typing A & B		Yellow-top (ACD) tubes; do not freeze or refrigerate; ethnic origin must be included	Disease association, bone marrow, platelet capability, liver or heart transplant
Human chorionic gonadotropin	HCG		Pregnancy, testicular cancer
Immunoglobulins-IgA IgG IgM			Measurement of proteins capable of becoming antibodies, chronic liver disease, myeloma
Iron, total	Fe	Draw in AM, should be fasting; avoid hemolysis	Iron toxicity
Lactate/lactic acid		Plasma-gray top; do not use a tourniquet during phlebotomy or allow patient to clench their fist	Glucose metabolism
Lactic dehydrogenase	LDH	Serum, avoid hemolysis—do not freeze	Cardiac injury & other muscle damage
Lead	Pb	Royal blue EDTA or tan-top lead-free tube; do not centrifuge	Lead toxicity
Lipase		Refrigerate serum	Pancreatic disease

Test	Abbreviation	Special Considerations	Clinical Correlation
Lipoproteins- High-density lipoprotein	HDL	Must be fasting a minimum of 12 hours	Evaluates lipid disorders and coronary artery disease risk
Low-density lipoprotein	LDL	Must be fasting a minimum of 12 hours	Evaluates lipid disorders and coronary artery disease risk
Magnesium	Mg		Mineral metabolism, kidney function
Phosphorus	P		Thyroid function, bone disorders, and kidney disease
Prostatic specific antigen	PSA	Refrigerate serum; draw before rectal examination or biopsy	Prostate cancer
Serum protein electrophoresis	SPEP or PEP		Abnormal protein detection
Sweat electrolytes (Iontophoresis)	Sweat chloride	Fluid collected is sweat	Cystic fibrosis
Thyroid studies	T_3, T_4, TSH		Hyper or hypothyroid conditions
Total iron binding capacity & Fe	TIBC & Fe	Drawn in AM, should be fasting	
Triglycerides		Fasting 12–14 hours is required	Atherosclerosis and heart disease
Troponin			
Uric acid			Gout
Zinc	Zn	Royal blue, no additive	Liver dysfunction

Department	Tube Type		
Hematology	Lavender—ethylenediaminetetraacetate (EDTA) Green—sodium heparin		

Test	Abbreviation	Special Considerations	Clinical Correlation
Complete Blood Count	CBC	Lavender tube invert gently 6–8 times; includes WBC, RBC, hgb, hct, indices, platelets and diff	Blood dyscrasias
Differential	Diff	Blood smear stained with Wright's stain	Classifying types of leukocytes, describing erythrocytes, and estimation of platelets
Eosinophil Count	Eos. ct.	Lavender tube; invert gently 6–8 times	Allergy studies

Test	Abbreviation	Special Considerations	Clinical Correlation
Erythrocyte sedimentation rate	ESR, sed rate	Lavender tube; invert gently 6–8 times	Abnormal protein linkage
Hematocrit	Hct	Lavender tube; invert gently 6–8 times	Anemia
Hemoglobin	Hgb or Hb	Lavender tube; invert gently 6–8 times	Anemia
Hemoglobin electrophoresis		Lavender tube; invert gently 6–8 times	Abnormal hemoglobin
Indices	MCV, MCH, MCHC	Lavender tube; invert gently 6–8 times	Indicate mean cell hemoglobin concentration and mean cell volume
Lupus erythematosus cell prep	LE prep	Green tube to lab immediately	Screen for LE disease
Platelet count	Plt. ct.	Lavender tube; invert gently 6–8 times	Bleeding disorders
Red cell count	RBC	Lavender tube; invert gently 6–8 times	Anemia
Reticulocyte count	Retic ct.	Lavender tube; invert gently 6–8 times	Anemia
White cell count	WBC	Lavender tube; invert gently 6–8 times	Infection (viral or bacterial)

Department	Tube Type
Coagulation	Light blue—sodium citrate Tube must be completely filled by vacuum for all tests

Test	Abbreviation	Special Considerations	Clinical Correlation
Activated clotting time	ACT		Clotting factor deficiency
Antithrombin III			Clotting factor deficiency
D-Dimer	D-D1	Completely fill blue-top tube; centrifuge; separate and freeze if not performed immediately	DIC and thrombotic episodes such as pulmonary emboli
Disseminated intravascular coagulation	DIC screen	On ice or frozen if not tested immediately	Distortion of the normal coagulation and fibrinolytic mechanisms
Factor assay		Place on ice immediately	To determine the actual percentage of a specific coagulation factor
Fibrinogen		Centrifuge; separate and place on ice immediately	

Test	Abbreviation	Special Considerations	Clinical Correlation
Fibrin split products/ Fibrin degradation product	FSP/FDP	1 mL of blood in special blue-top tube containing thrombin and soybean trypsin inhibitor; do not refrigerate or freeze	DIC and thrombotic episodes, valuable early diagnositc sign of increased rate of fibrin deposition
Platelet aggregation			Hemostasis and thrombus formation
Plasminogen		Centrifuge; separate and place on ice immediately—specimen in glass vials will not be accepted	Fibrin clot formation prevention
Prothrombin Time	PT	Do not freeze	Clotting factor deficiency, monitoring warfarin therapy
Partial thromboplastin time (Activated PTT)	PTT (APPT)	Do not freeze	Clotting factor deficiency, monitoring heparin therapy

Department	Tube Type
Immunology/Serology	Red—no additive Red/gray—clot activator & inert silicon gel Gold—clot activator & inert silicon gel

Test	Abbreviation	Special Considerations	Clinical Correlation
Antinuclear antibodies	ANA (screen or titer)	Avoid hemolysis & lipemia	Systemic lupus erythematosus and other autoimmune connective tissue diseases
Antistreptolysin O test	ASO	Refrigerate or freeze if not performed immediately	Group A streptococcal infection
Cold agglutinins		Do NOT refrigerate	Viral and atypical pneumonia
Chlamydia antibody panel		Refrigerate serum	For trachoma, psittacosis, LGV and pneumoniae
C-reactive protein	CRP	Freeze if test will be delayed longer than 72 hours	Chronic inflammation
Cytomegalovirus Screen	CMV	Refrigerate serum	Screens donors and blood products for transplant programs
Epstein-Barr Virus	EBV		Mononucleosis

Test	Abbreviation	Special Considerations	Clinical Correlation
Febrile agglutinins			Screens for Salmonella, Tularemia, Proteus, and Brucella
Fluorescent treponemal antibody	FTA		Syphilis
Hepatitis B surface antibody	HBs/Ab		Determination of previous infection and immunity by hepatitis B
Hepatitis B surface antigen	HBsAg		Diagnosis of acute or some chronic stages of infection and carrier status of hepatitis B
Human immunodeficient virus	HIV Ab		HIV
Mono-Test or monospot			Infectious mononucleosis
Radioallergosorbent test	RAST		Allergies
Rheumatoid arthritis	RA		Arthritic condition
Rapid plasmin reagin	RPR		Syphilis
Viral antibody titer			Adenovirus, herpes simplex, Coxsackie B, cytomegalovirus

Department	Tube Type
Immunohematology/Blood Bank	Plain red—no additive Lavender—ethylenediaminetetraacetate (EDTA)

Test	Abbreviation	Special Considerations	Clinical Correlation
Antibody screen		Special ID procedure	Identify any atypical antibodies present
Blood group & Rh type		Special ID procedure	ABO group & type
Cord Blood			Group and type baby's blood to detect the presence of incompatibilities, or mother for possible Rh immune globulin
Direct antiglobulin test	DAT	Special ID procedure	Detects antibodies attached to the red cells
Indirect antiglobulin test	IAT (Coombs)	Special ID procedure	Detects antibody sensitization, either acquired or inherited, which is present in serum

Test	Abbreviation	Special Considerations	Clinical Correlation
Rh immune globulin	Rhogam workup	Special ID procedure	Administered to Rh-negative mothers to prevent Rh immunization
Type & screen		Special ID procedure	Group & type and detect atypical antbodies for prenatal screen or crossmatch
Type & crossmatch		Special ID procedure	Group & type and cross-match with donor unit

Department	Tube Type
Microbiology	Yellow—sodium polyanetholesulfonate Isolator—lysing agent, anticoagulant, HIV inactivator

Test	Abbreviation	Special Considerations	Clinical Correlation
Acid fast bacillus smear	AFB smear	True sputum—early AM best specimen	Tuberculosis
Blood cultures	BC	2 blood culture bottles: 1 anaerobic and 1 aerobic	Septicemia
Culture & sensitivity	C & S		Identification of infective agent and appropriate antibiotic treatment
Screen			
Gonorrhea	GC	Submit culturette	Sexually transmitted disease
Streptococcus	Strep	Throat swab in culturette	Strep throat
Sputum		True sputum—early AM sample	TB

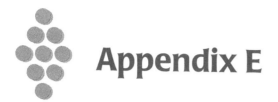

Appendix E

Conditions Requiring Work Restrictions for Health Care Employees

Condition	Work Restriction
Chicken pox (Varicella)	Off work until 7 days after appearance of first eruption and lesions are dry and crusted
Hepatitis A	Off work until cleared by a physician
Hepatitis B	Off work until cleared by a physician
Herpes zoster	May work if no patient contact
Influenza	Work status determined by Employee Health Department depending on work area
Impetigo	Off work or no patient contact until crusts are gone
Measles	Off work until rash is gone (minimum 4 days)
Mononucleosis	Off work until cleared by a physician
MRSA (methicillin-resistant *Staphylococcus aureus*)	May work, but no patient care until treatment is successful
Pink eye (acute conjunctivitis)	Off work until treatment is successful
Positive PPD test	May work depending upon evaualtion and follow-up by Employee Health Department
Pregnancy	May work, but avoid contact with patients with rickettsial or viral infections, patients in isolation, and patients being treated with radioactive isotopes. Avoid areas with radioactive hazard symbol.
Tuberculosis (active)	Off work until treated and AFB smears are negative for 2 weeks
Rubella (German measles)	Off work until rash is gone (minimum 5 days)
Salmonella	Varies depending on symptoms, treatment results, and Employee Health Department evaluation

Condition	Work Restriction
Scabies	Off work until treated
Shigella	Varies depending on symptoms, treatment results, and Employee Health Department evaluation
Strep throat (group A)	Off work until 24 hours after antibiotic therapy is started and symptoms are gone
URI (upper respiratory infection)	Work status determined by Employee Health Department

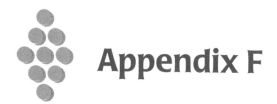

Appendix F

Procedure Evaluation Checklists

VENIPUNCTURE PROCEDURE EVALUATION

Name:_____ Date:_____ Total points:_____

Rating system:
2 = Meets or exceeds standards
1 = Opportunity for improvement
0 = Unsatisfactory performance
Total points possible = 50

Procedure Step	Rating	Comments
1. Prepare paperwork and review test requisition		
2. Introduce yourself and identify patient		
3. Verify diet restrictions if indicated		
4. Wash hands and put on gloves		
5. Assemble equipment and supplies		
6. Reassure and position patient		
7. Apply tourniquet		
8. Select venipuncture site		
9. Release tourniquet		
10. Cleanse venipuncture site and allow to air dry		
11. Verify equipment and tube selection		
12. Reapply tourniquet		
13. Anchor vein		
14. Insert needle into vein		
15. Place and fill tubes following proper order of draw		
16. Release tourniquet within 1 minute of application		
17. Remove tubes from holder and mix if applicable		
18. Place gauze, withdraw needle, and apply pressure to site		
19. Dispose of needle		
20. Label tubes and follow specimen handling instructions		
21. Check the patient's arm and apply bandage		
22. Dispose of used materials and gather equipment		
23. Thank patient		
24. Remove gloves and wash hands		
25. Complete paperwork and transport specimen to the lab		
Total points		

NEEDLE AND SYRINGE VENIPUNCTURE PROCEDURE EVALUATION

Name: _____ Date: _____ Total points: _____

Rating system:
2 = Meets or exceeds standards
1 = Opportunity for improvement
0 = Unsatisfactory performance
Total points possible = 50

Procedure Step	Rating	Comments
1. Prepare paperwork and review test requisition		
2. Introduce yourself, identify patient, and verify any diet restrictions		
3. Wash hands and put on gloves		
4. Reassure and position patient		
5. Apply tourniquet		
6. Select venipuncture site		
7. Release tourniquet; clean venipuncture site and allow to air dry		
8. Verify tube selection and place tubes in test rack		
9. Assemble needle and syringe		
10. Pull and reseat syringe plunger to ensure free movement		
11. Reapply tourniquet		
12. Remove needle cap		
13. Grasp arm and pull skin taut to anchor vein		
14. Insert needle into vein until flash of blood appears in needle hub		
15. Pull back on syringe plunger until the barrel fills with blood		
16. Release tourniquet within 1 minute of application		
17. Place gauze, withdraw needle, and apply pressure to site		
18. Penetrate tube stopper with syringe needle		
19. Fill tubes following syringe order of draw		
20. Dispose of needle and syringe as one unit		
21. Label tubes and follow specimen handling instructions		
22. Check the patient's arm and apply bandage		
23. Dispose of used materials, gather equipment, and thank patient		
24. Remove gloves and wash hands		
25. Complete paperwork and transport specimen to the lab		
Total points		

HAND VEIN VENIPUNCTURE USING A BUTTERFLY PROCEDURE EVALUATION

Name:_____ Date:_____ Total points:_____

Rating system:
2 = Meets or exceeds standards
1 = Opportunity for improvement
0 = Unsatisfactory performance
Total points possible = 50

Procedure Step	Rating	Comments
1. Prepare paperwork and review test requisition		
2. Introduce yourself, identify patient, and verify diet restrictions		
3. Wash hands and put on gloves		
4. Assemble equipment and supplies, verify tube selection		
5. Reassure patient and position patient's hand		
6. Apply tourniquet just beyond wrist bone		
7. Select venipuncture site and release tourniquet		
8. Cleanse venipuncture site and allow to air dry		
9. Attach butterfly to syringe or tube holder		
10. Stretch tubing slightly to minimize recoil		
11. Reapply tourniquet		
12. Have patient make a fist and anchor the vein		
13. Hold butterfly wings and insert needle into vein		
14. Advance needle until flash of blood appears in the tubing		
15. Anchor needle to prevent it from spinning out of the vein		
16. Place and fill tubes following proper order of draw		
17. Release tourniquet within 1 minute of application		
18. Remove tubes from holder and mix if applicable		
19. Place gauze, withdraw needle, and apply pressure to site		
20. Release needle and tubing from holder into sharps container		
21. Label tubes and follow specimen handling instructions		
22. Check the patient's arm and apply bandage		
23. Thank patient, discard used materials, and gather equipment		
24. Remove gloves and wash hands		
25. Complete paperwork and transport specimen to the lab		
Total points		

FINGER PUNCTURE PROCEDURE EVALUATION

Name:_____ Date:_____ Total points:_____

Rating system:

2 = Meets or exceeds standards
1 = Opportunity for improvement
0 = Unsatisfactory performance

Total points possible = 50

Procedure Step	Rating	Comments
1. Prepare paperwork and review test requisition		
2. Introduce yourself and identify patient		
3. Explain procedure and verify any diet restrictions		
4. Wash hands and put on gloves		
5. Assemble equipment and supplies		
6. Reassure patient and position patient's hand		
7. Select puncture site and warm site if indicated		
8. Cleanse puncture site and allow to air dry		
9. Hold patient's finger between your thumb and forefinger		
10. Perform puncture perpendicular to fingerprint whorls		
11. Discard puncture device in sharps container		
12. Wipe away first drop of blood		
13. Apply and release pressure to aid blood flow		
14. Collect microhematocrit specimens without air bubbles		
15. Collect bullets without scooping or scraping		
16. Collect specimens following proper order of draw		
17. Seal collection containers		
18. Mix anticoagulant containers to prevent clotting		
19. Place gauze apply pressure to site		
20. Label containers and follow specimen handling instructions		
21. Check site and apply bandage		
22. Dispose of used materials and gather equipment		
23. Thank patient		
24. Remove gloves and wash hands		
25. Complete paperwork and transport specimen to the lab		
Total points		

OUTPATIENT INFANT PKU COLLECTION EVALUATION

Name:_____ Date:_____ Total points:_____

Rating system:
2 = Meets or exceeds standards
1 = Opportunity for improvement
0 = Unsatisfactory performance
Total points possible = 38

Procedure Step	Rating	Comments
1. Prepare paperwork and review test requisition		
2. Identify patient and explain procedure to parent		
3. Wash hands and put on gloves		
4. Assemble equipment		
5. Position infant and apply warming device to infant's heel		
6. Remove warming device and select puncture site		
7. Clean site with alcohol and allow to air dry		
8. Prepare incision device		
9. Grasp heel with index finger supporting the arch		
10. Perform puncture in safe area of the heel		
11. Discard incision device in sharps container		
12. Apply pressure to encourage blood flow		
13. Wipe away the first drop of blood		
14. Apply blood to filter paper circles evenly without layering		
15. Fill circles completely, from one side of the paper only		
16. Place gauze and hold pressure until bleeding stops		
17. Discard used items, finish paperwork and dismiss patient		
18. Place filter paper in horizontal position to dry		
19. Remove gloves and wash hands		
Total points		

BLOOD SMEAR PREPARATION EVALUATION

Name:_____ Date:_____ Total points:_____

Rating system:
2 = Meets or exceeds standards
1 = Opportunity for improvement
0 = Unsatisfactory performance
Total points possible = 20

Procedure Step	Rating	Comments
1. Put on gloves		
2. Wipe two clean slides with gauze to remove fingerprints or residue		
3. Apply medium size drop of blood to appropriate area of the slide		
4. Position spreader in front of drop at correct angle		
5. Pull spreader slide back until it just touches the drop of blood		
6. Allow blood to spread the width of the spreader slide		
7. Push the spreader slide forward with one smooth motion		
8. Examine resulting blood smear for acceptability		
9. Label slide		
10. Remove gloves and wash hands		
Total points		

BLOOD CULTURE PROCEDURE EVALUATION

Name:_____ Date:_____ Total points:_____

Rating system:

2 = Meets or exceeds standards
1 = Opportunity for improvement
0 = Unsatisfactory performance

Total points possible = 50

Procedure Step	Rating	Comments
1. Prepare paperwork and review test requisition		
2. Introduce yourself and identify patient		
3. Wash hands and put on gloves		
4. Reassure and position patient		
5. Apply tourniquet		
6. Select venipuncture site		
7. Release tourniquet		
8. Clean site with alcohol to remove dirt and surface debris		
9. Scrub site with povidone–iodine or equivalent for 2 minutes		
10. Clean site with povidone–iodine using concentric circles		
11. Allow site to air dry completely		
12. Clean tops of blood culture bottles or tubes		
13. Assemble blood collection equipment		
14. Reapply tourniquet, being careful not to touch collection site		
15. Perform venipuncture		
16. Fill blood culture containers in proper order for collection method		
17. Mix blood culture containers gently		
18. Place gauze and withdraw needle		
19. Apply pressure to site		
20. Dispose of needle or needle and syringe		
21. Label blood culture containers with required information		
22. Check the patient's arm and apply bandage		
23. Dispose of used materials, gather equipment, and thank patient		
24. Remove gloves and wash hands		
25. Transport specimen to the lab		
Total points		

BLEEDING TIME PROCEDURE EVALUATION

Name:_____ Date:_____ Total points:_____

Rating system:
2 = Meets or exceeds standards
1 = Opportunity for improvement
0 = Unsatisfactory performance
Total points possible = 40

Procedure Step	*Rating*	*Comments*
1. Review test requisition		
2. Introduce yourself and identify patient		
3. Explain procedure and ask about interfering medications		
4. Wash hands and put on gloves		
5. Reassure patient and position arm on firm surface		
6. Select incision site		
7. Assemble equipment and prepare incision device		
8. Clean incision site with alcohol and allow to air dry		
9. Place blood pressure cuff around arm and inflate to 40 mm Hg		
10. Perform puncture and simultaneously start stop watch or timer		
11. Discard puncture device in sharps container		
12. Wick blood with filter paper 30 seconds after timing starts		
13. Continue wicking every 30 seconds until end point is determined		
14. Discard contaminated filter paper in biohazard waste container		
15. Record end point time		
16. Remove blood pressure cuff		
17. Clean site, apply butterfly bandage, and cover with sterile dressing		
18. Instruct patient on how to care for site and when to remove bandage		
19. Dispose of used materials, gather equipment, and thank patient		
20. Remove gloves and wash hands		
Total points		

RADIAL ARTERY PUNCTURE PROCEDURE EVALUATION

Name:_____ Date:_____ Total points:_____

Rating system:
2 = Meets or exceeds standards
1 = Opportunity for improvement
0 = Unsatisfactory performance
Total points possible = 50

Procedure Step	Rating	Comments
1. Receive and review test requisition and gather ABG equipment		
2. Introduce yourself, identify patient, and explain procedure		
3. Verify "steady state" and log metabolic and oxygen therapy data		
4. Wash hands and put on gloves		
5. Reassure patient and position patient's arm, palm up		
6. Determine presence of collateral circulation		
7. Prepare ABG syringe, and anesthetic syringe if applicable		
8. Locate radial artery using your index and middle fingers		
9. Palpate radial artery to judge size, depth, and direction		
10. Clean puncture site with alcohol and allow to air dry		
11. Clean puncture site with povidone–iodine and allow to air dry		
12. Clean gloved finger in the same manner		
13. Administer anesthetic if indicated and wait 2 minutes		
14. Locate artery with index finger of nondominant hand		
15. Insert needle into skin and advance until a flash of blood appears		
16. Allow arterial pressure to fill syringe		
17. Place gauze, remove needle, and apply pressure for 5 minutes		
18. Expel air bubbles from syringe and embed needle in latex cube		
19. Mix specimen, remove and discard needle, and cap syringe		
20. Label specimen and place in crushed ice slurry		
21. Check site for swelling or bruising; check pulse distal to site		
22. If site appears normal, apply pressure bandage		
23. Dispose of used materials, gather equipment, and thank patient		
24. Remove gloves and wash hands		
25. Transport specimen to the lab ASAP		
Total points		

MODIFIED ALLEN TEST PROCEDURE EVALUATION

Name:_____ Date:_____ Total points:_____

Rating system:
2 = Meets or exceeds standards
1 = Opportunity for improvement
0 = Unsatisfactory performance
Total points possible = 20

Procedure Step	Rating	Comments
1. Explain procedure to patient		
2. Have patient extend wrist and make a fist		
3. Use appropriate fingers to locate radial and ulnar arteries		
4. Simultaneously compress and occlude both arteries		
5. Maintain pressure while patient slowly opens and closes hand		
6. Lower patient's hand and release pressure on the ulnar artery		
7. Observe color of patient's hand		
8. Record results as positive or negative		
9. Explain the significance of a positive result		
10. Explain the significance of a negative result		
Total points		

Index

Note: Page numbers followed by *f* indicate figures; those followed by *t* indicate tables.

A

AAAHP (American Association of Allied Health Professionals, Inc.), 7, 8, 369
Abbreviations, 50, 50t–54t
Abdominal cavity, 60, 60f
ABO blood group system, 103–104, 104t, 369
Accepting assignment, of health care costs, 23, 369
Accession number, 354–355, 369
Accreditation, of educational programs, 7–8, 369
Acid citrate dextrose, in tubes, 164
ACTH (adrenocorticotropic hormone), 70
Activated coagulation time test definition of, 369
  point-of-care, 273–274, 275f
  specimen warming for, 332
Activated partial thromboplastin time test, 32, 34t, 107
  point-of-care, 277, 278f
Adapters, in evacuated tube system, 158, 159f, 160, 160f, 162
Additives, for tubes, 163–165, 369
  carryover of, order of draw and, 166–167, 168t, 169
  definition of, 383
  mixing of, 215–216
Adhesives, allergies to, 186
Administrators, laboratory, duties of, 41–42
Admission, routine tests in, 180
Adrenal glands, 70, 70f
  disorders of, 72
Adrenocorticotropic hormone, 70
Aerobic collection, 259, 369
Aerosols, formation of, in specimen processing, 331, 335
  definition of, 369
Age, basal state and, 176
Agglutination, 103
  in blood type mismatch, 256
  at cool temperatures, 264–265, 264t, 265f
  definition of, 369

Agglutinins, 103, 369
Agranulocytes, 102–103, 369
Airborne precautions, in isolation, 128, 133t, 134f, 369
Airborne transmission
  of biohazards, 133
  of infections, 116
Air bubbles, in arterial blood specimen, 303
Airway obstruction, first aid for, 148–149, 148f
Albumin, 101, 369
Alcohol, tests for, 269
Alcohol prep pad, 212
Aldosterone, 71
Aliquots
  definition of, 333, 369
  preparation of, 335, 336f
Alkalosis, 83
Allen test, 299, 300f
  definition of, 369
  procedure evaluation checklist for, 414
Allergies, 185–186
Alpha-fetoprotein, in amniotic fluid, 314
Alternate site testing. *See* Point-of-care testing
Altitude, basal state and, 176
Aluminum foil, in light protection, 263, 264f
Alveoli, 81, 81f, 369
Ambulatory care, 20, 369
American Association of Allied Health Professionals, Inc., 7, 8, 369
American Medical Technologists, 7, 8, 369
American Society for Clinical Laboratory Sciences, 370
American Society for Medical Technology, 370
American Society for Phlebotomy Technicians, 7, 8, 370
American Society of Clinical Pathologists, 7, 8, 370
Ammonium oxalate, in tubes, 164

Amniotic fluid, 314, 369
AMT (American Medical Technologists), 7, 8, 369
Anabolism, 61, 369
Anaerobic collection, 259, 369
Analyte, definition of, 369
Analyzers, point-of-care, 279, 280f
Anatomic position, 58, 370
Anatomy
  cavities in, 60, 60f, 315
  definition of, 58
  directional terms in, 59–60, 59f
  planes in, 58, 59f
  position in, 58
Anchoring, of vein, 214
Ancillary blood glucose testing, 283, 283f, 370
Anemia, 370
Anesthetic, local, for arterial puncture, 299, 301
Aneurysm, 370
Ankle, venipuncture in, 99, 99f, 212
Antebrachial vein, 98f
Antecubital fossa, 98–99, 98f, 370
Antecubital veins, 98, 98f, 370
  in pediatric patients, 227
Anterior direction, 59, 59f, 370
Antibiotic susceptibility
  definition of, 370
  testing for, of urine bacteria, 309
Antibodies
  definition of, 370
  in plasma, 101
Anticoagulants, 105
  for arterial puncture, 298, 304
  definition of, 370
  for evacuated tubes, 164–165
  reflux of, in blood collection, 188–189
Antidiuretic hormone (vasopressin), 70
Antigens, definition of, 370
Antiglycolytic agents, 165, 370
Antimicrobial removal device, 262, 370

Antimicrobial therapy, definition of, 370
Antisepsis and antiseptics
 allergies to, 185–186
 for blood collection, 154–155, 259–261, 260f, 261f
 definition of, 370
 skin, 259–261, 260f, 261f, 381
Anuclear cells, definition of, 101, 370
Aorta, 93f, 94, 370
Aortic valve, 90
Appearance, communication through, 343–344
Approval, of educational program, 7–8, 370
ARD (antimicrobial removal device), 263, 370
Arizona Health Care Cost Containment System, 24
Arm
 arteries of, 295f
 veins of, for venipuncture, 98–99, 98f
Arrhythmias, cardiac, 90, 370
Arterial blood gases
 definition of, 370
 evaluation of
  arterial puncture for. *See* Arterial puncture
  point-of-care, 277–278
Arterialized specimen, in skin puncture, 242, 249–250
Arterial puncture, 100
 accidental, 188
 Allen test in, 299, 300f, A-30
 anesthetic for, 299, 301
 brachial, 295–296, 295f
 collection devices for, 209
 complications of, 303
 equipment for, 296–298, 297f
 femoral, 295f, 296, 297f
 historical review of, 294
 personnel for, 294
 preparation for, 298–299, 300f
 procedure for, evaluation checklist for, A-29
 radial, 294–295, 295f, 299, 301–302, 301f, 302f
 reasons for, 293–294
 sampling errors in, 303–304
 site care after, 302
 site selection for, 294–296, 295f, 297f
 specimen rejection in, 304
Arteries, 93–94, 93f. *See also* specific arteries
 of arm, 295f
 catheters in, blood collection from, 183
 definition of, 370
 of hand, 295f
 of leg, 297f

puncture of. *See* Arterial puncture
 spasm of, after puncture, 303
 structure of, 95–96, 95f
Arterioles, 94, 95f, 370
Arteriosclerosis, 370
Arteriospasm, 303, 370
Arteriovenous shunt, 371
 blood collection from, 185, 186f
ASAP tests, 179, 370
ASCLS (American Society for Clinical Laboratory Sciences), 370
ASCP (American Society of Clinical Pathologists), 7, 8, 370
ASMT (American Society for Medical Technology), 370
Aspiration
 of gastric contents, 315
 suprapubic, 382
ASPT (American Society for Phlebotomy Technicians), 7, 8, 370
Assault, 10, 370
Assignment, of health care costs, 23, 369
Atherosclerosis, 370
Atria, 88, 370
Atrioventricular bundle, 371
Atrioventricular node, 89, 90f, 370
Atrioventricular valves, 88, 370
Autologous blood donation, 259, 371
Autonomic nervous system, 76
Avascular, definition of, 78, 371
A-V shunt, 371

B
Bacteremia, 371
 blood culture in, 259
Bactericidal agents, 371
Bacteriostatic agents, 371
Bandages, 154, 217
Barcodes
 in patient identification, 325, 326f
 in specimen identification, 325, 326f
 in test requisitions, 195, 195f
Barriers
 in communication, 340
 definition of, 371
 in infection control, 138
Basal state
 definition of, 175, 371
 factors affecting, 176–178
Basilic vein, 98f, 99, 371
Basophils, 102, 371
Battery, 10, 371
Bed rails, venipuncture with, 206
Bedside manner, 202, 371
Bevel, of needle, 157, 371
Bicarbonate ion
 point-of-care tests for, 279
 in respiratory system, 82–83, 82f

Biconcave shape, 101, 371
Bilirubin
 light degradation of, 263
 test for, skin puncture for, 250–251
Bill of Rights, Patient's, 9, 379, A-7–A-8
Biohazards, 133–139
 bloodborne pathogens. *See* Bloodborne pathogens
 definition of, 133, 371
 disposal of, 138
 entry routes for, 133–134
 exposure control plan for, 138–139
 exposure incident management in, 135, 137
 spill clean-up, 137–138
 surface decontamination for, 137
 symbol for, 133, 137f
Biopsy, tissue specimen from, 318
Bladder, 77–78, 77f
 urine specimen collection from, 313–314
Bleeding
 after venipuncture, 217
 excessive, 187
 first aid for, 145–146
Bleeding time test, 34t
 definition of, 371
 point-of-care, 274–277, 275f, 276f
 procedures for, evaluation checklist for, 412
Blood, 100–106
 components of, 101–103
 diagnostic tests for, 106
 disorders of, 105–106
 formed elements in, 101–103, Color Plate 3
 occult
  point-of-care test for, 284–285, 285f
  in stool, 316
 oxygen carrying capacity of, 82–83, 82f
 spilled, clean-up procedure for, 137–138
 transfusions of. *See* Transfusions
 types of, 103–105, 104t
 volume of, 101
 whole, 105
Blood alcohol tests, 269
Blood banking, 40, 40t, 257–259. *See also* Transfusions
 autologous blood collection in, 259, 371
 donor blood collection in, 257–259
 specimens for, 256–257, 257f
 tests performed in, 400–401
Bloodborne pathogens, 118–119
 body substance isolation procedures for, 125–126, 125f, 127f, 128f

definition of, 371
occupational exposure to, 135, 137
universal precautions with, 125, 131f
Blood collection
    antiseptics in, 153–154
    arterial. *See* Arterial puncture
    from arteriovenous shunt, 185, 186f
    for blood alcohol test, 269
    for blood banking, 257–259, 257f, 258f
    blood-drawing station for, 152, 152f
    carts for, 152–153
    for coagulation studies, 263–265, 263f, 264t, 265f
    complications of, 185–191
        affecting patient, 185–189
        affecting specimen integrity, 189–191
    for culture, 158, 159f, 259–262, 260f, 261f, 411
    disinfectants in, 154
    disposal containers for, 154, 155f
    dressings for, 154
    for drug screening, 269, 271, 271t
    for epinephrine tolerance test, 268
    equipment for, 151–155, 152f, 153f, 155f. *See also*
        Needle(s); Tube(s)
    for forensic studies, 269, 270f
    gloves in, 153
    for glucagon tolerance test, 268
    for glucose testing
        postprandial, 265–266
        tolerance, 266–268, 267f
    from heparin lock, 183–184, 185f
    for lactose tolerance test, 268–269
    for paternity/parentage testing, 265
    pen for, 154
    physiologic factors in, 175–178
    from saline lock, 183–184, 185f
    site selection for, 180–182
    slides for, 154
    test status in, 178–180
    for therapeutic drug monitoring, 272–273, 272f
    for therapeutic phlebotomy, 266
    for tolerance tests, 266–269, 267f
    for toxicology studies, 269–273, 270f, 271t, 272f
    for trace element measurement, 273
    trays for, 153, 153f
    from vascular access device, 182–183, 183f–184f
    by venipuncture. *See* Venipuncture

Blood culture, specimen collection for, 158, 159f, 259–262, 260f, 261f
    procedure evaluation checklist for, A-27
Blood film preparation
    evaluation checklist for, A-26
    routine, 245–248, 247f, 248f, 249t
    thick, 248–249
Blood flow, 96, 97f
Blood gases
    arterial. *See* Arterial blood gases
    capillary
        definition of, 372
        skin puncture for, 236–237, 237f, 249–250
Blood-Loc Safety System, for transfusions, 257, 258f
Blood pressure, 91, 371
Blood smears
    definition of, 371
    preparation of
        evaluation checklist for, A-26
        routine, 245–248, 247f, 248f, 249t
        thick, 248–249
Blood specimens
    collection of. *See* Blood collection
    cooling of, 263, 263f, 264t
    integrity of, collection techniques and, 189–191
    light-sensitive, 263, 264f, 264t
    transport of, 219
    types of, 105, 106f
Blood vessels, 92–96. *See also*
    Arteries; Veins; *specific vessels*
    structure of, 95–96, 95f
    types of, 93–95, 93f–95f
Blood volume
    adult, 366
    calculations with, 366–367
    definition of, 371
    infant, 367
B lymphocytes, 103, 371
Body
    cavities of, 60, 60f, 371
        fluid specimens from, 315
    directional terms for, 59–60, 59f
    functions of, 61
    organization of, 61–62, 62f
    planes of, 58, 59f, 371
    positions of, 58
    systems of, 62–84
        circulatory. *See* Circulatory system; *specific components*
        digestive, 68–69, 68f
        endocrine, 69–73, 70f
        integumentary, 78–80, 79f
        muscles, 64–66, 65f
        nervous, 73, 74f, 75f, 76
        reproductive, 66, 67f

        respiratory, 80–84, 81f, 83f
        skeletal, 62–64, 63f
        urinary, 76–78, 77f
Body fluids
    pathogens in, 118–119
    body substance isolation procedures for, 125–126, 125f, 127f, 128f
    universal precautions with, 125
    tests for, 34t
Body language, 342–344, 342f, 343f
Body substance isolation, 125–126, 125f, 127f, 128f, 371
Bone marrow, tests for, 34t
Bones, 62–64
    diagnostic tests for, 64
    disorders of, 64
    functions of, 62–63, 63f
Bracelet, identification, 199–200, 200f
    for transfusions, 256–257, 257f, 258f
Brachial artery
    definition of, 371
    puncture of, 100, 295–296, 295f
Bradycardia, 90, 371
Brain, 73, 74f
Breach of confidentiality, 15, 371
Bronchi, 81, 81f
BSI (body substance isolation), 125–126, 125f, 127f, 128f, 371
Bubbles, in arterial blood specimen, 303
Buffy coat, 105, 106f
Bundle of His, 371
Burns, site selection in, 180
BURPP mnemonic, in skin puncture, 242
Butterfly needle set, 170–171, 171f, 172f
    procedure with, 220, 221f, 222–223
        evaluation checklist for, 407

C

Calcaneus, 371
    protection of, in heelstick, 239–240, 240f
Calcitonin, 70
Calcium, 371
    ionized, point-of-care tests for, 279
Cannula
    arteriovenous, blood collection from, 185, 186f
    definition of, 371
CAP (College of American Pathologists), 8, 371
Capillaries
    blood, 95, 95f, 96f, 371
    lymph, 110–111

Capillary action, 236, 372
Capillary blood gases
 definition of, 372
 skin puncture for, 236–237, 237f,
  249–250
Capitation, as reimbursement
 method, 23–24, 372
Caraway tubes, 236, 372
Carbaminohemoglobin, 82, 372
Carbon dioxide
 exchange of, in respiratory system, 82–83, 82f
 partial pressure of, measurement of, 277–278
Cardiac cycle, 89, 372
Cardiac muscle, 64, 65f
Cardiac output, 90, 372
Cardiac troponin T, point-of-care
 tests for, 279, 281f
Cardiopulmonary resuscitation,
 148–149, 148f, 372
Carotene, light degradation of, 263
Carryover, of additives, order of
 draw and, 166–167, 168t,
 169
Carts, for blood collection, 152–153
Catabolism, 61, 372
Category-specific isolation, 125,
 126t
Catheters
 blood collection from
  arterial, 183
  central venous, 182, 183f,
   184f
 definition of, 372
 urine collection from, 313
Caudal cavity, 60, 60f
Caudal direction, 59f, 60
Cavities, body, 60, 60f, 371
 fluid specimens from, 315
CDC. See Centers for Disease
 Control
Cells, 61, 62f
Celsius scale, 363, 364f, 372
Centers for Disease Control, 114,
 372
 infection control guidelines of,
  118
 isolation guidelines of, 126–129,
  130f–131f, 132t, 133t,
  134f–136f
Centigrade scale, 363, 364f
Central nervous system, 73, 74f
Central processing, of specimens,
 333–336, 334f–336f, 372
Central processing unit, com-
 puter, 350, 351f, 373
Central supply service, 30
Central venous catheter, blood
 collection from, 182, 183f,
 184f

Centrifugation, 332, 333f, 372
 blood separation in, 105, 106f
 clotting before, 333–334
 procedure for, 334
 specimen preparation for, 334,
  334f
Centrioles, 61, 62f
Cephalic vein, 98, 98f
 definition of, 372
 location of, in obesity, 181
Cerebrospinal fluid, 73, 314–315,
 372
Certification, 6–7, 372
Certified Laboratory Phlebotomist,
 7
Certified Phlebotomy Technician,
 7
CEU (continuing education
 units), 8, 327, 373
Chain of custody, 372
 for forensic specimens, 269, 270f
Chain of infection, 114–117, 114f,
 372
Chair, for blood drawing, 152,
 152f, 206, 206f
Checklists, for procedure evaluation, 405–414
Chemical safety
 chemical identification in,
  142–143, 144t–145t,
  145f–146f
 decontamination equipment in,
  143, 147f
Chemical spills, clean-up procedure for, 143, 147f
Chemistry analyzers, point-of-
 care, 279, 280f
Chemistry department, 34,
 35t–37t
 tests performed in, A-9–A-13
Children. See Pediatric patients
Chiropractor, 27t
Chloride
 point-of-care tests for, 279
 in sweat, in cystic fibrosis,
  316–317, 382
Cholesterol, point-of-care tests
 for, 281
Chordae tendineae, 372
Circulation, 96, 97f
 collateral
  Allen test for, 299, 300f, 414
  definition of, 373
 pulmonary, 92, 96, 97f, 380
 systemic, 92, 96, 97f, 382
Circulatory system, 87–112. See
 also Arteries; Blood; Veins
 definition of, 372
 heart in, 88–92, 90f, 91f, Color
  Plate 1
 hemostasis and, 107, 108f, 109

lymphatic system in, 109–111,
 110f
 overview of, 84
Citrate, in tubes, 164
Civil law, 10, 372
Clean-catch urine specimen,
 312–313, 372
Cleaning and cleansing
 of contaminated surfaces,
  137–138, 143, 147f
 of skin
  for blood collection, 154–155,
   212
  for blood culture specimen,
   259–261, 260f, 261f
  for skin puncture, 242
Clergy visit, venipuncture dur-
 ing, 199
CLIA (Clinical Laboratory
 Improvement Act of 1988),
 43, 372
Clinical laboratory assistants, 42
Clinical Laboratory Improvement
 Act of 1988, 43, 372
Clinical Laboratory Phlebotomist,
 7
Clinical laboratory scientist, 42
Clinical laboratory technicians, 42
Clock, twenty-four hour, 362, 363f
Clot activators, 165, 333–334, 372
Clothing, protective. See Protective
 clothing and equipment
CoaguChek system, 277, 278f
Coagulation. See also Hemostasis
 definition of, 372
 platelets in, 103
Coagulation cascade, 107, 108f, 109
Coagulation department, 33, 34t
 tests performed in, 398–399
Coagulation factors, 107, 108f
Coagulation tests
 point-of-care, 273–277, 275f,
  276f, 278f
 specimen collection for,
  263–265, 263f–265f, 264t
Coccidioidomycosis test, 287
Coinsurance, 23, 372
Cold agglutinin, 265, 372
Collateral circulation
 Allen test for, 299, 300f, 369, A-30
 definition of, 373
Collection. See Blood collection;
 Specimen collection
College of American Pathologists
 definition of, 371
 drug interference guidelines of,
  177
 standards of, 8
Combining forms, in terminol-
 ogy, 49, 373
Combining vowels, in terminology, 48–49, 373

Comfort, zones of, 343, 384
Communicable diseases, 114
Communication
  barriers in, 340
  in computer networks, 349, 350f,
    351f
  computers in. *See* Computer(s);
    Information management
  definition of, 340
  elements of, 344–346
  listening in, 340, 342
  nonverbal, 342–344, 342f, 343f
  Spanish-English equivalents
    for, A-3–A-6
  telephone, 346, 347t
  verbal, 340, 341f
Compatibility, of blood groups,
  103–105, 104t, 256, 373
Complete blood count, 32, 32f, 32t
Complications, of blood collec-
    tion, 185–191
  affecting patient, 185–189
  affecting specimen integrity,
    189–191
  by arterial puncture, 303
Computer(s), 346–357
  classification of, 348–349
  components of, 349–350, 351f,
    352
  elements of, 352–353, 352f
  future applications of, 357
  in Laboratory Information
    Management System,
    353–355, 355f, 356f
  laboratory uses of, 353
  literacy in, 347
  networking of, 349, 350f, 351f
  skills for, 353–354
  terminology of, 348, 348t
  in test requisition, 194–195, 195f
Computerized axial tomography,
  58
Concentric circles, in skin
    cleansing, 261f, 373
Conduction system, of heart, 89,
  90f
Confidentiality, 14–15
  breach of, 15, 371
  in HIV testing, 15
Confirmation, in communication,
  345–346
Connective tissue, 61
Consent
  expressed, 13, 374
  implied, 13, 376
  informed, 9, 13, 202–204, 376
Contact precautions, 129, 133t,
  136f, 373
Contact transmission, of infec-
    tions, 116

Contamination, of specimen,
    190–191
  with additive, 166–167, 168t, 169
Continuing education, 8, 373
  in quality control, 327
Continuous quality improve-
    ment, definition of, 373
Control, in communication, 345
Conversation, Spanish-English
    equivalents for, A-3–A-6
Conversions, of measurement
    units, 361–363, 361t, 362t,
    363f
Cooling, of specimens, 263, 263f,
    264t, 331–332
  arterial blood, 298, 303
Coring, of tissue, 373
Coronal plane, 58
Coronary arteries, 89, 373
Cortisol, 71
Cost shifting, 373
Cotton balls, 154
CPR (cardiopulmonary resuscita-
    tion), 148–149, 148f, 372
CPU (central processing unit),
    350, 351f, 373
CQI (continuous quality
    improvement), 373
Cranial cavity, 60, 60f
Cranial direction, 59f, 60
Criminal law, 10
Crossmatching, of blood groups,
    103–105, 104t, 256–257,
    257f, 258f, 373
CRT (cathode ray tube), 373
CRUD acronym, for interfering
    substances, 177
Cryofibrinogen, 265
Cryoglobulin, 265
Cubital veins, 98, 98f
  median, 98, 98f, 377
Culture
  blood, specimen collection for,
    158, 159f, 259–262, 260f,
    261f
    procedure evaluation check-
      list for, 411
  nasopharyngeal, 315, 378
  throat, 317, 317f
Culture and sensitivity test, 309,
    309f, 373
Cupping, 3–4, 3f
Cursor, on computer screen, 353,
    373
Cutaneous nerve, median, injury
    of, in venipuncture, 100
Cutdown, site selection in, 180
Cyanosis, 373
  skin puncture and, 239
Cystic fibrosis, sweat chloride test
    in, 316–317, 382

Cytogenetics department, 41
Cytology, urine, 309–310
Cytology department, 41
Cytoplasm, 61, 62f

D
Data
  definition of, 373
  entering of, on computer, 353
  evaluation of, in quality assur-
    ance, 323
Decimal system, 373
Decontamination, of surfaces,
    137–138
Deep (internal) direction, 59
Dehydration, basal state and, 176
Department of Health and
    Human Services, Public
    Health Service, 22, 22t
Department of Transportation,
    hazardous material label-
    ing system of, 143,
    144t–145t, 145f
Dermis, 78, 79f, 373
Diabetes insipidus, 373
Diabetes mellitus, 72, 373
Diagnostic-related groups, 23, 373
Diapedesis, 102
Diaphragm, 60
Diarrhea, infection control in, 132t
Diastole, 89, 373
Diastolic blood pressure, 91, 373
Dick test, 287
Diet
  basal state and, 176
  restrictions of, verification of, 203
Dietary service, 30
Differential count, 33t, 373
  smear preparation for, 246–247,
    247f, 248f
Digestive system, 68–69, 68f
Dilutions
  calculations with, 366
  micropipet, in skin puncture,
    237, 238f
Diplomacy, 9
Direction, body, 59, 59f
Discard tube, 263, 373
Disease-specific isolation, 125, 126t
Disinfectants, 155, 374
Disposal
  of biohazardous waste, 138
  of needles, 131f, 154, 155f, 160,
    161f–163f, 162, 213f, 218
  of sharps, 154, 155f
Distal direction, 59f, 60, 374
Diurnal variations, 70, 374
  basal state and, 176
Documentation, in quality assur-
    ance, 327–329, 328f

Donation, blood
  autologous, 371
  collection of, 257–259
Do not resuscitate order, 197–198
Dorsal cavities, 60, 60f, 374
Dorsal (posterior) direction, 59, 59f, 374
Draw, order of, in venipuncture, 166–170, 168t, 170f, 378–379
Droplet precautions, 374
  in isolation, 129, 133t, 135f
Droplet transmission, of infections, 116
Drugs
  basal state and, 176–177
  screening for, 260, 271–272, 271t
    in urine, 310
  therapeutic monitoring of, 272–273, 272f, 382
Duke bleeding time test, 275

E
Edema
  definition of, 374
  site selection in, 181
  skin puncture and, 239
Education
  continuing, 8, 327, 373
  program for, accreditation of, 7–8, 369
Electrical safety, 139, 374
Electrocardiography, 30, 30f, 89, 91f, 281–283, 281f, 374
Electrolytes, 77
  definition of, 374
  in plasma, 101
  point-of-care tests for, 278–279
Electroneurodiagnostics, 30–31, 30f
Embolism, 100, 374
Embolus, 100, 374
Emergency department, 29
  identification procedures for, 201
Empathy, in communication, 344–345, 374
Employee screening, in infection control, 119–120
Endocardium, 88, 374
Endocrine system, 69–73
  diagnostic tests for, 73
  disorders of, 71–73
  functions of, 69, 70f
  glands of, 70–71, 71f
Endoplasmic reticulum, 61, 62f
Engineering controls, in exposure control, 138, 374
English system of measurement, 361–362, 361t
Entitlement programs, 24, 374
Environment, basal state and, 177
Environmental services, 30

Enzyme immunoassays, 35–36
Eosinophil(s), 102, 374
Eosinophil count, 34t
Epicardium, 88, 374
Epidermis, 78, 79f, 374
Epiglottis, 81, 81f
Epinephrine, 71
Epinephrine tolerance test, 268
Epithelial tissue, 61
Equipment
  for arterial puncture, 296–298, 297f
  for blood collection, 151–155, 152f, 153f, 155f. *See also* Needle(s); Tube(s)
  history of, 2–4, 2f, 3f
  checking of, forms for, 329
  for point-of-care testing. *See* Point-of-care testing
  protective. *See* Protective clothing and equipment
  quality control of, 325
  for venipuncture. *See under* Venipuncture
Errors
  in arterial blood specimen handling, 302–304
  correction of, on computer, 354
Erythema, 287, 374
Erythrocytes, 101, 374
Erythrocyte sedimentation rate, 34t
Erythropoietin, 71, 374
Essentials, of educational programs, 7, 374
Estrogen, 71
Ethanol
  definition of, 374
  tests for, 269
Ethics, 9
Ethylenediaminetetraacetic acid, in tubes, 164
  contamination by, 167–168, 168t
Evacuated tubes
  additives for, 163–166
  color coding of, 165–166
    order of draw and, 168–169
  definition of, 374
  description of, 162–166
  quality control of, 325
  standards for, 325
  stoppers for, 165–166, 167f, Color Plate 2
  transfer from syringe, 225, 225f
Evacuated tube system, 157–162, 157f
  holders in, 158, 159f, 160, 160f, 205, 205f
  needle disposal systems in, 160, 161f–163f, 162
  needles in, 158
  order of draw in, 166–169, 168t
Exercise, basal state and, 177

Exposure control plan, for bio-hazards, 138–139
Expressed consent, 13, 374
External (superficial) direction, 59
External respiration, 80, 374
Extinguishers, fire, 140, 141f
Extrasystoles, 90
Extravascular location, 374
Extrinsic pathway, of coagulation cascade, 107, 108f, 374
Eye contact, in communication, 343, 343f
Eye wash stations, 143, 147f

F
Face shields, 121
Fahrenheit scale, 363, 364f, 374
Fainting, 187
Family, handling of, 199, 227
Fasting, 374
  for specimen collection, 179, 203
Feather, on slide, 247, 249t, 374
Feces specimen, 316, 316f
Feedback, in communication, 340, 341f
Fee-for-service, 23
Female
  clean-catch urine specimen from, 312–313
  reproductive system of, 66, 67f
Femoral artery, 375
  puncture of, 100, 295f, 296, 297f
Femoral vein, 99, 99f
Fever of unknown origin, blood culture in, 259
Fibrillations, heart, 90
Fibrin, 375
Fibrin clot, formation of, 107
Fibrin degradation products, 34t, 109, 375
Fibrinogen, 101, 105, 375
Fibrinogen test, 34t
Fibrinolysis, 108f, 109, 375
Financing, health care. *See under* Health care
Finger stick procedure, 241, 242f, 243, 245, 244f, 246f
  evaluation checklist for, 408
Fire extinguishers, 140, 141f
Fire safety, 139–141, 141f
First aid, 145–146, 148–149, 148f
First morning urine specimen collection, 310
Fistula, 375
  arteriovenous, blood collection from, 185, 186f
Flanges, definition of, 158, 375
Fleas (metal stirrers), in capillary blood gas specimen collection, 237, 375

Floor book, 375
Folate, light degradation of, 263
Follicle stimulating hormone, 70
Fomites, 116, 375
Foot, veins of, for venipuncture, 99, 99f
Forensic specimens, 269, 270f, 375
Formed elements, in blood, 101–103, Color Plate 3
Forms, for quality assurance, 329
Fractional (double-voided) urine specimen, 311–312
Fraud, 11, 375
Frontal plane, 58, 59f, 375
FUO (fever of unknown origin), blood culture in, 259

G
Gas exchange, in respiratory system, 82–83, 82f
Gastric analysis, 315, 375
Gatekeeper, primary care physician as, 25, 375
Gauge, 157, 375
Gauze pads, 154
Gel separator tubes, 165, 382
Gender, basal state and, 177
Germicides, 375
Glands. *See* Endocrine system
Global capitation, as reimbursement method, 24
Glomeruli, 77
Gloves, 121–122, 123f, 124f, 130f, 154
    donning, 205
    removal of, 219
Glucagon, 71
Glucagon tolerance test, 268
Glucose, definition of, 375
Glucose testing
    ancillary, 283, 283f, 370
    monitoring, 375
    point-of-care, 283, 283f
    postprandial, 265–266
    specimen stability in, 332
    tolerance, 375
        specimen collection for, 266–268, 267f
        urine specimens for, 310–311
Glycogen storage, epinephrine tolerance test of, 268
Glycolysis, 165, 375
Goggles, 121
Golgi apparatus, 61, 62f
Gowns, protective, 121–123, 124f, 130f
Gram, metric system based on, 359–360, 360t, 375
Granulocytes, 102, 375
Growth hormone, 70

Guaiac test, 316, 375
    point-of-care, 284–285, 285f
Guideline for Isolation Precautions in Hospitals, 126–129, 130f–131f, 132t, 133t, 134f–136f

H
Hair, 78, 79
Hand
    arteries of, 295f
    veins of, 98f
        butterfly needle use in, 220, 221f, 222–223
        in pediatric patients, 228, 228f
        venipuncture of, procedure evaluation checklist for, A-23
Handling, of specimens, 329–336
    in blood bank, A-16–A-17
    in chemistry department, A-9–A-13
    in coagulation department, A-14–A-15
    errors in, 302–304
    guidelines for, 331, 332
    in hematology department, A-13–A-14
    in immunohematology department, A-16–A-17
    in immunology department, A-15–A-16
    importance of, 329, 331
    light protection in, 331
    in microbiology department, A-17
    nonblood, 308
    routine, 331
    in serology department, A-15–A-16
    special, 331–332
    temperature considerations in, 331–332
    time constraints on, 332, 333f
    tissue, 318
Handwashing, 120–121, 130f, 205
Hardware, computer, 352, 352f, 375
Hazardous Communication Standard (OSHA), 143, 375
Health care
    facilities for. *See also* Hospital(s)
        classification of, 20–21, 21t
        inpatient, 20–21
        outpatient, 20
        Public Health Service, 22, 22t
    financing of, 22–27
        changes in, 24–25
        employment status and, 24
        managed care plans in, 25–26, 26t

payment methods for, 23
    reimbursement methods in, 23–24
    third-party payers in, 22–24
Health maintenance organizations, 25, 375
Health unit clerk or secretary, 194, 194f
Heart, 88–92
    chambers of, 88
    conduction system of, 89, 90f
    diagnostic tests for, 92
    disorders of, 92
    function of, 89–91, 90f, 91f
    layers of, 88
    structure of, 88–89, Color Plate 1
    valves of, 88–89
Heart attack, 89
Heart beat, 90
Heart rate, 90
Heart sounds, 90
Heating devices, for specimens, 264–265, 264t, 265f
Heelstick procedure, 239–240, 240f, 241f, 243, 245, 245f, 246f
    evaluation checklist for, 409
Hematocrit
    definition of, 33t, 375
    point-of-care test for, 284, 284f
Hematology department, 33, 33f, 32t, 33t
    tests performed in, A-13–A-14
Hematoma
    from arterial puncture, 303
    definition of, 375
    site selection in, 181
    from venipuncture, 187
Hemochromatosis, 266, 375
Hemochron system, 274, 275f
Hemoconcentration
    definition of, 375
    in dehydration, 176
    specimen integrity and, 189
HemoCue hemoglobin system, 284, 284f
Hemogard closure tubes, 335, 335f
Hemoglobin, 101
    definition of, 375
    oxygen carrying capacity of, 82–83
    point-of-care test for, 284, 284f
    test for, 33t
Hemolysis, of specimen, 190, 375–376
Hemopoiesis, 62–63
Hemorrhage. *See* Bleeding
Hemostasis, 61
    definition of, 107, 376
    diagnostic tests for, 109
    disorders of, 109
    primary, 107, 380
    secondary, 107, 108f, 109, 381

Hemostatic plug, 109, 376
Heparin
    in arterial puncture, 299
    in tubes, 164
        contamination by, 167–168,
            168t
Heparin lock, 376
    blood collection from, 183–184,
        185f
Hepatitis, definition of, 376
Hepatitis B
    definition of, 376
    immunization for, 138
    occupational exposure to, 135,
        137
    transmission of, 118
    viral viability in, 116
Histology department, 40
Histoplasmosis test, 287
HMOs (health maintenance orga-
    nizations), 25, 375
Holders, in evacuated tube sys-
    tem, 158, 159f, 160, 160f,
    162, 205, 205f
Homeostasis, 61, 376
Hormones. *See* Endocrine system
Hospital(s). *See also* Laboratory,
        clinical
    classification of, 20–21, 21t
    infections acquired in, 114
    organization of, 21, 27, 28f, 29f
    secondary care in, 20
    services of
        clinical laboratory. *See* Labo-
            ratory, clinical
        nursing, 27, 29–30
        outpatient, 20
        professional, 30–31, 30f, 31f
        radiology, 31
        support, 30
Hospital Infection Control Prac-
        tices Advisory Committee,
        114, 376
Housekeeping, in exposure con-
        trol, 138
Human chorionic gonadotropin,
        in pregnancy testing, 285,
        286f, 376
Human immunodeficiency virus
        infection
    definition of, 376
    occupational exposure to, 135,
        137
    testing for
        confidentiality in, 15
        consent for, 13
    transmission of, 118
    viral viability in, 116
Hyperglycemia, 376
    glucose tolerance test for,
        266–268, 267f

Hypoglycemia, 376
    glucose tolerance test for,
        266–268, 267f
Hypothyroidism screening, skin
    puncture for, 251

I
ID. *See* Identification
Identification
    patient
        bands for, 376
        cards for, 376
        definition of, 379
        discrepancies in, 201
        in emergency room, 201
        in forensic studies, 269, 270f
        missing, 201
        outpatient, 202
        pediatric, 201
        in quality control, 325, 326f
        verification of, 199–200, 200f
    specimen. *See also* Labels and
            labeling
        for blood bank, 256–257,
            257f, 258f
        in forensic studies, 269, 270f
Illness, work restrictions in, 403–404
Imaging services, 31
Immunity, 117
Immunization, in infection control,
        119–120
Immunoassays, 35–36
Immunoglobulins, 376
Immunohematology department,
        40, 40t
    tests performed in, 400–401
Immunology department, 34, 37t,
        37
    tests performed in, A-15–A-16
Implanted port, blood collection
        from, 182, 184f
Implied consent, 13, 376
Incident reports
    for exposures, 135, 137
    form for, 16f, 17
    in quality assurance, 329
Indemnity insurance, 23, 376
Induration, definition of, 376
Indwelling lines, 376
    blood collection from, 182–183,
        183f–184f
Infants. *See* Pediatric patients
Infections. *See also specific infections*
    after blood collection, 188
    bloodborne, 118–119
        occupational exposure to,
            135, 137
        universal precautions with,
            125, 131f
    causative agents of, 114

chain of, 114–117, 114f, 372
communicable, 114
control of
    breaking chain of infection in,
        117
    handwashing in, 120–121,
        130f, 205
    isolation in. *See* Isolation
    in nursery, 123–124
    programs for, 119–120
    protective clothing in,
        121–123, 122f–124f
    regulations on, 117–118
definition of, 114, 376
local, 114
nosocomial, 114, 378
sources of, 115–116, 115f
susceptibility to, 115, 115f, 117
systemic, 114
transmission of, 115, 115f,
    116–117
    bloodborne, 118–119, 125,
        131f, 135, 137
urinary tract, culture and sensi-
    tivity test in, 309, 309f
work restrictions in, 403–404
Inferior direction, 60, 376
Inflammation, definition of, 376
Information, patient's right to, 9
Information management, 29. *See
    also* Computer(s)
    systems for, 353–355, 355f, 356f
    of test requisition, 194–195,
        195f–196f
Informed consent, 13, 376
    as patient's right, 9
    for venipuncture, 202–204
Ingestion, of biohazards, 133–134
Inpatient care, 20–21, 376
Input, computer, 349, 376
Insulin, 71
Insurance
    health care
        changing conditions in, 24–25
        institution reimbursements in,
            24
        payment methods in, 23
        provider reimbursements in,
            23–24
        types of, 22–23
    indemnity, 23, 376
    malpractice, 12
    service, 23, 381
Integumentary system
    definition of, 376
    diagnostic tests for, 80
    disorders of, 80
    functions of, 78, 79f
    skin in. *See* Skin
Intensive care unit, 29
    neonatal, infection control in,
        123–124
Internal (deep) direction, 59

Internal respiration, 81, 376
Internet, 349, 351f
Interstitial fluid, 376
   in skin puncture specimen, 238
Intracellular fluid, 376
   in skin puncture specimen, 238
Intravascular, definition of, 376
Intravenous therapy, site selection in, 181–182
Intrinsic pathway, of coagulation cascade, 107, 108f, 376
Invasion of privacy, 15, 376–377
Iontophoresis, 376
   in sweat chloride test, 317
IRMA instrument, 279, 280f
Ischemia, 89, 376
Islets of Langerhans, 70, 70f
Isolation, 124–129
   body substance, 125–126, 125f, 127f, 128f, 371
   category-specific, 125, 126t
   definition of, 376
   disease-specific, 125
   guidelines for, 126–129, 130f–131f, 132t, 133t, 134f–136f
   protective (reverse), 125
   universal precautions in, 125
i-STAT instrument, 279, 280f
Ivy bleeding time test, 275–276, 276f, 377

J
Jaundice, monitoring of, skin puncture for, 250–251
Joint Commission on Accreditation of Healthcare Organizations (JCAHO), 8, 320, 322, 377

K
Keloids, 377
Kidney, 77–78, 77f
   endocrine function of, 71
Kinesics, 342–343, 342f, 343f, 377
Kinesic slip, 342, 377

L
Labels and labeling. *See also* Identification
   computer generation of, 194–195, 195f, 355, 355f
   of specimen, 216–217
      for blood bank, 256
      computerized, 194–195, 195f
      nonblood, 308
      pen for, 154
      quality control of, 327

warning
   for biohazards, 138
   for chemical hazards, 143, 144t–145t, 145f, 146f
   for radiation hazards, 141–142, 142f
Laboratory
   clinical, 30
      departments in, 31–40, 32f, 33t–40t, 36f
      mathematics in. *See* Mathematics
      personnel in, 42–43
      safety in. *See* Biohazards; Safety
   reference, 380
Laboratory director, duties of, 41
Laboratory Information Management Systems, 353–355, 355f, 356f
Laboratory procedure manuals, 328–329, 330f
Laboratory user manuals, 325
Lactose tolerance test, 268–269
Lancets, 234–235, 234f
   definition of, 377
   disposal of, 154, 155f
   quality control of, 325
Larynx, 80, 81f
Lateral direction, 59, 377
Latex, allergies to, 186
Latex block, for arterial blood specimen collection, 298
Leeching, 2f, 3
Leg
   arteries of, 297f
   veins for, for venipuncture, 99, 99f
Legal considerations, 10–17
   confidentiality, 14–15
   consent, 13
   criminal vs. civil law in, 10
   in forensic specimens, 269, 270f
   malpractice, 12–13, 377
   medical records and, 14
   negligence, 11
   respondeat superior, 11–12
   risk management, 15, 16f, 17
   standard of care, 12
   statute of limitations, 14–15
   tort law in, 10–11
   vicarious liability, 14
Leukemia, 105, 377
Leukocytes, 102, 377
Leukocytosis, 106, 377
Leukopenia, 106, 377
Liability, vicarious, 14, 384
Licensure, 7, 377
Light
   specimen degradation in, 263, 264t, 264f
   specimen protection from, 331

Lipemia, 377
   after meals, 176
Lipoproteins, point-of-care tests for, 281
Listening, in communication, 340, 342
Liter, metric system based on, 377, 359–360, 360t
Lithium iodoacetate, in tubes, 165
Litigation, avoidance of, risk management in, 15, 16f, 17
Liver, in hemostasis, 109
Local, definition of, 114, 377
Local anesthetic, for arterial puncture, 299, 301
Logging on computer, 353
Luer adapter, 222, 377
Lumen
   of blood vessels, 96
   definition of, 377
   of needle, 157
Lung, 81, 81f
Lupus erythematosus cells, 34t
Lymph, 110
Lymphatic system
   diagnostic tests for, 111
   disorders of, 111
   function of, 109
   structure of, 110–111, 110f
Lymph nodes, 110–111, 110f
Lymphocytes, 103, 377
Lymphostasis, 181, 377
Lysis, 377
   in blood type mismatch, 256
Lysosomes, 61, 62f

M
Magnet, in capillary blood gas specimen collection, 237
Magnetic resonance imaging, 58
Mainframe computers, 349
Male
   clean-catch urine specimen from, 312–313
   reproductive system of, 66, 67f
Malpractice, 12–13, 377
Managed care, 25–27, 26t, 27t, 377
Manual requisitions, 195, 196f
Manuals
   laboratory procedure, 328–329, 330f
   laboratory user, 325
   in quality assurance, 327–329, 328f
Masks, 121, 122, 124f, 130f
Mastectomy, site selection in, 181
Material Safety Data Sheets, 143, 377
Mathematics, 359–368
   blood volume, 366–367
   dilutions, 366

Mathematics (*continued*)
  metric system, 359–362, 360t–362t
  military time, 362, 363f
  percent, 365–366
  Roman numerals, 363–365
  temperature measurement, 363, 364f
Mean corpuscular hemoglobin, 33t
Mean corpuscular hemoglobin concentration, 33t
Mean corpuscular volume, 33t
Measurement systems
  English, 361–362, 361t
  metric, 359–362, 360t–362t
  military time, 362, 363f
  temperature, 363, 364f
Medial direction, 59, 377
Median cubital vein, 98, 98f, 377
Median cutaneous nerve, 100, 377
Medicaid, 8, 24, 377
Medical emergency tests, 179, 377
Medical laboratory technicians, duties of, 42
Medical record, 14, 30
  number of, 377
    on identification band, 200
  of occupational exposures, 139
Medical specialties, 26, 26t
Medical technologist, duties of, 42
Medical terminology. *See* Terminology
Medicare, 8, 24, 377
Megakaryocytes, 103, 377
Melatonin, 70
Meningitis, infection control in, 132t
Menu, on computer, 377
Metabolism, 61, 378
Metacarpal vein, 98f
Meter, metric system based on, 359–360, 360t, 378
Metric system, 359–362, 360t–362t, 378
Microbes, 114, 378
Microbiology department, 39, 39f, 39t
  tests performed in, A-17
Microcollection containers, 378
  in skin puncture, 235–236, 235f
Microcomputers, 348
Microhematocrit tubes, 378
  in skin puncture, 236, 236f
Micropipet dilution system, in skin puncture, 237, 238f
Midsagittal plane, 58, 59f
Midstream clean-catch urine collection, 312–313
Midstream urine collection, 312, 378
Military time, 362, 363f, 378
Milliliter, 360t, 378
Minerals, in plasma, 101
Minicomputers, 348–349
Mitochondria, 61, 62f

Mitosis, 61
Mitral valve, 88
Mixing
  of additives, 215–216
  of arterial blood specimen, 304
  of capillary blood gas samples, 246, 250
Mnemonics
  in computer use, 354–355
  definition of, 378
Modes of transmission, definition of, 116, 378
Monocytes, 102–103, 378
Motor nerves, 74f
MSDSs (Material Safety Data Sheets), 143, 377
Mucous membrane
  biohazard contact with, 134
  bloodborne pathogens transmission through, 119
Multidrug-resistant organisms, precautions with, 132t
Multiple samples, collection of
  syringe procedure in, 223, 225
  with tubes, 166–170, 168t, 170f
Murmurs, heart, 90
Muscular system
  diagnostic tests for, 65–66
  disorders of, 65
  functions of, 64
  muscles in, 64, 65f
Myocardium
  description of, 89
  infarction and ischemia of, 89, 378

N

NAACLS (National Accrediting Agency for Clinical Laboratory Sciences), 8, 378
Naeturopath, definition of, 27t
Nails, 78, 79
Nasopharyngeal culture, 315, 378
Natelson tubes, 236, 236f, 378
National Accrediting Agency for Clinical Laboratory Sciences, 8, 378
National Certification Agency for Medical Laboratory Personnel, 7, 378
National Committee for Clinical Laboratory Standards, 8, 378
  evacuated tube standards of, 325
National Fire Protection Association
  fire classification of, 140
  hazardous material labeling system of, 143, 146f
National Institute on Drug Abuse, collection procedures of, 271–272

National Phlebotomy Association, 7, 8
National standards, 8
Nausea, in blood collection, 188
NCA (National Certification Agency for Medical Laboratory Personnel), 7, 378
NCCLS (National Committee for Clinical Laboratory Standards), 8, 378
  evacuated tube standards of, 325
NCMLP (National Certification Agency for Medical Laboratory Personnel), 7, 378
Needle(s)
  for arterial puncture, 298
  butterfly, 170–171, 171f, 172f
    procedure with, 220, 221f, 222–223, 407
  depth of, 218–219, 219f
  disposal of, 131f, 154, 155f, 160, 161f–163f, 162, 211f, 216
  in evacuated tube system, 158
  gauge of, 157
  holders for, 158, 159f, 160, 160f, 162, 205, 205f
  insertion of, 210f, 214–215
  multisample, 158
  parts of, 157
  position of, 218–220, 219f
  quality control of, 325
  reinsertion of, 219–220
  resheathing of, 381
  sheath of, 378
    removal of, 214
  syringe, 169, 170f
  types of, 156–157
  winged infusion, 170–171, 171f, 172f
  withdrawal of, 211f, 216
Needlesticks, accidental
  OSHA procedures for, 135, 137
  prevention of, 160, 160f, 171, 171f, 172f
Negligence, 11, 378
Neonatal intensive care unit, infection control in, 123–124
Neonates
  bilirubin testing in, skin puncture for, 250–251
  screening in, 251, 252f, 378
Nephrons, 77
Nerves, injury of, in blood collection, 188
Nervous system
  diagnostic tests for, 76
  disorders of, 76
  functions of, 73, 74f, 75f
  structures in, 73, 76
Networks, computer, 349, 350f, 351f
Neurons, 73, 74f, 75f
Neutrophils, 102, 378

Newborns. *See* Neonates
Nonblood specimens. *See under*
    Specimen collection
Noninvasive procedures, defini-
    tion of, 378
Nonverbal communication,
    342–344, 342f, 343f
Norepinephrine, 71
Nose, function of, 80, 81f
Nosocomial infections, 114, 378
NPA (National Phlebotomy Asso-
    ciation), 7, 8
Nucleus, of cell, 61
Nursery, infection control in,
    123–124
Nursing services, 27, 29–30

O
Obesity, site selection in, 181
Occlusion, definition of, 378
Occult blood test
    point-of-care, 284–285, 285f
    of stool, 316
Occupational exposure, definition
    of, 378
Occupational Safety and Health
    Administration
    Bloodborne Pathogens Stan-
        dard of, 118, 119, 131f, 371
    definition of, 379
    Hazardous Communication
        Standard of, 143
    infection control regulations of,
        118, 119
    safety mandates of, 129
    specimen processing regula-
        tions of, 333, 335
Occupational therapy, 31
Occurrence reports, in quality
    assurance, 329
ONE TOUCH II blood glucose
    meter, 283, 283f
On-line, definition of, 348, 378
Order of draw, in venipuncture,
    166–170, 168t, 170f,
    378–379
Organelles, 61, 62f
Organs, definition of, 62
OSHA. *See* Occupational Safety
    and Health Administration
Osmotic fragility test, 34t
Osteochondritis, 379
    from heel puncture, 239
Osteomyelitis, 379
    from heel puncture, 239
Outpatients, 20
    identification of, 202
Output, computer, 352, 379
Ova and parasite specimens, 316,
    316f, 379
Ovary, 70, 70f

Oxalates, in tubes, 164
    contamination by, 168, 168t
Oxygen, partial pressure of, mea-
    surement of, 277–278
Oxygen exchange, in respiratory
    system, 82–83, 82f
Oxyhemoglobin, 82, 379

P
Pain
    in blood collection, 188
    in venipuncture, 205
Palmar surface, definition of, 379
Palpation
    definition of, 379
    of vein, 210, 211f
Pancreas, 70, 70f
    disorders of, 72–73
    functions of, 70, 70f
Parasites, in stool, 316, 316f, 379
Parathyroid glands, 70, 70f
    disorders of, 72
Parenteral route, definition of, 379
Parenteral transmission, of blood-
    borne pathogens, 119
Password, for computer users, 354
Patency, definition of, 189, 379
Paternity/parentage testing, 265,
    379
Pathogens, 114
    bloodborne. *See* Bloodborne
        pathogens
    definition of, 379
Pathologist, duties of, 41
Pathology department, 40–41
Patient(s)
    contact with, 197–199, 198f
    identification of. *See* Identification
Patient care technicians and assis-
    tants, 29
Patient's Bill of Rights, 9, 379,
    A-7–A-8
Peak levels, drug, 272, 272f, 379
Pediatric patients
    blood volume of, 367
    identification of, 201
    skin puncture in, in pediatric
        patients, 239–240, 241f,
        250–251, 252f
    tubes for, 379
    urine collection from, 314
    venipuncture in, 225–228, 227f,
        228f
Pelvic cavity, 60, 60f
Percent, calculations with, 365–366
Percutaneous, definition of, 379
Pericardial fluid, 315, 379
Pericardium, 88, 379
Peripheral catheter, blood collec-
    tion from, 182, 184f
Peripheral nervous system, 73,
    74f, 76
Peritoneal fluid, 315, 379

Personal computers, 348
Personal protective equipment.
        See Protective clothing and
        equipment, personal
Personal territory, 343
Petechiae, 379
    in blood collection, 188
pH, blood, measurement of,
    277–278
Phagocytosis, 102, 379
Pharmacy, 31
Pharynx, 80, 81f
Phenylketonuria, 379
    screening for, skin puncture
        for, 251
    evaluation checklist for, A-25
Phlebitis, 100, 379
Phlebotomist
    duties of, 4–5, 42–43
        multi skilled, 5
    professionalism of, 5–8
    in public relations, 9
Phlebotomy
    definition of, 379
    history of, 2–4, 2f, 3f
    procedures for
        current, 4
        early, 2–4, 2f, 3f
    therapeutic, 2–4, 2f, 3f, 266, 382
Phlebotomy Technician, 7
Phlebotomy therapeutic, definition
    of, 382
Physical therapy, 31
Physician visit, venipuncture
    during, 199
Physiology
    of body systems. *See* Body,
        systems of
    definition of, 58
Pineal gland, 70, 70f
Pituitary gland, 70, 70f
    disorders of, 71–72
PKU (phenylketonuria), 379
    screening for, skin puncture
        for, 251
    evaluation checklist for, A-25
Planes, body, 58, 59f, 371
Plantar surface
    definition of, 379
    of heel, puncture of, 239–240, 241f
Plasma
    composition of, 101
    definition of, 379
    description of, 105, 106f
    specimens of, processing of, 333
Plastic closures, in capillary blood
        gas specimen collection, 237
Platelet(s), 103
    adhesion of, 107, 379
    aggregation of, 107, 379
    in hemostasis, 107
    plug formation from, 107, 379

Platelet count, 33t
Pleural fluid, 315, 379
Plural endings, 49, 50t
PMNs (polymorphonuclear neu-
    trophils), 102
Pneumatic tube system, 380
Podiatrist, definition of, 27t
Point-of-care testing, 273–285
    analyzers for, 279, 280f
    for arterial blood gases, 277–278
    for cardiac troponin T, 279, 281f
    for cholesterol, 281
    for coagulation monitoring,
        273–277, 275f, 276f, 278f
    definition of, 379
    electrocardiography, 281–283,
        281f, 282f
    for electrolytes, 278–279
    equipment for, 273
    for glucose, 283, 283f
    for hematocrit, 284, 284f
    for hemoglobin, 284
    for lipoproteins, 281
    for occult blood, 284–285, 285f
    personnel for, 273
    for pregnancy, 285, 286f
Polycythemia, 266, 379
Polymorphonuclear cells, 102, 379
Popliteal vein, 99f
Porphyrins, light degradation of,
    263
Port, implanted, blood collection
    from, 182, 184f
Positions
    anatomic, 58, 370
    basal state and, 178
    body, 58
    for venipuncture, 205–208, 206f
Posterior direction, 59, 59f, 380
Post-op tests, 180
Postprandial, definition of, 380
Postprandial glucose testing,
    265–266
Potassium, 380
    point-of-care tests for, 278
Potassium oxalate, in tubes, 164
    contamination by, 168, 168t
Povidone iodine, in skin antisep-
    sis, 261–262, 261f
PPOs (preferred provider organi-
    zations), 25, 380
PPSs (prospective payment sys-
    tems), 25, 380
Preferred provider organizations,
    25, 380
Prefixes, 380
    general, 46–47, 47t
    in metric system, 360, 360t
Pregnancy, basal state and, 178
Pre-op tests, 180, 380
Primary care, definition of, 380
Primary care physicians, 20
    as gatekeepers, 25

Privacy, invasion of, 11, 376–377
Procedure manuals, 328–329,
    330f, 380
Processing, of specimens, 333–336
    additive mixing in, 215–216, 331
    aliquot preparation in, 335, 336f
    central area for, 333–336,
        334f–336f
    centrifugation in. *See* Centrifu-
        gation
    OSHA regulations on, 333
    plasma, 333
    precautions in, 334
    serum, 333–334
    stopper removal in, 335, 335f
    transport in, 218, 331
    work flow sheet for, 356f
Professionalism, 5–8, 380
    accreditation of educational
        program in, 7–8, 369
    bedside manner and, 202, 371
    certification in, 6–7, 372
    continuing education in, 8, 327
    definition of, 5
    image of, 6
    licensure in, 7
    national standards in, 8
Professional services, in hospitals,
    30–31, 30f, 31f
Progesterone, 71
Prone position, 58, 380
Prospective payment systems, 25,
    380
Protective clothing and equip-
    ment, personal, 121–123,
    122f–124f, 130f
    in arterial puncture, 297
    definition of, 379
    in exposure control, 138
Protective isolation, 125
Prothrombin, 108f, 380
Prothrombin time test, 32, 34t
    point-of-care, 277, 278f
Proxemics, 343, 380
Proximal direction, 60, 380
Psychologist, definition of, 27t
Psychoneuroimmunology, 178,
    380
Public Health Service, 22, 22t
Public relations, 9
Pulmonary artery, 88
Pulmonary circulation, 92, 96, 97f,
    380
Pulmonary valve, 89
Pulmonary veins, 88
Pulse, 91, 380
Pumping, of fist, 210, 380
Puncture
    arterial. *See* Arterial puncture
    skin. *See* Skin puncture
    venous. *See* Venipuncture
Purkinje fibers, 89, 90f

Q
Quality assurance, 319–329
    definition of, 322, 380
    forms for, 324f, 329
    historical aspects of, 320
    indicators of, 322–323, 324f, 380
    Joint Commission on Accredi-
        tation of Healthcare Orga-
        nizations and, 320, 322
    monitoring and evaluation
        process in, 323
    performance dimensions in,
        320–321
    quality control in. *See* Quality
        control
    vs. quality control, 325
    thresholds in, 323
    total quality management in,
        321–322, 383
Quality control
    definition of, 325, 380
    documentation of, 327–329,
        328f, 330f
    in patient preparation, 325
    in specimen collection, 325,
        326f, 327
Quantity not sufficient (QNS),
    336, 380

R
RACE mnemonic, for fire action,
    141
Radial artery, 380
    puncture of, 100, 299, 301–302,
        301f, 302f
        advantages of, 294
        disadvantages of, 295
        evaluation checklist for, 413
        location for, 295, 295f
Radial vein, 98f
Radiation safety, 141–142, 142f
Radiation therapy, 31
Radioimmunoassays, 35–36
Random Access Memory (RAM),
    350, 380
Random urine specimens, 310
Read Only Memory, 350, 380
Reassurance, patient, 205
Reciprocity, 380
    in certification, 7
Record keeping. *See* Documenta-
    tion; Information manage-
    ment
Red blood cell(s) (erythrocytes), 101
Red blood cell count, 33t
Reference accounts, in clinical
    laboratory, 41
Reference laboratory, 380
    log book for, 327–328
Reference values
    based on basal state, 175
    definition of, 381
    for skin puncture, 238–239

Reflectance meter glucose test, 283, 283f
Reflux, 381
  from tubes, 188–189
Registered Phlebotomy Technician, 7
Registration, of phlebotomist, 7
Reimbursement
  of institutions, 24
  of providers, 23–24
  salaried, 24
Rejection, of specimens, 336
Renin, 71
Reproductive system, 66, 67f
Requisitions, test, 194, 194f
  computer, 194–195, 195f
  definition of, 382
  information for, 197
  manual, 195, 196f
  receipt of, 197
  review of, 204
Resheathing, of needle, 381
Respiration, 80, 82–83, 82f
  external, 80, 374
  internal, 81, 376
Respirators, 121, 122f
Respiratory system, 80–84
  diagnostic tests for, 83–84
  disorders of, 83
  functions of, 82–83, 82f
  infections of, infection control in, 132t
  structures in, 80–82, 81f
Respiratory therapy, 31
Respondeat superior, 11–12, 381
Restraints, in venipuncture, 226–227, 227f
Reticulocyte(s), 101, 381
Reticulocyte count, 34t
Reverse isolation, 125
Rh blood group system, 105, 381
Rh immunoglobulins, 381
Ribosomes, 61, 62f
Right to refuse treatment, 9
Risk management, 15, 16f, 17, 381
ROM (Read Only Memory), 350, 380
Roman numerals, 363–365, 381
Routine tests, 180

S
Safety, 129–143
  in arterial puncture, 297
  with biohazards, 133–139, 137f
  chemical, 142–143, 144t–145t, 145f–147f
  electrical, 139, 374
  fire, 139–141, 141f
  first aid in, 145–146, 148–149, 148f
  in laboratory, general rules for, 129
  in needle disposal, 160, 161f–163f, 162

  in needle use, 171, 171f, 172f
  in patient rooms and areas, 129, 131
  radiation, 141–142, 142f
Safety showers, 143
Sagittal plane, 58, 381
Salaried reimbursement, of providers, 24
Saline lock, blood collection from, 183–184, 185f
Saphenous vein, 99f
  great, 94f, 95, 375
Scarificator, 3–4, 3f
Scars, site selection in, 180
Schick test, 287
Schnapper, 3–4, 3f
Sclerosis, 381
  venous, 209
Sealants, tube, in capillary blood gas specimen collection, 237
Sebaceous glands, 79
Secondary care, definition of, 381
Seizures, in blood collection, 189
Semen analysis, 315–316, 381
Semilunar valves, 88, 381
Sensory nerves, 74f
Septicemia, 381
  blood culture in, 259
Serology department, 34, 37t, 37
  tests performed in, A-15–A-16
Serum
  definition of, 381
  description of, 105
  specimens of, processing of, 333–334
Service insurance, 23, 381
Sexually transmitted diseases, 381
Sharps
  containers for, 381
  disposal of, 131f, 154, 155f
Sheaths, needle, 378
  removal of, 214
Shock
  electrical, actions in, 139
  prevention of, 148
Showers, safety, 143
Sickle cell count, 34t
Signs
  biohazard, 137f
  body substance isolation, 127f
  chemical hazards, 145f, 146f
  informational, watching for, 197–198
  precaution, 128f, 130f–131f
    airborne, 134f
    contact, 136f
    droplet, 135f
    radiation hazard, 142f
Sinoatrial node, 89, 90f, 381
Site, for specimen collection
  cleansing of, for venipuncture, 212

selection of
  for arterial puncture, 294–296, 295f, 297f
  factors in, 180–182
  for skin puncture, 239–241, 240f–242f
  for venipuncture, 180–182, 209, 212, 213f
Skeletal system, 62–64
  bones in, 63
  diagnostic tests for, 64
  disorders of, 64
  functions of, 62–63, 63f
Skin
  antisepsis for, 259–261, 260f, 261f, 381
  biohazard contact with, 134, 135
  bloodborne pathogens transmission through, 119
  cleansing of
    for blood collection, 154–155
    for blood culture specimen, 259–261, 260f, 261f
  functions of, 78
  infections of, precautions with, 132t
  layers of, 78–79, 79f
  structure of, 79–80
Skin puncture, 233–253
  arterialized specimen in, 242, 249–250
  blood composition in, 238
  for capillary blood gas test, 236–237, 237f, 249–250
  collection devices for, 235–237, 235f–238f
    quality control of, 325
  definition of, 381
  dilution system for, 237, 238f
  equipment for, 234–238, 234f–238f
  finger stick, 241, 242f, 243, 245, 244f, 246f
  heelstick, 239–240, 240f, 241f, 243, 244f, 245, 246f
    evaluation checklist for, 409
  indications for, 239
  lancets for, 234–235, 234f
  in newborn screening, 251, 252f
  in pediatric patients, 239–240, 241f, 250–251, 252f
  principles of, 238–241, 240f–242f
  procedure for, 241–245, 244f–246f
    in bilirubin testing, 250–251
    in blood smear preparation, 245–248, 247f, 248f, 249t
    in capillary blood gas determination, 236–237, 237f, 249–250
    evaluation checklist for, A-24

Skin puncture (*continued*)
  reference values for, 238–239
  site cleaning in, 242
  site selection for, 239–241,
    240f–242f
  tests not performed by, 239
  warming for, 237f, 238, 242
Skin tests, 285, 287, 288f, 381
Sleep, venipuncture during, 198
Slides, 154
  for smear preparation, 246–247,
    247f, 248f, 410
Smear preparation
  evaluation checklist for, A-26
  routine, 245–248, 247f, 248f, 249t
  thick, 248–249
Smoking, basal state and, 178
Smooth muscle, 64, 65f
Sodium, 381
  point-of-care tests for, 278
Sodium citrate, in tubes, 164
Sodium fluoride, in tubes, 165
  contamination by, 168
Sodium polyanethol sulfonate, in
    tubes, 165
Software
  computer, 352
  definition of, 381
Solutes, in plasma, 101, 381
Spanish-English conversational
    phrases, A-3–A-5
Special chemistry division, 35
Specialties
  medical, 26, 26t
  non-medical, 27t
Specimen(s)
  blood. *See* Blood collection;
    Blood specimens
  collection of. *See* Specimen col-
    lection
  cooling of, 263, 263f, 264t,
    331–332
    arterial blood, 298, 303
  forensic, 375
  handling of. *See* Handling, of
    specimens
  processing of. *See* Processing
  rejection of, 336
  warming of, 332
Specimen collection. *See also*
    Blood collection
  nonblood
    amniotic fluid, 314
    body cavity fluids, 315
    cerebrospinal fluid, 314–315
    gastric contents, 315
    nasopharyngeal, 315
    semen, 315–316
    stool, 316, 316f
    sweat, 316–317
    throat, 317, 317f
    tissue, 318
    urine. *See* Urine specimens,
      collection of

patient preparation for, 325
priorities in, 327
procedures for, quality control
  of, 325, 326f, 327
timed, 179
Sphygmomanometer, 91, 381
Spills, clean-up procedure for
  blood, 137–138
  chemical, 143, 147f
Spinal cavity, 60, 60f
Spinal cord, 73, 74f
Standard of care, 12, 381
Standard precautions, 381–382
  in isolation, 127–128, 130f–131f
Standards, national, 8
Station, for blood drawing, 152, 152f
STAT tests, 179, 382
Statute of limitations, 15, 382
Steady state, 382
  in arterial puncture, 298–299
Stirrers, metal, in capillary blood
  gas specimen collection, 237
Stomach contents, specimen of, 315
Stool collection, 316, 316f
Stoppers, tube
  evacuated, 165–166, 167f, Color
    Plate 2
  precautions with, 334
  removal of, 335, 335f
Storage, of information, in com-
  puter, 353
Strep testing, 288, 288f
Stress, basal state and, 178
Striated muscle, 64, 65f
Subcutaneous layer, 79, 382
Suffixes, 47–48, 48t, 382
Sugar. *See* Glucose
Supercomputers, 349
Superficial (external) direction, 59
Superior direction, 59f, 60, 382
Supine position, 58, 382
  venipuncture in, 206
Support services, in hospitals, 30
Suprapubic aspiration, of urine,
  313–314, 382
Surfactant, respiratory, 81–82
Susceptibility
  antibiotic, definition of, 370
  to infections, 115, 115f, 117, 382
Sweat chloride test, 316–317, 382
Sweat glands, 79
Sweating, 78
Sweeps, definition of, 197, 382
Symbols, 50, 50t–54t
Syncope, 198, 382
Synovial fluid, 315, 382
Syringe(s), 170, 170f
  for specimen collection
    arterial blood, 298, 304
    needles for, 169, 170f
    procedure evaluation check-
      list for, 406

Syringe system
  multiple samples with, 223, 225
  order of draw in, 169–170, 170f
  procedure for, 223, 224f,
    225–226, 225f
Systemic circulation, 92, 96, 97f, 382
Systole, 89, 382
Systolic blood pressure, 91, 382

T
Tachycardia, 90
Tech code, for computer users,
    354, 382
Technical supervisor, duties of, 42
Telephone communication, 346,
    347t
Temperature
  measurement of, 363, 364f
  specimen sensitivity to,
    264–265, 264t, 265f
Terminology, 45–55
  abbreviations in, 50, 50t–54t
  combining forms in, 49, 373
  combining vowels in, 48–49, 373
  computer, 348, 348t
  plural endings in, 49, 50t
  prefixes in, 46–47, 47t
  reminders for, 49
  suffixes in, 47–48, 48t
  symbols in, 50, 50t–54t
  word roots in, 45–46, 46t
Tertiary care, 20, 382
Test(s)
  in blood bank, A-16–A-17
  in chemistry department,
    A-9–A-13
  in coagulation department,
    A-14–A-15
  in hematology department,
    A-13–A-14
  in immunohematology depart-
    ment, A-16–A-17
  in immunology department,
    A-15–A-16
  in microbiology department,
    A-17
  patient inquiry about, 203
  requisitions for. *See* Requisitions
  right to refuse, 9
  in serology department,
    A-15–A-16
  status of, 178–180
Testis, 70, 70f
Testosterone, 71
Test panel groupings, 37t
Therapeutic monitoring, of drugs,
    272–273, 272f, 382
Therapeutic phlebotomy, 2–4, 2f,
    3f, 266
Third party payers
  coverage under, 22–23
  definition of, 382

payment methods of, 22–23
social entitlement programs, 24
Thixotropic gel separators, 165, 382
Thoracic cavity, 60, 60f
Thoracic duct, 110f, 111
Threshold values
definition of, 382
in quality assurance, 323
Throat culture collection, 317, 317f
Thrombin, 108f, 382
Thrombin time, 34t
Thrombocytes, 103, 382
Thrombocytopenia, 106, 382
Thrombocytosis, 106, 382
Thrombophlebitis, 382
Thrombosis, venous, 209
Thrombus
definition of, 382
formation of, in arterial puncture, 303
Thymus gland, 70, 70f
Thyroid gland, 70, 70f
disorders of, 72
Thyroid stimulating hormone, 70
Thyroxine, 70
Tibial veins, 99f
Time
constraints on, in specimen delivery, 332, 333f
military, 362, 363f, 378
Timed specimen collection, 179
of urine, 310
Tissues, 61–62
specimens of, 318
T lymphocytes, 103, 383
Tolerance tests
definition of, 383
specimen collection for, 266–269, 267f
urine, 310–311
Tort law, 10–11, 383
Total Quality Management, 320, 383
Total quality management, themes of, 321–322
Touch, in communication, 344
Tourniquet
application of, 208–209, 207f–208f, 210f–211f
release of, 215
types of, 155–156, 156f
Toxicology studies, 269–273, 270f, 271f, 272f
Trace elements
definition of, 383
measurement of, 273
Training, for exposure control, 139
Transfusions. *See also* Blood banking
autologous, 259, 371
crossmatching in, 104–105, 256–257, 257f, 258f
reactions in, 103, 383

typing in, 103–105, 104t, 256–257, 257f, 258f
universal recipients and donors in, 104
Transmission, of infections, 115–117, 115f
Transmission-based precautions, 383
in isolation, 127–129, 132t, 133t, 134f
Transport, of specimens, 218, 331
media for, 383
Transverse plane, 58, 59f, 383
Trays, for blood collection, 153, 153f
Treatment, right to refuse, 9
Tricuspid valve, 88
Troponin T, cardiac, point-of-care tests for, 279, 281f
Trough levels, in drug monitoring, 272, 272f, 383
Trust, in communication, 345
Tube(s)
additives for. *See* Additives
adjustment of, 218
anticoagulant reflux from, 188–189
barcodes on, 326f
for blood alcohol test, 269
for blood bank, A-16
Caraway, 236, 372
for chemistry department, A-9
for coagulation department, A-14
discard, 373
evacuated. *See* Evacuated tubes; Evacuated tube system
filling of, 210f, 215–216
for hematology department, A-13
holders for, 158, 159f, 160, 160f, 162, 205, 205f
for immunohematology department, A-16
for immunology department, A-15
labeling of, 218
for microbiology department, A-16
microhematocrit, 236, 236f, 378
multisample collection with, 166–170, 168t, 170f
Natelson, 236, 236f, 378
partially filled, specimen integrity and, 190
pediatric, 379
sealants for, 237
selection of, 212
for serology department, A-15
for skin puncture specimen collection, 235–237, 235f–237f

stoppers for
evacuated, 165–166, 167f, Color Plate 2
precautions with, 334
removal of, 335, 335f
for trace element specimens, 273
Tuberculin test, 287, 383
Tuberculosis, 383
Tunica adventitia, 95, 95f, 383
Tunica intima, 95f, 96, 383
Tunica media, 95f, 96, 383
Turn-around-time, 383
Twenty-four hour urine collection, 311, 312f
Typenex Blood Recipient Identification Band, 256–257, 257f, 383
Typing, of blood
specimen collection for, 256–257, 257f, 258f
systems for, 103–105, 104t

U
Ulnar artery, evaluation of, before arterial puncture (Allen test), 299, 300f, 369, 414
Unconsciousness, venipuncture during, 198
United Nations hazard classes, 144t–145t
Units, of measurement
English system, 361–362, 361t
metric system, 359–362, 360t–362t
military time, 362, 363f
temperature, 363, 364f
Universal precautions, 125, 383
Urethra, 77–78, 77f
Urinalysis
definition of, 383
point-of-care, 289, 289f
routine, 308–309
Urinalysis department, 37–38, 38t
Urinary system
diagnostic tests for, 78
disorders of, 77–78
functions of, 76–77, 77f
infections of, culture and sensitivity test in, 309, 309f
Urine
culture and sensitivity test of, 309, 309f
cytology studies of, 309–310
drug screening tests for, 310
specimen of, catheterized, 372
tests for, 308–310, 309f
Urine specimens
collection of
catheterized, 313
containers for, 309, 312f
first morning (8-hour), 310
fractional (double-voided), 311–312

Urine specimens, collection of
    (*continued*)
    methods for, 312–314
    midstream, 312, 378
    midstream clean catch, 312–313
    patient instructions for, 308
    pediatric, 314
    random, 310
    regular voiding in, 312
    suprapubic, 313–314
    timed, 310
    for tolerance tests, 310–311
    twenty-four hour, 311, 312f
    types of, 310–312, 312f
User manuals, 327, 328f, 383
UTI (urinary tract infection), cul-
    ture and sensitivity test in,
    309, 309f

V
Vacuum tubes. *See* Evacuated tubes
Valves
    heart, 88–89
    venous, 95, 95f, 96
Vascular access devices
    blood collection from, 182–183,
        183f–184f
    definition of, 383
Vascular system, 92–100
    blood flow in, 96–97, 97f
    blood vessels in, 92–96. *See also*
        Arteries; Veins
        structure of, 95–96, 95f
        types of, 93–95, 93f–95f
        for venipuncture, 98–100,
            98f, 99f
    diagnostic tests for, 100
    disorders of, 100
    functions of, 92
Vasoconstriction, 383
    in hemostasis, 107
Vasopressin (antidiuretic
    hormone), 70
Vasospasm, after arterial punc-
    ture, 303
Vector transmission, 383
    of infections, 117
Vehicle transmission, 383
    of infections, 117
Veins, 94–95, 94f. *See also specific
    veins*
    anchoring of, 214
    of arm, 98–99, 98f
    collapse of, 372
        in blood collection, 189, 220
    damaged, site selection in,
        180–181
    definition of, 383
    hand, 98f
        venipuncture of, procedure
            evaluation checklist for, A-23
    injury of, in blood collection,
        189

of leg, 9, 99f
location of, 155, 156f
    in obesity, 181
palpation of, 209, 210f
puncture of. *See* Venipuncture
sclerosed, 209
structure of, 95–96, 95f
thrombosed, 209
Vena cavae, 71, 88, 383
Venesection, 384
Venipuncture
    absent patient and, 199
    during arterial puncture
        attempt, 304
    during clergy visit, 199
    definition of, 384
    in difficult persons, 202
    equipment for, 151–171, 152f,
        153f, 155f
        antiseptics, 153–154
        assembly of, 204–205, 204f, 205f
        blood-drawing station, 152,
            152f
        carts, 152–153
        disinfectants, 154
        disposal containers, 154, 155f
        dressings, 154
        gloves, 153
        needles. *See* Needle(s)
        pediatric, 227
        pen, 154
        slides, 154
        tourniquet, 155–156, 156f
        trays, 153, 153f
        tubes. *See* Tube(s)
        vein locating device, 155, 156f
        winged infusion set, 170–171,
            171f, 172f
    explanation of, 202–203
    family present during, 199
    order of draw in, 166–170, 168t,
        170f
    during physician visit, 199
    physiologic factors in, 175–178
    positions for, 205–208, 206f
    problems with, 218–220, 219f
    procedure for, 204–220
        bandage application in, 217
        butterfly needle set in, 220,
            221f, 222–223
        dietary restriction verifica-
            tion in, 204
        disposal measures in, 217
        equipment assembly in,
            204–205, 204f, 205f
        equipment verification in, 214
        evaluation checklists for,
            A-21–A-23
        failure of, 218–220, 219f
        glove donning in, 205
        glove removal in, 217–218
        handwashing in, 205
        needle disposal in, 211f, 216

needle insertion in, 210f,
    214–215
needle sheath removal in, 212,
    214
needle withdrawal in, 211f,
    216
patient contact in, 197–199, 198f
patient identification for,
    199–202, 200f, 204
patient preparation for,
    202–203
patient reassurance in, 205
pediatric, 225–228, 227f, 228f
positioning for, 205–208, 206f
record keeping in, 218
repeat after failure, 220
site selection for, 180–182,
    209, 212, 213f
specimen transport in, 218
syringe system in, 223, 224f,
    225, 225f, A-21
test request for, 194–197,
    194f–196f
test requisition review in, 204
tourniquet application in,
    207f–208f, 208–209,
    210f–211f, 214
tourniquet release in, 212
tube filling in, 210f, 215–216
tube labeling in, 211f, 216
tube selection for, 212
vein anchoring in, 214
during sleep, 198
test status in, 178–180
during unconsciousness, 198
in uncooperative patient, 203
veins for
    in arm, 98–99, 98f
    in leg, 99, 99f
Venoscope, 155, 156f
Venous stasis, 384
    specimen integrity and, 189
Ventral cavities, 60, 60f, 384
Ventral (anterior) direction, 59, 59f,
    384
Ventricles, 88, 384
Venules, 95, 95f, 384
Verbal communication, 340, 341f
Viability, of microbes, 115–116
Vicarious liability, 14, 384
Virulence, of microbes, 116, 384
Visceral muscle muscle, 64, 65f
Visitors, handling of, 199
Vitamin B$_{12}$, light degradation of,
    263
Vomiting, in blood collection, 188

W
Warming
    in skin puncture, 237f, 238, 242
    of specimens, 332
Warning signs. *See* Signs

Waste, biohazardous, disposal of, 138
White blood cell(s) (leukocytes), 102
White blood cell count, 33t
Whole blood, 105
Whorls, 241, 384

Winged infusion set. *See* Butterfly needle set
Word roots, 45–46, 46t, 384
Work practice controls, in exposure control, 138
Work restrictions, conditions requiring, A-19–A-20

Wright's stain, for leukocytes, 102

Z
Zones of comfort, 343, 384